Nursing older people
Issues and innovations

Nursing older people

Issues and innovations

SECOND EDITION

Rhonda Nay

Professor/Director Gerontic Nursing Clinical School
Director Australian Centre for Evidence Based Aged Care
La Trobe University and Bundoora Extended Care Centre

Sally Garratt

Adjunct Associate Professor Gerontic Nursing Clinical School
La Trobe University and Bundoora Extended Care Centre

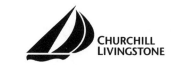

Sydney Edinburgh London New York
Philadelphia St Louis Toronto

ELSEVIER

Churchill Livingstone
is an imprint of Elsevier

Elsevier Australia
30–52 Smidmore Street, Marrickville, NSW 2204

This edition © 2004 Elsevier Australia
(a division of Reed International Books Australia Pty Ltd)
ACN 001 002 357

National Library of Australia Cataloguing-in-Publication Data

---

Nursing older people: issues and innovations.

 2nd ed.
 Bibliography.
 Includes index.
 ISBN 0 7295 3751 X

 1. Geriatric nursing. 2. Geriatric nursing—Australia.
 3. Aged—Care—Australia. I. Nay, Rhonda. II. Garratt, Sally.

610.73650994

Publisher: Vaughn Curtis
Publishing Editor: Meg O'Hanlon
Edited and project managed by Kay Waters
Internal design by Pamela Horsnell, Juno Creative Services
Cover design by Modern Art Production Group
Typesetting by Arc Typography
Proofread by Pamela Dunne
Index by Russell Brooks
Printed & bound in Australia by Southwood Press Pty Ltd

Dedications

To my Mum and Dad, whose examples of ageing optimistically will always inspire me.

Rhonda

For Emily, who I am sure will carry on the tradition and example of her great, great grandmother; also Emily, as a woman of courage and feisty commitment to ageing positively.

Sally

Contents

Foreword

As the demography of the Australian population changes, with a large cohort moving inexorably into being classified as aged, the issues around ageing explored in this book are certain to become more prominent.

The group which will move into being aged—the so-called 'baby boomers'—are used to being able to command what they need, whether by political pressure or by the mere fact that they are financially better off than the generation before them, and they are more articulate and more skilled at manipulating the political culture. It is therefore certain that as clients or patients, they will be more demanding about how their aged-care needs are to be met.

While it is very difficult to describe or provide generic health-care solutions for this complex variety of health-care requirements, there is little doubt that nursing can contribute greatly to the design of the best care for each individual aged person.

Nurses now deliver the great majority of care to the aged, whether the setting be an aged-care facility, acute-care hospital or the community. Future demographic changes and major shifts in the epidemiology and cultural expectations of this group will mean that the nursing role in both direct care provision and policy analysis, policy development and policy implementation will become even more important.

Any nurse involved in this area of health care will benefit from becoming more familiar with the issues canvassed and debated in this book. The editors have assembled a wide range of experts to build on the reputation established by the first edition of this book. I congratulate both the editors and the contributors on the production of such a valuable reference.

Rosemary Bryant FRCNA

Preface

Since the first edition of this book (1999), a lot has happened in relation to the care of older people. Ageing in all its facets has finally appeared on major government agendas. We have, for example, a National Strategy for an Ageing Australia, an Intergenerational Report informing the National Budget, processes in place to build an ageing research agenda, and recognition of ageing as a priority area for funding, accreditation in aged care (which has been accepted and even applauded by many), and aged-care scholarships to attract nurses to develop their educational and career pathways in this important specialty. Numerous State and Federal projects have been undertaken in relation to recruitment and retention of nursing staff. It is also being recognised that older people make up the majority of clients in acute care.

This second edition of *Nursing Older People* aims to reflect these contemporary issues. It remains a book about issues (not a text about diseases) that immediately affect nurses and that nurses tell us are important to them. In most cases it draws upon research undertaken by the authors and situates our work within the international context. While most chapters are written by nurses, significant contributions to the book have come from other disciplines in recognition of the multidisciplinary teamwork imperative to good care of older people.

Like the first edition, it celebrates the many innovations in aged care through vignettes (included in most chapters), which provide examples from practice.

ORGANISATION OF THE VOLUME

This book is organised into three sections. The first deals with the broader issues that affect care: funding, quality, staffing, legal and ethical issues and the need to recognise diversity in the client population. It also explores important contextual influences such as care in the community, acute care of older people and the significant influences on providing care in rural communities.

The second section concentrates on more specific care issues. In the third section, the need for an evidence base to care is acknowledged and some examples of current and future research trends are identified.

Part 1 Contextual issues and innovations

Changes in residential aged-care policy and funding are outlined by **Courtney, Abbey** and **Abbey**, and the impact of these changes on internal management is explored.

Duckett and **Jackson** continue their analysis of acute-care costs and provide further evidence that older people do not cost more despite the continuing ageist assumptions which pervade the acute-care sector. Continuous quality improvement is the aim of all good health-care providers. **Percival** reports on recent work in the aged-care sector.

Nursing shortages are challenging the health-care system internationally. **Nay** draws on her own work and that of recent studies to examine the issues and opportunities that these shortages bring. With litigation expected to become increasingly common in nursing practice, **Field** and **Garratt** look at legalities relating to aged care and the emphasis of Australian law on rights. Practice issues pertaining to various rights are looked at from a nursing viewpoint, and ethical dilemmas in practice are addressed.

Australia is a country that embraces a diversity of cultures. **Stein** explores issues relating to the delivery of health care to older people from Indigenous and culturally and linguistically diverse backgrounds. The implications for care delivery are addressed and an example is provided of where staff understanding of a resident and her family's cultural beliefs was essential in dealing with the family.

Brooke and **Kendig** provide insight into the care of older people who receive nursing care in the community, such as at home or in community-based facilities. The roles and issues for nurses in community care are explored and case studies are presented. **Lavender** and **Keleher** also focus on a subpopulation of older people— those living in rural areas. Older people living in rural regions of Australia are said to experience poorer health and poorer access to health-care services. The need for nursing education programs to address rural and remote health issues is explored.

Another domain in which older people receive health care is in hospital. **Street** provides a geriatrician's perspective on the experience of older people in acute care. He acknowledges the increased presence of aged-care staff in acute wards in Australian hospitals compared with the previous decade, and anticipates that strategies to manage age-related conditions will assume greater importance.

Fiveash and **Watts** focus on the older person being participatory in their health care and maintaining control, known as client-managed care. This approach has the client taking charge of their own health care, a contrast with stereotypical associations of old age with dependency and compliance with health-care requests.

Part 2 Clinical issues and innovations

Much has been written about the ageing of the Australian population and the associated predicted increases in the incidence of age-related conditions. **Garratt** continues her exploration of issues associated with formally assessing mental ill health in older people. Cultural differences and not knowing the status of the person's cognition before they grew old can lead to misinterpretation of test results. Her discussion includes possible factors to assist in preventing deterioration in mental health. **Mott** and **Kingsley** call for the residential aged-care industry to address issues of abuse relating to dementia, mental illness and aged care in general. Protocols and attention to resident and staff mix are recommended as areas that need to be considered in providing an optimal environment.

Chronic illness is typically associated with those aged over sixty years. **FitzGerald** and **Horton** take a phenomenological approach in attempting to understand what it is like to be an older person and have chronic illness. Details of their study of eighteen people with chronic illness are presented, in which these people provide an insight into their experiences which may assist nurses to take new perspectives and better understand their older clients. The consumption of both prescription and over-the-counter medications is common in older people, because of chronic illness and/or co-morbidities. **Baker** and **Tiziani** discuss the physiological changes associated with ageing that may affect the manner in which the body of an older person responds to medication, sometimes with detrimental effects.

The issue of using restraint on older people in aged-care facilities has received considerable attention of late. **Susan Koch** reports on changes to restraint use, brought about by both local and international policy review. Challenges to minimising restraint use and alternatives to applying restraint are presented.

Another issue which has also received the recent attention of policy makers is palliative care in residential aged-care settings. **Abbey** looks at what constitutes palliative care and the dilemmas associated with introducing palliative care for a person without a malignancy and/or known time trajectory.

While some issues have received much attention lately, one issue pertinent to older people which has not is sexuality. **Nay** looks at the relationship between sexuality and identity, and societal attitudes towards sex and older people. Barriers to sexual expression for older people are explored and an example of a sexual rights policy for use in residential aged-care facilities is presented.

In **Bill Koch**'s chapter, computerised care planning is explored through evaluation data collected from aged-care facilities that have adopted a computer-based approach. A timeline of the developmental process, from the original paper-based model, to the PC-based version, through to the current internet-based care plan system is also presented.

Part 3 Research issues and innovations

This section concentrates on research strategies and visions for the future in gerontic nursing research. **Pearson** looks at the link between quality improvement and the practical application of research findings. He expands on developments in Australasia which are currently contributing greatly to international knowledge of evidence-based practice in aged care. **Street** continues her focus on action research and its relevance to gerontic nursing. An example of its application to an issue of concern to gerontic nurses is presented. **Koch** and **Tiziani** report on an Australian study, where academic staff from schools of nursing were asked to provide details about their current research in gerontic nursing and their thoughts on what issues should be addressed in the future.

This book draws on the expertise of academics from a broad spectrum of nursing-related domains. Insight is given into some of the issues and challenges facing those working in aged care. With Australia's ageing population, it is an optimal time for individual nurses to view these challenges as opportunities and to develop innovative strategies that enable them to contribute meaningfully to the care of the older sector of society and provide them with the quality care they deserve.

Acknowledgements

Jenny Curtis and Debbie Lee were central to the publication of the first edition of this book, and encouraged and supported a second edition.

Elsevier, and in particular Vaughn Curtis, adopted the book into their 'stable' and immediately emphasised and demonstrated their enthusiastic support for a continuing partnership.

We thank the chapter authors, whose cooperation and expertise—despite all having other demands on their time—enabled us to deliver another great book!

We also sincerely thank the hundreds of older people who have inspired and taught us over the years—and the clinicians who never, ever give up aspiring to better care and showing in so many ways that with passion and commitment anything is possible.

This book would not have been delivered on time if it had not been for the diligent, insightful and constant support provided by Jacinda Wilson. For her research assistance, attention to detail, follow-up, editorial work and professional approach we are indeed indebted!

Vale

Elizabeth (Beth) Jean Kingsley RN, PhD, FRCNA

14 December 1943 – 15 September 2003

Beth graduated as a registered nurse in 1964 from the Royal Perth Hospital. She worked in the university sector, nursing homes, hospitals, Council of the Ageing, the Health Department, in Australia and overseas.

The focus of Beth's work was always on the care and well-being of the community. Among the personal achievements of which Beth was very proud were: being awarded an ANZAC Fellowship to study aged care and nursing education programs throughout New Zealand; and being the inaugural recipient of the Curtin University School of Social Sciences and Asian Studies Alumni Medal for academic excellence and outstanding contribution to the community. Beth was well known as an elder abuse activist, at the forefront of efforts to combat this social crime. She was involved in aged care in both a professional and voluntary capacity and conducted many education programs for older people and their carers. A community project dear to Beth's heart was her involvement in the book *Songs of Strength: Sixteen Women Talk About Cancer*, in which these women told their stories of living—and sometimes dying—with cancer, in an attempt to help and empower other women with cancer.

Beth was, and is, an inspiration to others to live full lives, follow their hearts and speak out on the hard issues. She is survived by her dearly loved husband John and sons Simon and Stuart.

Sarah Mott

Contributors

EDITORS

Rhonda Nay RN, BA (UNE), MLitt (UNE), PhD (UNSW), FRCNA, FCN (NSW), FAAG

Professor/Director, Gerontic Nursing Clinical School, and Director, Australian Centre for Evidence Based Aged Care (ACEBAC), La Trobe University and Bundoora Extended Care Centre, Melbourne, Victoria

Rhonda Nay is Foundation Professor of Gerontic Nursing and Director of the Gerontic Nursing Clinical School and ACEBAC, based at La Trobe University and Bundoora Extended Care Centre. She has been involved in aged care for over thirty years through practice, education and research. She is president of the AAG (Victorian Division). Rhonda serves on numerous committees including the National Advisory Committee on Ageing.

Sally Garratt RN, CertMidwifery, DipAppSc(Nurs Ed), BEd, MScN (Colorado), FRCNA

Adjunct Associate Professor, Gerontic Nursing Professorial Unit and Clinical School, La Trobe University and Bundoora Extended Care Centre, and Director, Royal Freemasons Homes for the Aged, Victoria

Prior to her retirement in 2003, Sally Garratt held a joint position between Caulfield General Medical Centre and the Gerontic Nursing Clinical School, La Trobe University, as an Associate Professor of Gerontic Nursing. Her most recent involvement was in the delivery of nursing education programs and research. She has served on numerous government committees concerned with aged-care matters and is a Director of Royal Freemasons Homes of Victoria. Sally has presented over sixty papers at conferences and co-edited three books on aged-care nursing. Her main interests are dementia care and person–environment interaction.

AUTHORS

Brian Abbey BA, MEd(Admin)

Research Assistant, School of Nursing, Queensland University of Technology, Brisbane, Queensland

Brian Abbey has experience in teaching and researching political science and public policy at Monash University and the University of Adelaide. He has also served in administrative roles at the University of Adelaide, Flinders University and the University of New England. He has published and lectured widely on a range of subjects in the field of social theory and public policy and most recently has been engaged as a consultant in quality and compliance audits of health services.

Jennifer Abbey RN, PhD, FRCNA

Professor of Nursing (Aged Care), School of Nursing, Queensland University of Technology, Brisbane, Queensland

Jenny Abbey was appointed as Queensland's first Professor of Nursing (Aged Care) in March 2003. The position is a joint appointment between three partners: Queensland University of Technology's School of Nursing, The Prince Charles Hospital Health Service District and the Kedron-Wavell Services Club. Professor Abbey has been a hands-on-nurse practitioner, a union organiser, Assistant Dean, Research, at Flinders University and a health-care consultant. The needs of people with dementia has been an interest of hers for at least two decades. Her present research interests are assessing pain in people with end-stage-dementia, the introduction of a structured hospice approach for people with end-stage dementia in residential aged-care facilities, contributions to compression of morbidity in the older person, the use of advance directives by the older person, investigations of feeding difficulties for people with dementia, the impact of aged care clinical placements on undergraduate students and the effects of ageing in place.

Helen Baker RN, BNurs(Hons), PhD, FCN (NSW), FRCNA

Professor of Nursing, Faculty of Human Development, School of Nursing and Midwifery, Victoria University, Melbourne, Victoria

Helen Baker's interests include clinical nursing—in particular, care of older people in acute-care settings, nurses and medications, and quality use of medications by nurses. She has a clinical background in operating rooms, infection control and quality assurance.

Libby Brooke RN, MA, PhD

Research Director, Centre for Business Work and Ageing, Swinburne University of Technology, Melbourne, Victoria

Dr Libby Brooke is the Research Director of the Centre for Business Work and Ageing, Swinburne University of Technology, Melbourne and is currently conducting research projects on employment issues and the ageing population. She has a particular interest in the experience of older people as consumers of care by professionals and the relationship between their personal stories, the communities to which they are related and their interpretation of the care they receive. Previously Dr Brooke was based at Lincoln Gerontology Centre at La Trobe University, where she conducted a range of social gerontology research projects including community care, housing and care, social support and social isolation, and examined models of service delivery in the residential and community sectors.

Mary Courtney RN, BAdmin(Acc), MHP, PhD, FRCNA, AFCHSE

Professsor of Nursing and Director of Research, School of Nursing, Queensland University of Technology, Brisbane, Queensland

Mary Courtney has research and teaching interests in the area of aged and community care and health-services management. Her PhD research was entitled Quality and Policy in Nursing Homes in Australia: A Critical Discourse Analysis. Her present research interests include leading an ARC SPIRT grant to evaluate in-home health assessment for older people over the age of 75 years who live alone in the community. In July 2003 she completed a Principles Paper for the Commonwealth Department of Health and Ageing to explore aged-care content in undergraduate nursing curricula and at the time of writing is undertaking a Paperwork Review of the RCS—Independent Assessor Trial. She is also widely known for her work in health-services management education, and authored *Financial Management in Health Service* (MacLennan & Petty).

Stephen Duckett BEc (ANU), MHA, PhD (NSW), FCHSE

Professor of Health Policy, Dean, Faculty of Health Sciences, and Pro Vice-Chancellor (Health Development), La Trobe University, Melbourne, Victoria

From 1994 to March 1996 Stephen Duckett was Secretary of the then Commonwealth Department of Human Services and Health. From 1983 to 1993, he held various operational and policy positions in the Victorian Department of Health and Community Services and its predecessors, including Regional Director of the Western Metropolitan Region and Director of Acute Health Services. He is an economist with a Masters degree and PhD in Health Administration from the University of New South Wales. He is a Fellow of the Australian College of Health Service Executives. In 1999–2000 Stephen was Chair of the Victorian Ministerial Review of Health Care Networks. He is currently Chair of the Board of Directors of Bayside Health (the metropolitan health service responsible for The Alfred, Caulfield and Sandringham hospitals), Chair of the Board of Directors of the Brotherhood of St Laurence and Convenor of the Council of Deans of Health Sciences. His research principally concentrates on the economics of hospital care, including development and use of casemix measures and methods of financing hospital care.

John Field RN, BLegSt, ADNE, FRCNA, FCN (NSW)

Solicitor of the Supreme Court of NSW, and Senior Lecturer and Director, International Programs and Strategic Alliances, School of Nursing and Midwifery, La Trobe University, Melbourne, Victoria

John Field has been involved in nursing for more than 25 years and holds qualifications in nursing, law, education and management. He has been engaged in teaching law and ethics to nurses, other health professionals and health-service managers since 1980. His professional experience includes 11 years of psychiatric-nursing practice and several years as a nurse educator. John's research interests principally involve the relationship between law and nursing, including the legal and ethical implications of developments such as evidence-based practice and outcomes-based quality measures and the ethical domain of qualitative research. For the past eight years he has been increasingly involved in developing international and offshore nursing education at all levels from undergraduate to doctoral programs.

Mary FitzGerald RN, DipN (Lond), CertEd, MN (Wales), PhD (UNE)

Professor of Nursing, The University of Newcastle, Newcastle, NSW, and Central Coast Health

Mary FitzGerald has had a long career in clinical nursing. Her interest in chronic illness stems from working with people in a medical ward of a district general hospital. Her research into the experience of chronic illness was undertaken as a postgraduate student at the University of New England. Her current research is in the broad area of aged care and clinical practice development.

Barb Fiveash RN, DNE (ACAE), BHlthSc (CSU), MN (Flinders)

Senior Lecturer, University of Ballarat, Ballarat, Victoria

Barb Fiveash teaches mental health and aged care. Using a range of qualitative methods, Barb has conducted research in the areas of mental health, aged care and consumer control over health care. One paper, titled 'Needs of carers of elderly people with dementia living in the community', was published in the *Australasian Journal on Ageing* (2001, 20(3) pp 133–8). Other papers include 'The experience of nursing home life' (*International Journal of Nursing Practice* 1998, 4(3) pp 166–75), 'Client-managed care' (*European Nurse* 1998, 3(3) pp 209–16) and 'The articulate resident's perspective on nursing home life' (*Lincoln Papers in Gerontology* 1997, No. 36, April).

Eleanor Horton RN, AND, CertAdultTchg, BHlthSc(Nsg), MHlthSc(Nsg), PhD candidate

Lecturer, School of Nursing and Midwifery, University of Newcastle, Newcastle, NSW

Eleanor Horton's interest in chronic illness evolved from many years of working in New Zealand with the Indigenous population and being involved with the development of cultural safety in nursing. Her recent experience in Australia has been in the not-for-profit sector and aged-care facilities.

Terri Jackson MA (Alberta), PhD (Brandeis, USA)

Senior Research Fellow, School of Public Health, La Trobe University, Melbourne, Victoria

Terri Jackson has been a leading Australian casemix researcher for the past decade, pioneering the use of patient-level cost data from management information systems to estimate DRG cost weights. Since 1993, she has provided research advice to six of the eight Victorian Cost Weight Studies, and devised and tested the VACS classification system which Victoria uses to pay for public hospital outpatient care. At the national level, she has provided advice on issues of technology assessment and economic evaluation. In 1998, she was appointed by the Minister for Health as health economist on the new Medicare Services Advisory Committee (MSAC), having served on its predecessor, the Australian Health Technology Advisory Committee, since 1993. Her current research projects include evaluations of the costs and consequences of PET scanning for a range of cancer indications, of therapeutic alternatives in the management of miscarriage, of diagnostic pathways in the treatment of appendicitis, and of within-DRG variation in cost.

Helen Keleher RN, BA, MA(HlthSt), PhD, FRCNA

Senior Lecturer in Public Health, Deakin University, Burwood, Victoria

Helen Keleher is a public health nurse with particular interest in policy. Her expertise is in population health models that deal with the social and environmental determinants of health, especially in relation to social and health inequities, health promotion and primary health care as strategies to tackle inequities, and rural health systems and services. Helen has served on significant scientific committees for public health including the National Public Health Partnership and in governance of health services. She is convenor of the Australian Women's Health Network and the National Committee for Women's Health.

Hal Kendig AB (University of California, Davis), MPI, PhD (University of Southern California), FASSA

Professor/Dean, Faculty of Health Sciences, University of Sydney, Sydney, NSW

Before his current position as Dean of the Faculty of Health Sciences at the University of Sydney, Hal Kendig served as Director of the Lincoln Gerontology Centre, a Key Centre of the Australian Research Council at La Trobe University, and he led the ANU Ageing and the Family Project. He is a Fellow of the Academy of Social Sciences in Australia, Honorary Life Fellow of the Australian Council on the Ageing, and Co-Chair of the Social Research and Planning Section, Asia-Oceania, International Association of Gerontology. His collaborative research includes a longitudinal survey of healthy ageing and studies of caregivers, falls prevention, housing and aged-care policies. Recent publications include *Who Should Care for the Elderly?* (Singapore University Press 2000), co-edited with William Liu, and *Australian Directions in Aged Care*, co-authored with Stephen Duckett (Australian Health Policy Institute 2001).

Beth Kingsley RN, MMedSc, PhD, ANZAC Fellow, FRCNA

Former Lecturer in the School of Nursing, Curtin University of Technology, Western Australia

Beth Kingsley has comprehensive expertise in the area of elder abuse, from both the community and institutional perspectives, on which she is a prolific educator and public speaker. She has developed protocols for responding to elder abuse, co-developed a program to work with the perpetrators of elder abuse and was awarded the 1997 Aged Care Australia National Meritorious Award for her contribution to the field of elder abuse.

Bill Koch RN, RNT, BSc (Stirling), MSc (Edinburgh), PhD (RMIT), MRCNA

Senior Lecturer in Information Technology, School of Nursing and Midwifery, La Trobe University, Melbourne, Victoria

Bill Koch graduated as a registered nurse at Stirling & Falkirk School of Nursing in Scotland in 1976. His clinical experience is mainly in the areas of surgical nursing and urology. He completed a BSc in Biology at the University of Stirling, graduating in 1981, after which he undertook a Master of Science in Nursing Education at the University of Edinburgh, graduating in 1983. He subsequently worked as a nurse educator in Scotland, before moving to Australia in 1987. His PhD was undertaken between 1996 and 1999. His thesis, ongoing research interests and publications are mainly focused on the use of information technology solutions to care planning and documentation problems within gerontic nursing, with a particular interest in the implementation and evaluation of decision support software for nurses.

Susan Koch RN, RCNT (Glasgow), BA(EducStud), DipProfStud, MN, PhD (La Trobe), FRCNA, FAAG

Senior Lecturer, School of Nursing, La Trobe University, Melbourne, Victoria

Susan Koch completed her nursing course at Glasgow Royal Infirmary, Scotland in 1975, Bachelor of Educational Studies at the University of Stirling in 1988 and Master of Nursing (Research) in 1995 at RMIT, Melbourne, and was awarded her PhD in 2003 from La Trobe University. She has been a senior lecturer in the School of Nursing at La Trobe University since 1997. Her practice, research and teaching have been predominantly in the area of aged care. She has received funding for research projects including: elder abuse of people with dementia and their carers; the use of restraints on older people; the retraining of circadian sleep/wake cycles; using computer-assisted learning to teach nurses mental health status assessment of elderly clients; experiences of people living with dementia after referral to a geriatric assessment team; the effect of reminiscence groups on fatigue, affect and life satisfaction in older Australian women; and the carer's experience of caring for someone with a dementia. Susan has been invited by Residential Care Rights and the Office of the Public Advocate to assist in resolving care issues involving older people in residential care, their families and staff.

Elizabeth Lavender RN, CertWardMgt&Tch, BSocSc(Nurs), MedSt (Monash), MRCNA

Deputy Dean, Faculty of Health Sciences and Senior Lecturer, School of Nursing and Midwifery, La Trobe University, Melbourne, Victoria

From 1990 to 1999 Elizabeth Lavender was responsible for the nursing programs at the regional campuses of La Trobe University at Albury/Wodonga and Shepparton. Her research interests at the time focused on rural nursing practice and education. She was a member of the Board of the Co-ordinating Unit Rural Health Education, Victoria (CURHEV). She also has long experience in teaching gerontic nursing in undergraduate and postgraduate nursing programs.

Sarah Mott RN, RMHN, PhD, FRCNA

Professor of Rehabilitation Nursing, University of Western Sydney, and Director, Rehabilitation Nursing Research and Development Unit, Royal Rehabilitation Centre, Sydney, NSW

Sarah Mott is Australia's first Professor of Rehabilitation Nursing, a joint appointment with the Royal Rehabilitation Centre, Sydney and the University of Western Sydney. Sarah has extensive experience in clinical practice, education and research in the areas of rehabilitation and aged care in Australia, the United States and England. She has many areas of research interest, including: the rehabilitative role of nurses; optimal well-being of people (primary health care to tertiary settings); mental health aspects of chronic illness and disability; aged care mental health; precursors to and management of aggressive behaviour; and leisure and recreation for people in residential care. She is editor-in-chief of the *Journal of the Australasian Rehabilitation Nurses Association* and is on the editorial boards of the *Australasian Journal of Ageing* and the *International Journal of Therapy and Rehabilitation*.

Alan Pearson RN, ONC, DipNEd (CAN), DANS, MSc (Manch), PhD (London), FINA, FCN (NSW), FRCNA, FAAG, FRCN

Professor of Nursing, and Director, Nursing Studies Unit, School of Nursing and Midwifery, Faculty of Health Sciences, La Trobe University, Melbourne, Victoria; Executive Director, Joanna Briggs Institute for Evidence Based Nursing and Midwifery, Royal Adelaide Hospital; and Adjunct Professor, School of Medicine, The University of Adelaide, Adelaide, South Australia

Alan Pearson has extensive experience in nursing practice, nursing research and academic nursing. He is editor of the *International Journal of Nursing Practice* and has published over thirty books and numerous journal articles. Since 1981 he has been an active researcher and is known internationally for his pioneering work on the establishment and evaluation of nursing beds in Oxford (UK) from 1981 to 1986, as well as his ongoing work, which emphasises the centrality of practice, and his work in evidence transfer and utilisation. He is active in developing and promoting nursing at the State, national and international levels and is currently chairperson for the national Aged Care Complaints Resolution Scheme, Chairperson of the National Committee—Documentation Framework for Aged Care. He is a member of a number of editorial boards of international journals.

Elizabeth Percival RN, DipAppSc, BN, MSc (Flinders), FRCNA, FAICD, FAIM

International Nursing Consultant, and Adjunct Associate Professor, School of Nursing, University of Canberra, ACT

In her current position as a consultant, Elizabeth Percival has been involved in nursing projects at a national and international level. She has worked extensively in the Asia-Pacific region for the US-based Honor Society of Nursing, Sigma Theta Tau International. She has also undertaken projects for the International Council of Nurses, Geneva. In addition, her work involves national consultancies, including the coordination of a project for the Department of Health and Ageing to implement Clinical Quality of Care Committees in residential aged-care facilities. In her previous role as the executive director of the Royal College of Nursing Australia (1994–2000), she was involved in developing a program of self-regulatory activities for the Australian nursing profession. She has a background in aged care, both as a clinician and as a Director of Nursing. She also held the position of Chief Executive Officer of the Nurses Board of South Australia. Elizabeth has served on numerous government and professional committees at a national and State level. She has been a member of the NH&MRC, the Australian Pharmaceutical Advisory Council and the Australian Nursing Council, and she is currently a commissioner on the Safety Rehabilitation and Compensation Commission.

Irene Stein RN, BA, MA, BN, PhD

Clinical Services Coordinator, Baptist Community Services (NSW and ACT), Cojoint Professor of Nursing, School of Nursing, University of Newcastle, Newcastle, NSW

Irene Stein completed her general nursing certificate at Balmain Hospital, Bachelor and Masters of Arts degrees at Wollongong University, Bachelor of Nursing at Charles Sturt University, Gerontological Nursing Certificate at the NSW College of Nursing and PhD at Wollongong University. She has held several senior academic positions. Irene is currently the Clinical Services Coordinator for Baptist Community Services (NSW and ACT). She also holds a Visiting Professorial appointment at Victoria University and is a Senior Research Fellow at the University of Technology, Sydney. Her areas of practice and research relate to aged-care delivery methods and workforce planning. Irene has published in these areas and is a strong advocate for workplace reform. She has a prevailing interest in cross-cultural issues related to aged care.

Annette Street BEd(Hons), PhD

Professor of Cancer and Palliative Care Studies and Director, La Trobe Clinical School of Nursing, at Austin Health, Victoria

Annette Street has an international reputation developed over the past twenty years through collaborative research and publication with clinical nurses. Her research interests are primarily focused on exploring the nursing and psychosocial dimensions of cancer and end-of-life care across a variety of acute, community and aged-care settings using mixed methods, action research and qualitative methodologies. She has received grant support from major funding bodies in Australia, New Zealand and Thailand and is widely published and cited. Annette has received numerous international awards and has conducted research consultancies throughout Australia, New Zealand, Sweden, Canada, Thailand, the United Kingdom and the United States.

Philip Street MBBS, FRACP

Senior Geriatrician, Bundoora Extended Care Centre, Melbourne, Victoria

Philip Street is a geriatrician at Bundoora Extended Care Centre and Austin Health, Melbourne. He has had extensive clinical experience in the medical care of older people in the acute and post-acute settings. He was involved in the establishment and operation of an acute hospital-based hip-fracture service in the early 1990s and more recently has helped to develop a model of collaborative care of hip-fracture patients at Austin Health. He has conducted a number of projects on the interface between hospital and post-discharge community care for older people. His current clinical interests centre around the areas of continence problems in older people, and dementia. He continues to play an active role in the teaching of geriatric medicine at undergraduate and postgraduate level.

Adriana Tiziani RN, BSc, DipEd, MEdSt, MRCNA

Research Assistant, Gerontic Nursing Professorial Unit, La Trobe University, Melbourne, Victoria

Adriana Tiziani has had a varied career in nursing. She has worked in acute care, community education, nursing education and infection prevention. Her interest in aged care stems from working with carers of people with dementia and as a charge nurse of a medical unit that encompassed an aged-care assessment unit. She is also interested in the use of medications by nurses and has published a number of editions of *Harvard's Nursing Guide to Drugs*.

Robin Watts RN, Dip(N Ed), BA (Curtin), MHSc (McMaster), PhD (Colorado), FRCNA

Foundation Professor of Nursing, Curtin University of Technology, Perth, Western Australia; Director of the WA Centre for Evidence Based Nursing and Midwifery, a Collaborating Centre of the Joanna Briggs Institute; and General Manager, University Planning

Robin Watts has had international experience in Honduras, Thailand, Canada and the United States. Her research interests include community participation, community health nursing, rural nursing and evidence-based practice, with a particular focus on women's and children's health.

VIGNETTE CONTRIBUTORS

Phillip Abbott RN
Nurse Unit Manager, Glen Huntly Aged Care Unit, Caulfield General Medical Centre, Melbourne, Victoria

Regina Barry RN, GradDip AdultEd (Deakin), PG Cert Health Service
Management (ECU), Executive Care Manager, Marsfield Centre For Aged Care, Baptist Community Services (NSW and ACT)

Steven Demeye RN, BN(PostReg), PBGNC
Director of Nursing, Lyndoch Aged Care, Warrnambool, Victoria

Karen Glaetzer RN, BN, NP, GradCertHealth(Palliative Care), CertOnc, CertBioethics, MNG-Nurse Practitioner
Nursing Coordinator, Community Palliative Care Service, South Adelaide, Palliative Services

June Heinrich Primary Teacher's Cert (Balmain TC), BA(Hons) (Macquarie), MSc (Tennessee), DipEd (Newcastle)
Chief Executive Officer, Baptist Community Services (NSW and ACT)

Rosalie Hudson RN, BAppSc(AdvNurs), BTheol, MTheol, GradDipGer, PhD, FRCNA, AAG Fellow
Honorary Associate Professor, School of Nursing, Melbourne University, and Aged Care Consultant

Dianne Johnson RN (Div 1), Midwifery Cert, Critical Care Cert, GradCertGer
Nurse Unit Manager, Bundoora Extended Care Centre, Bundoora, Victoria

Craig Lockwood, RN, BN, GradDipClinNurs, MNSC
Deputy Director, Centre for Evidence-based Nursing South Australia (CENSA), a collaborating centre of The Joanna Briggs Institute, Royal Adelaide Hospital, South Australia

Maria McIntosh RN, BN, GradDipGerNurs
Clinical Nurse Consultant, Caulfield General Medical Centre, Melbourne, Victoria

Bart O'Brien RGN, PhD, MRCNA
Project Manager, Year of Clinical Focus, RDNS, South Australia

Daniel Olivieri RN, BEd, MEd, IDCert, GradCert(Ger Nurs)
Nurse Unit Manager, Bundoora Extended Care Centre, Bundoora, Victoria

Helen Page RN Div 1, BBus Mkt
Manager, RSL Park Hostel, Frankston, Victoria

Anne Pitcher RN, CM, PostGradDip(Ger Nurs)
Gerontic Nursing Professorial Unit and Clinical School, La Trobe University, Bundoora, Victoria

Barbara Potter AM, Hon. FRCNA, Hon. Member Alzheimer's Association of Victoria

Elizabeth Pringle BEd Adult Ed (HRM), MAEd Adult Ed (VET) UTS
General Manager, Education, The Aged Care Standards and Accreditation Agency

Suzanne Sawyer RN, RM, DipCommHealthNurs, BAppSc(Nurs)
Director of Nursing, Jindalee Nursing Home

Margaret Winbolt RN, PostGradDipAdvNurs(Ger Nurs), MRCNA
Clinical Nurse Consultant (Gerontic Nursing), Bundoora Extended Care Centre, Bundoora, Victoria

Part 1

Contextual issues and innovations

CHAPTER 1

Funding and policy in residential care in Australia

MARY COURTNEY, BRIAN ABBEY AND JENNY ABBEY

INTRODUCTION

From the early 1950s, when the Commonwealth Government first became involved in residential aged care, until the 1980s, the history of this sphere of aged-care nursing in Australia was a fragmented story of complex legislative and funding arrangements involving a shifting and obscure mix of Commonwealth and State responsibilities, all underpinning the rapid but haphazard growth in the number of nursing-home beds operated by State governments, commercial providers and not-for-profit church and charitable bodies. The engine of this growth, it is now clear, was a system of generous but ill-considered and sometimes contradictory Commonwealth financial incentives. Periods of sudden expansion alternated with periods of stagnation, driven not by need but by the size of the subsidies on offer. There was little coordination between the States and the Commonwealth, resulting in great variations in bed supply and the cost to the consumer from one State to another. Standards of management were, in general, poor; money was handed out with inadequate controls over what it bought, who benefited, and the quality of the services it supported (Craik 1981; Howe 1992; Palmer & Short 1989).

Since the early-to-middle 1980s there has been significant change and major reform on all these fronts, leading to the emergence of a more coherent and streamlined national approach. This chapter describes those changes and discusses where they are leading the industry and the aged people who do or will depend on it for care in their later years.

Residential aged care, once of interest only to a narrow range of health professionals and those members of the public directly concerned with their own or a relative's circumstances, is now a major topic of discussion in the media and the wider community. Undoubtedly the three major factors driving this change are, first, the occurrence of another phase in the community's awakening to the implications of Australia's changing demographic profile. Second, there have been consequential concerns, especially in government circles, over the budgetary impact of funding the future provision of aged care in the quantities likely to be needed. Third, the first and second factors have prompted a renewed questioning of when and how far community-based and home-delivered services can be substituted for full-time residential care, a question this chapter briefly returns to in closing.

Australia's changing demographic profile and the projected future costs of aged care provide our starting point. The chapter then briefly traces the confused course of residential care provision between about 1950 and 1980, a picture of abundant effort with little direction. We shall see how the ill-planned developments of that period caused problems necessitating successive waves of reforms culminating in the aged-care structural reforms of the mid-1980s and early 1990s, and the *Aged Care Act 1997*. The chapter closes by examining how far those reforms achieved their objectives and what problems can be expected to command our attention in the next ten or so years.

THE CHANGING DEMOGRAPHIC PROFILE, 1976–2041

It is well recognised that the Australian population is ageing, and that this trend is expected to increase right through the first half of this century. The rate of increase of the older population is significantly higher than that of the population as a whole, with the growth rate being highest among the very old (see Table 1.1). As recently as 1976, only 9% of the population (1.3 million people) were aged 65 years or over. However, by 1999, this age group made up 12% (2.3 million) of the total population; and projections suggest that by 2016 this will increase to 16% (3.6 million) and, by 2041, to 25% (6.2 million). Of even greater importance for aged-care planning is the number of people aged 80 years or more, since it is this group that requires most care. Here the growth rate is even more striking. In 1976, one in six older people (those aged 65 or above) was aged 80 or over; by 1999 it was one in five; by 2016 it is projected to be one in four; and by 2041 one in three older people will be aged over 80 years (Commonwealth Department of Health and Ageing [DOHA] 2000).

Table 1.1: Numbers of persons aged 65+ and 80+ years in the Australian population between 1976 and 2041

	Number (% total population)			
	1976	**1999**	**2016**	**2041**
Total Australian population	14,400,000	19,100,000	22,500,000	24,800,000
Aged 65+	1,300,000 (9%)	2,300,000 (12%)	3,600,000 (16%)	6,200,000 (25%)
Aged 80+	217,000 (1.5%)	460,000 (2.4%)	900,000 (4.0%)	2,067,000 (8.3%)

Source: adapted from DOHA 2000, ABS 1999, 2003 and Commonwealth Treasury 2002, p 22.

The increase in the total aged population can be expected to accelerate appreciably from about the end of the century's first decade, while the most rapid increase in the size of the cohort of people aged 80 and over will occur in the third decade (Australian Bureau of Statistics [ABS] 2000, cited by National Aged Care Alliance 2002, p 3).

If present trends in health status, capability for independent living and gender differentials continue as they now are (and we should never assume too readily that they will), there is a potential for the growth in the number of the 'old old' to impose some strain on Australia's resources. But the issue is more complex than this simple observation suggests. The truth is that Australia's population is still relatively young compared to those of other developed nations, and the situation confronting this country is by no means unique or even unusual. On the other hand, it is the speed with which this 'old old' group will grow in Australia that is unusual, and it is this need for us to adjust rapidly that may pose adjustment strains in policy settings, service provision and, just as important, in our cultural attitudes and our political and financial priorities.

Health expenditure on older people

As might be expected, average health expenditure per person is considerably higher for older persons than for younger persons because the former group seek more treatment and care. People aged over 65 years, for example, consume approximately four times the amount of health resources consumed by those under that age. The 65-and-above group are admitted to hospitals more often and stay longer, and their expenditure on pharmaceuticals is 2.5 times higher. This has been known and more or less consistent for some time. In 1993–94, even though older Australians made up only 12% of the total population, they used $11 billion (35%) of the $31 billion total health expenditure budget (Australian Institute of Health and Welfare [AIHW] 1997). This striking and persistent differential is largely explained by the correlation between ageing and expenditures on pharmaceuticals and, of course, residential care subsidies, which lump together both health and daily living costs. Moreover, the differential is even sharper when the expenditure for the 75+ group is compared to all others. Not surprisingly this heavier consumption of health services together with the demographic trajectory just described has given rise in some quarters to alarm about the impending budgetary impact of ageing and aged care. We shall return to examine the matter of costs in the final section of this chapter.

THE GROWTH IN RESIDENTIAL AGED CARE 1950–1995

The Commonwealth gets involved

The Commonwealth's involvement in modern residential aged care began in 1954 with the provision of subsidies to church and charitable bodies to build homes for the indigent aged who might otherwise have been homeless. This initiative was greeted with enthusiasm by various lobby groups and the Commonwealth's role soon broadened to include an expanding range of incentives offered by successive governments. The most dramatic spur to growth came in 1963 with the introduction of per-day nursing home benefits payable to each resident of an approved institution. In 1968, an additional per-day subsidy was introduced for those residents needing more intensive care. As a result of this system of benefits and other recurrent and capital incentives—some of which, it has been noted (Palmer & Short 1989, p 103), were at odds with one another—the nursing home sector grew explosively, especially between 1963 and 1971, when the number of nursing-home beds grew from a national average of 29 beds per thousand people aged 65+ to 46.5 per thousand (Sax 1990, p 97). At that time, national averages were misleading, however, because the rapid growth was scattered unevenly across the country, leading to very unequal access to residential care for citizens of different States (Commonwealth Department of Community Services and Health [CS&H] 1986, p 22). Nevertheless, although growth proceeded unevenly from year to year and from place to place, mainly depending on changes to the subsidy programs, it continued over two decades, with nursing home bed numbers rising by 165% between 1963 and 1983 (Sax 1990, p 99).

So rapid, haphazard and costly was this growth in the supply of nursing-home beds that government attempts to stimulate the level of provision of residential care were soon increasingly replaced, or at least supplemented, by various attempts to control and direct it. The three-part strategy that emerged at this point and was consolidated in the 1980s has formed the foundation of policy to the present. The key steps were, first, to impose controls on the creation of new nursing home beds; second, to tilt the balance of new provision towards the less expensive hostel model; and third, to increase the level of community-based and home-delivered services so as to slow the rate of institutionalisation.

Controls on the number of nursing-home beds introduced in 1971 slowed growth, but only for a while. Financial incentives were now used to stimulate the hostel sector, particularly between 1972 and 1975, thus creating a two-tier system and making beds available that were cheaper to create and maintain for those whose needs were more in the area of daily social and domestic support than around-the-clock nursing or personal care. The third part of the strategy was to expand subsidies to support domiciliary nursing and such services as home help and Meals on Wheels, both designed to make staying in the home more feasible for the infirm aged (Palmer & Short 1989, p 103). Some of the significant innovations of this type were gathered together under the auspices of the Home and Community Care (HACC) program announced in the 1994 Budget and implemented in the following year.

Thus, as the first half of the 1980s progressed, the Australian system for delivering aged residential care was undergoing fast but uneven and unplanned growth, with two distinct types of institutions—nursing homes (for higher-dependency residents) and hostels (for lower-dependency residents). It might have seemed that the system of residential aged care was beginning to mature and on the point of achieving some stability, but this was not so. Waves of change were about to break over the sector.

The pressure for further reform grows

As often happens, the inflow of public money and the higher sectoral profile resulting from its growth was accompanied by more sustained critical attention from all the parties involved—politicians, bureaucrats, providers and client groups. Coincidentally, these were the years of the most fundamental and systematic public sector reform that Australia has witnessed since the late 1940s; and so perhaps it is not surprising that calls for further, more comprehensive reform were soon coming from many directions and, what is more noteworthy, receiving a hearing in the highest echelons.

Palmer & Short (1989), writing at the end of the 1980s, noted the publication in the preceding eight years of no fewer than eight major Commonwealth reports examining all aspects of the aged-care residential industry, including its admini-stration, planning and funding, and providing 'many trenchant criticisms of the administration of the Commonwealth's program'(Palmer & Short 1989, pp 103–4). Central to these criticisms, made by a number of reports in this period, was concern at 'the absence of an adequate planning framework of the development of residen-tial programs costing over $1 billion per annum' (CS&H 1986, p 4). Indeed, most of what had occurred up to this turning point was described by one commentator as having been the outcome of 'policy by default' (Howe 1992, p 240).

So it was against this background that the process of beginning to lay the public policy foundations for the evolution of the aged-care residential system over the next ten or fifteen years began. The successive reports published during that time contain the landmark steps in the process. Among the tangible achievements of this phase of policy building were:

- the establishment of an explicit planning framework based on types of places available per 1000 people aged 70 or above;
- the decision to progressively re-balance the provision of high-care and low-care beds to better target needs and contain costs;
- devising and recommending measures to guard against premature institutionalisation of the aged;
- foreseeing the need for a progressively strengthened geriatric assessment system based on regional teams;
- anticipating the need to soften the demarcation between nursing homes and hostels;
- supporting a continuing expansion of community-based support services such as the HACC services that came into operation in 1985;
- recognising the need for dementia support;
- alerting the community to the need to define and protect consumer rights for those in residences; and
- increasing HACC funding, to further reduce reliance on residential care solutions for the frail aged.

Five or so years later, in 1990–91, with the intention of assessing the progress of the reform strategy and further extending its reach, the government launched the Aged Care Reform Strategy Mid-Term Review. The Stage I and II reports, published in September 1991 and October 1993 respectively and usually referred to as the Gregory reports (Commonwealth Department of Health, Housing and Community Services [HH&CS] 1991; Commonwealth Department of Health, Housing, Local Government and Community Services [HHLG&CS] 1993), highlighted the poor physical state of many nursing homes and their failure to meet either fire safety or local health requirements. Gregory pointed to the lack of incentives or capital funds for providers to maintain their facilities at a high standard, a point that was to be addressed by the 1997 Act. Gregory forecast that one of the likely effects of the shift towards hostel care, when coupled with the ageing dynamic, would be a much higher proportion of highly dependent people living in hostels. By the mid-1990s there was a growing recognition that some hostel residents, perhaps as many as 20% of them, were actually more dependent than some nursing home residents (AIHW 2002a, cited in AIHW, 2002b, p 2; CS&H 1986; Duckett 1995). But of course the funding system's different treatment of the two types of institutions prevented hostel residents from receiving the level of subsidy that would have purchased the sort of care they needed. Gregory, foreseeing the likelihood that this could worsen with time, suggested that a further review of the funding models and balance of care be conducted in about 1996, when the national age profile was expected to begin to curve sharply upwards (HH&CS 1991).

The collective impact of these successive reviews, agency research papers and a growing number of academic studies throughout the 1980s and early 1990s was twofold. First, they identified the issues that needed to be dealt with and the range of measures that might be employed. Second, that critical mass of research and debate marked the creation of a policy community focused on aged care, and the commencement of a coherent, ongoing dialogue over aged-care policy within government circles and between government and the various lobby groups and research institutions (Howe 1992). During these years we can trace the steps involved in:

- establishing a common, coherent and durable agenda for the sector;
- building mechanisms for interest articulation, debate and negotiation linking the various stakeholder interests;
- moving toward the creation of a single and much-simplified legislative framework; and
- fostering the growth of a culture of ongoing research and evaluation of the impact of policy.

It is fair to say that by the mid-1990s there was a substantial and mature reform agenda pressing for the attention of government and providers alike, and sufficient political pressure to ensure that it was addressed.

The importance of these developments, whether we are making policy or simply understanding it, becomes clearer after reading Palmer & Short's (2000) concise introduction (Chs 2 and 3) to the policy process as it applies in health care. Gregory's 1991 report also helps to give form and order to this process by including a 'Summary of Eight Stages of the Aged Care Reform Strategy' (HH&CS 1991, Appendix A.1); and Gibson's timeline of policy innovations also helps clarify the main steps (Gibson 1998, Appendix). With hindsight we can see that, with the agenda clear and the policy community close to consensus on the need for change, the stage was now set for the program of legislative reform that was to be introduced in 1997.

Residential-care bed provision prior to the 1997 reforms

One means of controlling nursing-home expansion and containing costs adopted in 1985 was to institute planning guidelines for ratios of different types of aged-care beds per 1000 people aged 70 and over. The total bed supply targeted at the aged, including both nursing home and hostel beds, expressed as a national average as at June 1985, stood at a ratio of 100 beds per 1000 persons aged 70 years or more (CS&H 1986, p 24). Originally these targets were set at 40 nursing-home places per 1000 people aged 70 years and older, and 60 hostel places per 1000 people aged 70 years and over. A subsequent modification, marking the rise of community-based alternatives, was to convert first five and then ten beds of the hostel allocation into equivalent funded home- and community-based services, promoting staying in the home.

Just prior to the 1997 reforms, there were a national total of 137,654 aged care long-term beds available in non-acute settings. Of these 75,009 were nursing-home beds—equivalent to 49.5 beds per 1000 persons aged 70 years and over—with 62,645 places within the hostel sector—equivalent to 41.4 places per 1000 persons aged 70 and over (AIHW 1999). This figure already represented a sharp change from the nursing home:hostel ratio of just a few years before, when government first began to swing the balance towards fewer of the former and more of the latter.

The nursing homes and hostels were operated by charitable and church bodies, by commercial 'for profit' enterprises and by State governments in what the AIHW has described as a 'mixed economy of care' (AIHW 1999). The parts played by the different types of providers in this two-tier system as it existed prior to the 1997 restructure can be represented thus:

- Private organisations—operating for profit—provided 47% of nursing-home beds and 2% of hostel places.
- Not-for-profit organisations provided 37% of nursing-home beds and 92% of hostel places.
- State governments provided 16% of nursing-home beds and 6% of hostel places (HH&CS 1991).

It is not easy to compare the situation before and after 1997 because of the changed terminology, but we do know that by mid-2002, across Australia, the three categories of providers shared provision of the beds as follows:

- private (for profit)—28%
- not-for-profit—63%
- State governments—9%

(Australian National Audit Office [ANAO] 2003).

State-to-State (Territories excluded) variations were marked. Victoria's beds were shared more equally between the three types of providers than in other States, with Victoria having the largest private and government sectors of all States. Tasmania had the least equally shared provision, with both its private and government sectors being smaller than in all other States (ANAO 2003, Fig 1.3, p 26).

It should be noted that the overall level of aged-care accommodation in Australia, while higher than in some natural comparators such as the United Kingdom, the United States and New Zealand, was not outstandingly high by, for example, some European standards. What was distinct about the Australian system was the heavy preponderance of nursing-home beds compared to, say, hostels or community-based services (CS&H 1986, p 24; Rowland 1991, p 99). As Palmer and Short explain:

The nursing home subsidy [begun in 1963 and expanded five years later] supplied the motive force behind the boom in the nursing home industry to the point where it dominated the development of Commonwealth policy for older persons.

Palmer & Short 2000, p 299

AGED-CARE STRUCTURAL REFORM 1996–97

Objectives of the aged-care structural reform strategy

In delivering its 1996 Budget, the Commonwealth Government announced a package of fundamental reforms directed at the main issues on the accumulating reform agenda. The aims of the package were to:

- bring hostels and nursing homes together in a unified system;
- devise a single funding model, sensitive to equity issues, and tied to residents' level of dependency rather than the category of home they live in;
- contain the future call on government recurrent and capital funding as the population ages, partly by more tightly targeting public subsidies;
- establish an element of user-pays in relation to both daily costs and capital raising for asset maintenance and expansion;
- allow 'ageing-in-place' so as to spare residents the disruption of a forced move to a different facility as their required care levels change;
- introduce an improved quality assurance process, with the results accessible to consumers, using a mix of inducements and sanctions to ensure the industry's adoption of a culture built upon continuous quality improvement in all spheres of activity;
- better recognise the impact of dementia and other behavioural problems on costs of care and resident amenity;
- enforce improved building and fit-out standards appropriate to the client's needs and capacity to pay;
- underpin the commercial stability of the industry and protect consumers' rights by some prudential oversight of each provider's asset backing and liquidity;
- further expand the range of community-based supports designed to buttress the care-at-home alternative to institutionalisation;
- rationalise the industry's provision of respite services;
- render staffing requirements more flexible and more focused on outcomes rather than inputs; and
- meet providers' demands for administrative streamlining and the professionals' demands for simplification of documentation and client record-keeping.

The heart of the legislative package was the merging of the two distinct streams of care—nursing homes and hostels—aimed at providing care determined by need for residents as they progressed through the range of dependencies within the one aged-care facility, with a single funding instrument allocating financial support.

It was expected that unification and the associated measures would rationalise and contain funding in the future, and allow 'ageing-in-place', thus avoiding the upset and distress of moving the elderly resident from one type of facility to a different type when a higher level of care was required and, in the process, separating him or her from friends and familiar surroundings, and possibly even from a spouse.

The Resident Classification Scale

A precondition of effective unification was the creation of a new single classification scheme focused on each resident's needs irrespective of where they lived, capable of facilitating a seamless transition from low-dependency to high-care needs. The new Resident Classification Instrument, which came into operation on 1 October 1997 and remains in effect at the time of writing, is called the Resident Classification Scale (RCS). The scale contains 22 questions and the weightings were formulated on the basis of a study of 20,000 residents in over 400 facilities, undertaken during February and March 1997. The RCS replaced the Resident Classification Instrument (RCI) previously used in nursing homes, and the Personal Care Assessment Instrument (PCAI) previously used in hostels. The RCS, still largely unchanged in mid-2003, forms the basis for Commonwealth subsidies for all aged-care facilities under the current funding arrangements.

The RCS, just like its predecessor, the RCI, requires that detailed documentation of care be maintained over a period of at least 21 days in order to classify a resident into a category, a requirement later to become the focus of much industry dissatisfaction. The 22 questions—presented in Table 1.2—are scored (and weighted) for each question, and then added together to give a total score for the resident. Level 1, a score of 81.00 or above, is the highest-dependency level and is entitled to the highest level of subsidy; while anyone scoring fewer than 10.6 points is rated Level 8 and is eligible for a Commonwealth subsidy unless or until their dependency is re-rated at a higher level.

The RCS introduced a greater weighting for behavioural questions than was the case with the previous RCI and PCAI tools, in order to meet the earlier criticism that classifications and funding did not adequately recognise the impact of dementia on an individual's care needs or the consequent burden imposed on the facility.

It was agreed by government at the time of the introduction of the 1997 reforms that a review of the functioning of the RCS would occur within twelve months of implementation (Gray 2001a, p 22). The outcome of that review and subsequent reviews will be examined later in this chapter.

Table 1.3 gives the range of points for each of the eight categories of care.

Cost containment and user-pays

As noted above, the amount of public subsidy is set by the resident's RCS classification. The resident's own contribution is made up of two parts, although how much each will be is decided by reference to Commonwealth-determined scales relating to the resident's income and assets. One part of the resident's (possible) liability is a contribution to the facility's capital costs, and this is further explained below. The other part potentially chargeable to the resident is known as a basic daily care charge and this is levied for the hotel costs which would accrue to the resident wherever she or he lived and the care provided. This charge may range up to a maximum specified by the Commonwealth, depending on the individual resident's income.

Table 1.2: RCS questions and weightings

Questions	A	B	C	D
1. Communication	0.00	0.28	0.36	0.83
2. Location change, mobility and transfers	0.00	1.19	1.54	1.82
3. Meals and drinks	0.00	0.67	0.75	2.65
4. Personal hygiene	0.00	5.34	14.17	14.61
5. Toileting	0.00	5.98	10.65	13.70
6. Continence—urinary	0.00	1.50	1.82	2.26
7. Continence—faecal	0.00	4.04	7.72	8.23
8. Comprehension/awareness	0.00	0.79	1.11	3.40
9. Wandering and absconding	0.00	0.44	0.83	1.35
10. Interfering with others and/or others' belongings	0.00	0.36	0.75	2.65
11. Noisy	0.00	0.91	1.35	3.17
12. Aggressive physically	0.00	2.34	2.69	3.05
13. Aggressive verbally	0.00	0.28	0.40	1.43
14. Extreme emotional dependence	0.00	0.28	1.50	3.84
15. Danger to self or others	0.00	1.11	1.54	1.98
16. Other behaviour	0.00	0.91	1.82	2.61
17. Social and human needs	0.00	0.95	1.98	3.01
18. Social and human needs—family and friends	0.00	0.28	0.55	0.91
19. Mediations	0.00	0.79	8.55	11.40
20. Technical and nursing procedures	0.00	1.54	5.54	11.16
21. Therapy—physiotherapy	0.00	3.64	6.10	7.01
22. Therapy—other	0.00	0.71	1.46	2.93

Source: Commonwealth Department of Health and Family Services 1997a, pp 5-3 and 5-4.

Table 1.3: Range of points for each category of care

Score range	Corresponding care category
> 81.01 points	Level 1
69.1–81.00 points	Level 2
56.01–69.60 points	Level 3
50.01–56.00 points	Level 4
39.81–50.00 points	Level 5
28.91–39.80 points	Level 6
10.61–28.90 points	Level 7
0–10.60 points	Level 8

Source: Commonwealth Department of Health and Family Services 1997a, p 5-4.

Capital raising for asset development: accommodation charges and bonds

Accommodation bonds were introduced into hostels in the late 1980s, and provided a flow of funds which enabled hostels to undertake capital-works programs that, prior to the 1997 reforms, usually allowed them to offer accommodation physically superior to that on offer by nursing homes. The Aged Care Act 1997 sought to eliminate this disparity by extending this capital-contribution arrangement to nursing homes. As from 1 October 1997, the Commonwealth Department of Health and Family Services (DH&FS) allowed nursing homes to charge accommodation bonds for all new residents entering their facility. Initially the government's plans were widely seen as placing little or no limit on how high such bonds might be and, it was said, might in many cases have virtually forced the sale of the family home to raise the required capital. Vehement public opposition caused the scheme to be withdrawn and replaced by a more politically acceptable scheme with safeguards over how much of the resident's assets might be claimed by the proprietor of the facility they were entering (Jones 1997–98; National Aged Care Alliance 2002, p 2). Accommodation charges and bonds depend on the assets test and remain fixed once they are established and agreed upon. This agreement is fixed, even if the resident moves from the low-band level of care (formerly hostel care) to the high-band level of care (formerly nursing-home care), or if the resident moves from one facility to another.

Accommodation charges applied to high-band (formerly nursing-home level) residents with sufficient assets from 6 November 1997. The size of the accommodation charge levied by the facility is set on a sliding scale determined by the government. At the time of writing (6 August 2003) this level is capped at a maximum of $45.07 per day for a resident whose annual income is in excess of $68,742 for a single person or $136,756 for a couple. If the resident's net assets are below $27,500, no accommodation charge is levied, and the resident is classified as a concessional resident. Residents with assets valued between these threshold amounts have their charge determined according to a sliding scale, based on the amount of their assets above $27,500 divided by five years. However, residents with assets between $27,500 and $44,000 cannot be charged more than $6.96 per day. These residents are classed as 'assisted residents' and this status can be counted under the concessional-resident ratio.

Accommodation bonds apply to low-band residents and are a revised version of the existing 'entry-contribution' scheme. There is no defined upper limit to the bond, and the level of the bond is mutually agreed between the resident and the provider. However, the resident must be left with minimum residual net assets of $27,500 and the maximum charge that may be 'drawn down' from the bond by the provider is $245.50 per month ($3054 per year) for five years. After that point the interest earned on the account flows to the provider but no more capital may be taken from the account. The resident receives a full refund of the balance, less the interest, when they leave the facility.

For purposes of asset determination, the resident's home is exempt—provided a spouse or carer has lived in the house for longer than two years. Furthermore, if one spouse from a married couple applies for residency, the amount of assets is divided by two (less the value of the house, if applicable). The Commonwealth Department of Health and Ageing provides a full up-to-date schedule of fees and charges on the following website: http://www.ageing.health.gov.au/finance/resfees.htm.

The quality assurance and accreditation framework

One of the frequently repeated criticisms of the aged-care residential system during the early and mid-1980s was its neglect of quality issues and the consequent lack of quality assurance mechanisms. In 1987 the government introduced Outcomes Standards for nursing homes and created Standards Monitoring Teams to carry out audits on site. This system was poorly regarded by providers, who complained that the teams were too often rigid in approach and somewhat punitive. The system also drew criticism from other quarters for its apparent inability to distinguish between one-off failures and systemic problems, or to deal effectively with poorly performing providers, and for failing to promote continuous quality improvement perspectives (Gray 2001a, pp 5, 86f). Braithwaite (2001) and some other scholars cited by Braithwaite provide a rather different assessment that points to strengths as well as weaknesses in the previous system.

During 1997, a new quality assurance and accreditation framework for the unified residential system was developed. The four main innovations included in the new quality system were:

- a single set of standards and expected outcomes applicable to all aged-care residences;
- four additional accreditation criteria aimed at important ancillary matters;
- a new independent agency for the conduct of periodic, scheduled quality audits; and
- publication of accreditation reports and measures to protect residents' rights.

Let us look at each of these in turn.

The Standards

A review of the previous Commonwealth Outcome Standards saw the formulation of four main Standards, with a total of 44 subordinate standards and expected outcomes which, as a whole, provide a new structured approach to the management of quality in residential-care facilities.

As shown in Table 1.4, the 44 Expected Outcomes are grouped into a matrix built around four basic Standards:

- management systems, staffing and organisational development;
- health and personal care;
- residential lifestyle; and
- physical environment and safe systems.

Table 1.4: Standards matrix

1.0 Management	2.0 Health	3.0 Lifestyle	4.0 Environment
1.1 Continuous	2.1 Continuous	3.1 Continuous	4.1 Continuous
1.2 Regulatory	2.2 Regulatory	3.2 Regulatory	4.2 Regulatory
1.3 Education	2.3 Education	3.3 Education	4.3 Education
1.4 Comments	2.4 Clinical	3.4 Emotional	4.4 Living
1.5 Planning	2.5 Specialised	3.5 Independence	4.5 OH and Safety
1.6 Human Res	2.6 Other	3.6 Privacy	4.6 Fire
1.7 Inventory	2.7 Medication	3.7 Leisure	4.7 Infection
1.8 Information	2.8 Pain	3.8 Cultural	4.8 Catering
1.9 External	2.9 Palliative	3.9 Choice	
	2.10 Nutrition	3.10 Tenure	
	2.11 Skin Care		
	2.12 Continence		
	2.13 Behaviour		
	2.14 Mobility		
	2.15 Dental Care		
	2.16 Sensory Loss		
	2.17 Sleep		

Source: DH&FS 1997b, p 10.

Significantly, three specific topics or themes—continuous improvement, regulatory compliance, and education and staff development—are common to all four basic standards in the matrix.

There are four parts to each of the standards:

- *Principle:* describes the purpose, intent, philosophy and rationale;
- *Expected outcome:* expands on the performance expectations;
- *Criteria:* tests for the policies and practices required for the outcome to be achieved during the time of audit assessment; and
- *Guidelines:* provide considerations to help in self-assessment.

To demonstrate the framework, an example is provided in Table 1.5.

Table 1.5: Draft standard

Standard 2.4 Clinical Care

Expected outcome: Residents receive appropriate clinical care.

Criteria: Policies and practices provide:
- each resident with their choice of doctor
- individual clinical care that is prescribed, assessed, documented and regularly monitored
- for a resident-care plan that is developed in partnership with each resident and/or his/her representative and the health-care team
- for access to emergency medical treatment at all times
- referral to medical and other associated health services
- a readily available record of assessment, diagnoses and treatment to enable other medical and health-care practitioners, in an emergency, to provide effective treatment
- regular review of clinical care
- prescribed treatment and medication to be correctly documented and administered.

Source: DH&FS 1997b, p 10.

Four additional accreditation criteria

In order to achieve accreditation, the facility must also satisfy requirements relating to certain other key operational matters in addition to meeting the care and service standards and expected outcomes referred to above.

- *Certification:* this is based on an assessment of the physical structure and plant of the facility, gauged against relevant legislation and practice codes.
- *Prudential arrangements:* these have been constructed in order to ensure that the facility has sufficient funds available to repay accommodation bonds as they fall due. This operates on a self-report format where the facility informs the Department of its status in relation to accommodation charge deposits.

- *Concessional resident ratio:* concessional residents are those who own assets valued at less than $27,500 in virtue of which they are excused of any liability for the accommodation bond or charge. A government subsidy is paid to the facility for such residents in lieu of the bond or charge. A mandatory concessional-resident ratio, set at 27% of the facility's beds, has been established in order to ensure access for financially disadvantaged persons. Sanctions apply to those facilities failing to meet the minimum, although the requirement can be relaxed for a time if a facility does not have a financially disadvantaged person waiting for admission.

- *User rights:* provision for user rights is included in the legislation via the Charter of Residents' Rights and Responsibilities, and is also manifest in resident agreements, complaint-resolution mechanisms, public access to accreditation reports, resident support from advocacy services, and via the Community Visitors Scheme.

The accreditation audit: the agency and the process

The *Aged Care Act 1997* sought to create a degree of independence from both government and the industry for the new monitoring agency, the Aged Care Standards and Accreditation Agency Ltd, by establishing it in 1998 as an independent company. The Agency is owned by government but operated by a seven-member board of directors comprising people from the industry, government, consumer peak groups and the wider community. It is charged with managing the accreditation process in accordance with the Accountability Principles, the Accreditation Grant Principles and the Act (*Aged Care Act 1997*; DH&AC 1999b). A little less than half the Agency's funding currently comes from government and the rest is earned as accreditation fees paid by facilities (ANAO 2003, p 34; Aged Care Standards and Accreditation Agency 1998).

Accreditation of each aged-care facility involves evaluation of the organisation's system of management against the Standards. A detailed account of the audit process may be found in the Australian National Audit Office document titled *Managing Residential Aged Care Accreditation* (ANAO 2003, Fig 1.4, p 29). In order to apply for accreditation, the facility will first conduct its own 'in-house' audit against the Aged Care Standards using a self-assessment tool designed by the Agency and available in its Accreditation Guide (downloadable from its website). Once the aged-care facility feels that it is ready for accreditation, it formally applies to the Agency, pays the relevant fee, and submits a copy of its self-evaluation. After a team is appointed by the Agency—the facility has the option of nominating one member to the team—the facility then undergoes two related (but distinct) auditing steps: the desktop audit (now renamed the 'self-assessment') and the compliance audit (now renamed the 'site audit').

The desktop audit will generally be conducted offsite and involves an examination of the facility's application and accompanying documentation. The compliance audit involves a site visit by the audit team. The auditors, known as 'quality assessors', observe processes, interview people within the facility and review appropriate documentation. This stage involves the collection of evidence to determine the level of compliance with the relevant Standard. At each stage the accreditation focuses on the design and performance of the systems used by the facility to achieve and monitor compliance with the Standards, and the extent to which a continuous quality improvement approach has been inculcated in the staff and entrenched in management procedures.

The initial target was to have all facilities undergo the accreditation process for the first time prior to 1 January 2001. Accreditation was to be given for either one or three years, and mechanisms were established whereby co-located facilities could undergo a single accreditation. During the first-round accreditations conducted between September 1999 and December 2000, each facility was awarded one of the following ratings:

- *Commendable:* the facility's policies and practices meet the expected outcome.
- *Satisfactory:* the facility's policies and practices generally meet the expected outcome; however, some minor deficiencies need to be rectified within an agreed timeframe.
- *Unacceptable:* the facility's policies and practices do not meet the expected outcome; there are major deficiencies which may take considerable time to rectify.
- *Critical:* a major health and/or safety risk has been identified which requires immediate corrective action.

Those ratings were re-worded in May 2002 to meet industry concerns, as we shall see later in this chapter when we review the other outcomes of the first accreditation round and some subsequent developments.

DEVELOPMENTS SINCE THE 1997 REFORMS

The swing to community-based care continues

Before examining how the reforms under the Aged Care Act contributed to the evolution of aged-care policy, it is perhaps appropriate to point out that, alongside these changes, the Commonwealth has continued the strategy of progressively raising the level of community supports that had begun to take shape with the formation of the Home and Community Care program in 1985 (HH&CS 1991, pp 5–7). A major post-1997 instance of the community supports strategy was the announcement of the Care and Support for Older Australians package by the federal government on 2 April 1998. This $270-million package, implemented over four years, included:

- expansion and/or modification of the community and aged-care package (CACPs) program introduced in 1992;
- continence management services;
- carer respite centres;
- residential respite services;
- community-based respite services for carers of people with dementia; and
- support services for ageing carers of an adult with a disability.

Impact of the Act

'Ageing-in-place'

Although not defined in the 1997 Act and not legally required of any provider, enabling residents to 'age-in-place' was a clear objective of the Act and was intended to be one of the significant benefits of unification of the aged care accommodation system. The concept has been defined thus:

> Ageing in place relates to the provision of responsible and flexible care in line with each individual's changing care needs in a familiar and appropriate environment.
>
> Commonwealth Department of Health and Ageing [DOHA] 2002, p 4

Gray, reviewing the extent to which providers had instituted ageing-in-place by mid-2000, found that 85% of homes had one or more residents classified in both the high-care and low-care RCS bands; and that, post-1997, up to 67% of residents originally admitted with low-care needs were still living in the same accommodation six months after being re-classified as needing high-level care, with 50% of them still in the same place after twelve months (Gray 2001a, pp 196–7). A more detailed study undertaken a year later by the highly respected Australian Institute for Health and Welfare (AIHW) confirmed Gray's report, finding:

> strong evidence that ageing in place has occurred, with one in five residents of former hostels now classified at the high-care or nursing home end of the reimbursement scale ... the majority [of these] have 'aged in place' (68% in 2001) ...
>
> There has also been a dramatic reduction in the number of hostel residents transferring to another facility as a result of increasing dependency.
>
> AIHW 2002c, p 8

Review of RCS and its outcomes

The first post-reforms review of the RCS was completed in July 1998 and reported on:

- the extent to which the RCS adequately describes care needs;
- its effectiveness in both high-care and low-care situations;
- the clarity of the tool; and
- the adequacy of the training materials and supports provided to facilities' management and staff.

Some consequential changes to the RCS system were adopted in November 1998. Departmental officers continued to carry out audits and other research into the accuracy of the providers' use of the tool and found error rates to be disturbingly high in the early days but reducing as familiarity with the tool increased (Gray 2001a, pp 128–31).

However, provider concerns, particularly to do with the administrative burdens imposed by the RCS, continued to be expressed forcibly through the various consultative and complaints channels created by the Department in the wake of the reforms. Accordingly, in August 2002, a full-scale review of the post-1997 classification system and payment tool was commissioned. The report, completed in February 2003

(DOHA 2003), contained twenty recommendations. The RCS Review (pp 3–7) found that:

- classification error rates remained high, with audits six times more likely to lead to an RCS downgrade than an upgrade to a higher classification;
- provider dissatisfaction was high, with the burden of documentation usually emphasised; and
- exploration of an alternative classification scheme, rather than further evolution of the RCS, was more likely to solve the shortcomings.

This latter recommendation in favour of further innovation was not universally welcomed by the industry (Young 2003, p 19). The largest provider peak group in Australia has claimed that the current system wastes 'at least four million hours of nurse time per annum in maintaining unnecessary validation documentation' and has costed this alleged waste at approximately $90 million per year (Young 2003). These allegations, it must be pointed out, come at a time when the industry is campaigning both for simpler reporting requirements and for increased subsidy levels. At the time of writing, research on possible simplification measures continues, but significant discontent is being expressed by the industry with the delays by the Minister and the Department in responding to the report (relevant materials are available from DOHA 2003).

Review of first-round accreditation

Despite the time pressure under which it operated and the teething problems (as were to be expected), the Agency completed all the first-round accreditations sought by providers by the deadline of 1 January 2001 (with about 20 exceptions, where some special circumstances applied), after which Commonwealth funding was withdrawn from unaccredited facilities. A total of 2938 facilities were accredited during the first round, with 93% of them receiving a three-year accreditation, a prima facie mark of sound compliance with the Standards.

Gray, who consulted widely during the conduct of the first-round accreditations while preparing his 2001 report, found that providers' concerns were concentrated on issues relating to the direct and indirect costs of accreditation, the apparent inconsistency of some judgements rendered by the assessors and what was perceived to be an undue focus on documentation and systems rather than what was described as 'actual care' (Gray 2001a, pp 90–1). Gray's report goes on to say, by way of reassurance, that 'the Department advised that ... there has been no failure of a home with sound, high quality practice, even where policies are not well documented' (Gray 2001a, p 91).

When that first round was completed, a working party made up of members of industry and consumer peak bodies was convened to consider the 'Lessons Learned from Accreditation'. It reported that 'while consultations and submissions indicated overwhelming support for the accreditation system, there was a general call for the refinement and revision of the current process' (Grenade & Boldy 2002; Working Group of the National Aged Care Forum 2002, p 1). The Working Group's main recommendations related to:

- improving accreditation reporting and consumer information;
- improving the integrity and consistency of the accreditation process by applying some quality monitoring measures to the Agency's work on an ongoing basis; and
- improving the education available to providers about the Standards and Outcomes (Working Group 2002, p 2).

A large amount of statistical information is provided in the Working Group's report, sufficient to suggest what might have been the areas of strength and weakness in the industry's performance at the time, but also provoking some questions about consistency of the assessment teams, especially between States. A searching examination of the Agency's performance was also carried out by the Australian National Audit Office, and the report (ANAO 2003, Ch 6) reinforced some of the findings of the Working Group relating to inexplicable variations in ratings, especially between States, and the need for improved training for assessors. A more theoretically informed assessment of the gains and losses under the new arrangements and of the performance of the Agency, which makes some serious criticisms, can be found in Braithwaite's (2001) work.

The second round of accreditations commenced in 2002 and was scheduled for completion in early 2003. As a result of industry feedback after the first round, the available ratings were changed in May 2002. The consensus was that those homes rated 'Satisfactory'—that is, the majority of homes—would be seen by consumers as having merely 'scraped through'. The new ratings are now either:

- Compliant,
- Not compliant, or
- Not compliant with serious risk

with two special higher ratings open to applicants:

- Commendable, or
- Accreditation with merit.

So far it seems safe to conclude with Gray (2001a, p 93) that the new accreditation regime has led to gains, among them the possibility of imposing more effective sanctions on poor-performing homes and the greater availability of useful performance information to assist consumer choice. A harsh critique of the actual quality of care in some duly accredited facilities, based on some first-hand accounts and compiled by an experienced investigative journalist (Legge 2003) should prevent any complacency, however.

Bed supply since the 1997 reforms

When introducing the 1997 reforms the government stated that it did not intend to reduce the overall bed:target population as a result of the reforms. The goal would remain 100 beds per 1000 people of 70 or more years of age, 40% of them high care, 50% of them low care and 10% community based, with 3% overall being available at any time for respite use (Gray 2001a, p 25). There was some scepticism in sections of the community about this claim (Lippert 1998), given that the changes followed the report of the National Commission of Audit, appointed shortly after a change of government to recommend on potential public sector savings. As with other questions concerning post-1997 changes confronted in this chapter, the readily accessible evidence leaves us without a definitive answer at the time of writing.

The total number of places available, including those funded through CACPs, was 143,582 in 1996; by mid-2001 this number had grown to 168,641—an increase of 17%. However, when these absolute figures are presented against the planning target of 100 places per 1000 people aged 70 and above, it is clear that at mid-2001 the ratio had fallen to one place for every 97.5 people aged 70 and over. Moreover, the targeted supply of places, according to the planning framework, should have contained 90% residential and 10% home- and community-based places, equivalent to 155,609 beds and 17,289 other places; whereas in fact there were only 144,012 beds and there were already 24,629 non-residential places. Clearly, the availability of residential care had at that stage fallen well below target, while community support, where most of the post-1997 growth was taking place, was making up more of the care supply than had been planned for. Against this, it must be recognised, first, that the available bed supply in a fast-ageing society is likely to fall behind target due to the delay between approval of new places and their being built and available for occupancy. Second, since 50% of separations from the CACPs program are admitted directly to high-care beds in residential facilities, while less than 1% of separations go to low-care beds (Gray 2001a, p 185), it could be argued that CACPs, far from being a poor substitute for a residential placement, are performing their allotted function in keeping people needing only basic or low-care support out of institutions as long as possible.

That there is a shortfall cannot be denied: but is that shortfall caused by the Aged Care Act reforms? The planning framework was introduced long before the 1997 reforms and therefore any pressure on access to places is not necessarily attributable to the impact of the 1997 Act. For instance, the under-supply was considerably worse in the decade prior to the reforms than it was at the time of the reforms (Gray 2001a, p 28, Table 1.2). It might be retorted that, when all that is allowed for, however, the Act did aim to improve access and therefore it must be charged with failing in this particular respect at least. Gray, after a balanced examination of the various factors, concluded that:

> overall the sector is under-supplied in terms of currently operating places, relative to the Department's planning targets, although not when new allocations are included … [However] the extent of under-supply across the sector has declined in the period since the reforms, and seems likely to decline further in the coming years as a result of the large recent release of new places.
>
> Gray 2001a, p 30

Staffing issues since 1997

Prior to the 1997 reforms, the funding component devoted to nursing and personal care in nursing homes was officially tied to that purpose alone, and expenditures of those funds had to be reported to the Commonwealth. By contrast, the Aged Care Act discontinued those staffing-mix controls, requiring only that the provider 'maintain an adequate number of appropriately skilled staff to ensure that the care needs of care recipients are met' (*Aged Care Act 1997*, Pt 4.1/Div 54.1). Under the Quality of Care Principles (Commonwealth Department of Health and Aged Care [DH&AC] 1999), supporting legislation meant to specify the requirements of the Act, there are general references to the types of tasks that should be carried out by registered nurses, and some references to relevant State and Territory laws, but no easily testable measure of the status, quality or quantity of staffing required. The basic assumption is that such specifications would be too rigid and that oversight and enforcement of any lapse on the part of providers would be dealt with by the accreditation procedures.

Predictably, this deregulation of staff mix requirements aroused strong feelings among stakeholder groups, including nursing unions, client groups and providers themselves, with the issues further obscured by differing approaches to nursing registration in different States. Several professional nursing bodies—including the NSW College of Nursing, Geriaction NSW and the Royal College of Nursing Australia—expressed their concerns to the Senate Community Affairs References Committee on the Funding of Aged Care Institutions. These concerns continue to be felt among various groups and find expression in the journals and newsletters relating to aged-care activities.

Staff and some consumer groups see the end of prescribed staff ratios as opening the door to de-skilling of the workforce, leading to higher profits but poorer care; and this just at a time when more residents are being classified as having complex nursing needs (Lippert 1998). Provider groups, on the other hand, focus on the difficulty of attracting and retaining high-quality staff in the middle of a protracted nursing staff shortage when the level of government funding is, in their eyes, too low to allow competitive salaries and incentives (Curtis 2002).

Gray's review (2001a, pp 94ff) of the first two years of operation of the 1997 reforms noted the politically charged nature of this issue and the paucity of good data. He declined to offer any conclusion beyond observing that, if it is accepted that achieving the Expected Outcomes against the Standards is a valid measure of good care, then the accreditation for three years of 93% of all operating homes gives grounds for thinking that the present system is working satisfactorily. Sensible and fair as far as it goes, this is unlikely to be the final word on this topic. Some considerable amount of further experience of the workings of the unregulated system, and perhaps some empirical research on the correlations, if any, between staff mix and care outcomes, is likely to be needed before all doubts on this score are silenced.

FUTURE ISSUES

Palliative care comes to RACFs

A significant policy development to have occurred since the 1997 reforms, affecting the nature and direction of care in facilities rather than the quantity or funding of it, concerns the projected introduction of a palliative care protocol into residential aged-care facilities. The Commonwealth Government engaged contractors to develop a set of guidelines governing the provision of palliative care in aged-care homes, and at the time of writing the draft guidelines are being refined in the light of expert comment. This development might be seen as flowing both from the implications of the age profile outlined earlier and from the government's need to create positive alternatives, given its recent opposition to attempts to liberalise the laws on when a patient may choose to end his or her life as a way of escaping intolerable pain. However that may be, the determination and implementation of policy on this issue will grow steadily in importance in the years following the publication of this work, if only because of the way the balance of public opinion has moved over recent decades. This brief notice of the issue must suffice, as the topic is covered in depth later in this book.

Is industry restructuring inevitable?

Substantive and procedural reforms of the kinds embodied in the *Aged Care Act 1997* have been seen in other industries and service sectors to prompt wholesale restructuring, impelled by new, stricter outcome standards and management requirements leading to higher physical and administrative infrastructure costs. As unit costs are pushed up, the pressure to get bigger or get out has been evident. The aged-care residential industry had begun to feel this pressure by the time the 1997 Act was implemented. Numerous providers, seeing the implications for them of the impending changes in terms of capital investment or the acquisition of new skills, sold their facilities or otherwise left the industry. There are those who see this trend as necessary to capture efficiency gains and lower overhead costs, allowing the savings to flow into direct care. The CEO of one large provider has confidently predicted that

> Industry restructuring will see within the next 10 years (sooner rather than later) a collapse of the sector whereby 1500 providers [operating through 3500 different facilities] will end up being only 100 providers.
>
> Ireland 2002, p 31

The most detailed study of these competitive pressures and how the new funding structures position facilities to meet them has been carried out by experts commissioned by Gray (2001a, Ch 5) and their findings make interesting reading. The research surveyed the overall viability of the industry and, separately, how individual homes of different types had been affected. As well as collecting the views of industry figures on the viability of the industry, the researchers examined the bidding competition among providers and prospective providers for places allocated by the Commonwealth. The upshot of the research is that the industry overall is viable and appears more securely profitable since the 1997 Act came into effect than was the case previously, with a widely achieved benchmark being a 12% annual return on capital invested. Distribution of the extra funding opportunities was not uniform across the sector, however, and so some types of homes—such as those in needy areas, in rural locations or those caring for especially costly clients such as people with severe dementia—appear less assured of a secure future. Gray saw the solution as lying in a relatively small and simple supplementary payments scheme directed to certain types of facilities, not unlike that already in limited operation.

It would be premature on the basis of Gray's evidence and findings to dismiss predictions of a torrent of takeovers and forced mergers of smaller providers with a single, stand-alone facility, similar to that quoted above. But if that scenario does eventuate it may take longer than some now believe. Caution in forecasting is appropriate here, however, because of the possible impact on future developments of the current pricing review, announced as part of the 2002/03 Commonwealth Budget and expected to report by the end of 2003 (Hogan 2002, pp 14–15).

How useful is the 1986 planning framework now?

The basic planning benchmark—the ratio of places per 1000 people over 70—that has guided policy since the mid-1980s has been mentioned frequently in this chapter, as have some potentially complicating factors such as the rapid growth in the numbers of the 'old old' (those aged 80 years or more) and the attendant rise in the RCS dependency level of those in aged-care accommodation. Taken together, these factors would seem likely to produce a shortfall in the number of beds overall and in high-care beds in particular. It seems clear that the question that lies beneath the surface of the debate is about the ways in which and the extent to which community support services can substitute for residential care.

There are those (McCallum et al 2001) who argue that the current system of planning, funding and accrediting serves to cement in place Australia's traditional focus on institutional bed supply.

> The number of beds becomes … a critical policy focus—rather than the number of older people receiving support, the number of carers receiving support, and the quality and quantity of that support.
>
> McCallum et al 2001, p 7

While acknowledging that

> Community Aged Care Packages, Extended Aged Care in the Home packages, Community Options services, all represent increasing flexibility in care options within and between the boundaries around the residential care service stream and community care service stream of the Australian Care system,

they go on to argue that

> these options are limited and fragmented and represent marginal measures rather than comprehensive improvements in the present system.
>
> McCallum et al 2001, p 11

They propose instead a system where subsidies follow the client rather than being attached to a building; where care and residence costs are distinguished; where the focus is on increasing choice for the client; and where a broader and more personalised assessment, possibly handled through a brokerage, determines the care package approved. They go on to insist that

> Decisions now have to be made in the face of a number of policy drivers: increasing capacity and preference for independent living in the community among older people, a rapidly changing interface with acute care, the need to strategically direct new funds to deal with the ageing population, and the need to deliver services more appropriately and effectively within current service mix and expenditure levels.
>
> McCallum et al 2001, p 14

Other commentators such as Gray (2001a,b) and Duckett (2000) are doubtful of the need for or practicability of major change to the underlying policy directions in the medium term. Gray observes that much of the policy debate in the years around the turn of the century has been about

> the provision of effective alternatives to residential care. This is influenced [Gray continues] by a widely held view that this is the preference of older people, and that the community alternative is less expensive.
>
> Gray 2001a,b pp 124–5

His own view is that the capacity of community-based care to provide genuine substitution remains uncertain. Noting the rapid increase in funding for such care since the mid-1980s, he observes that

> the care delivery system remains fragmented, and lacks clarity of purpose. ... There is universal opinion that a fix is required but resolution seems distant. In the meantime, it seems unlikely that the performance of an array of loosely related programs will produce the most effective support system for older people.

Duckett writes:

> Australia's long-term care policy has been relatively stable since the early 1980s: an emphasis on expanding HACC and reigning in growth of residential care. This policy has been remarkably successful and Australia is not facing an unsustainable increase in its institutionalised elderly population ... Dramatic change in policy settings is not required.
>
> Duckett 2000, p 218

Further debates about the costs of an ageing Australia

As we have seen, there are recurring waves of concern about the likely future costs of providing aged care. Such concerns surfaced in the early and mid-1980s, returned more sharply than before when the National Commission of Audit reported in 1996 and have been very apparent once again in the context of the 2003/04 Commonwealth Budget, chiefly due to the appearance of the Treasurer's Intergenerational Report (Commonwealth Treasury 2002). Current Treasury projections anticipate that the cost to the Commonwealth of residential care will rise from 0.58% of GDP in 2001/02 to 1.45% in 2041/42, and that community care for the aged will rise from 0.14% of GDP to 0.32% over the same four decades (Commonwealth Treasury 2002, p 39). That would mean that forty years from now, aged care in accommodation facilities and in the community will consume approximately 2.46 times the share of national income that it does now.

If this were to eventuate, it would be a daunting growth factor, but international comparisons suggest that it need not be met with alarm (ACIL 1999). Moreover— and this is a most important caution—such projections are notoriously dependent on the assumptions employed. Critics of the Treasury's forbidding forecast of ageing's economic burden on the taxpayer point out that it depends heavily on holding constant many variables—among them such measures as the average retirement age, the impact of improved public health policy on the care requirements of older age groups, fertility and immigration rates, male longevity, potential improvements to savings habits and reform of the superannuation industry, reducing welfare transfers to the well-off and so on—that are actually likely to vary or can be varied to achieve more positive outcomes (Barker 2001; Dowrick & McDonald 2002; Mitchell 2002).

Perhaps we can learn something from the past two decades, in which the population has been ageing and health's share of the GDP has gone from 7.8% in the mid-1980s to about 8.5% now, a rise of approximately one-tenth over fifteen years of rapidly increasing expenditure. Data from this period suggests that the key factor has been the rising real costs of health services rather than the impact of ageing (ACIL 1999, p 43). Technical consultants independent of Treasury who were asked to review the evidence on the costs of ageing reported:

> The conclusion we have reached about Australia's ability to cope with the progressive ageing of the population is that, even under current policy settings, the projected aged care bill will be affordable … However, just because the aged care bill is unlikely to be an unsustainable burden does not mean there is room for complacency.
>
> ACIL 1999, p 44

It is impossible to disentangle the threads of these debates here, with their complicated statistical calculations mixed sometimes with charges of 'complacency' and counter-charges of 'alarmism'. While this debate goes on, however, it is important to be aware of the influence of the assumptions chosen when such projections are being made, and aware also of the political implications of this debate, with the attendant possibility that political biases may play a part in the projections the protagonists put before us. We can expect to see these cost concerns subjected to further debate as the decades in which the 'old old' will emerge in numbers come closer.

CONCLUSION

This chapter has sought to trace the emergence of the present aged-care residential system since the 1950s and, intertwined with that, the emergence of an increasingly sophisticated policy dialogue involving the planning and research community and an array of lobby groups seeking to influence the course of public policy. We have seen how early government initiatives in the form of subsidies stimulated the activities of commercial interests and not-for-profit bodies, leading to an explosion over a couple of decades in the number of aged-care beds, mainly at first in nursing homes and only much later in hostel or low-care accommodation. The haphazard results of those stimulatory efforts necessitated a system of controls and planning targets based on beds per 1000 of the population over 70 years of age, as well as efforts to induce the frail aged to stay in their own homes, with community-based support services.

The most recent step along this path—the *Aged Care Act 1997*—has been drawn in detail and its early impact assessed. Some future issues have been canvassed and, in closing, we have returned to the debate over the costs of providing decent aged care to a fast-ageing population.

In the next decade or so, Australian voters will have to make sense of these issues and will register their views on how to balance the increasing financial costs of continuing to strive for an equitable and high-quality aged-care system against the social and ethical costs of moving away from what has been achieved in the past half-century.

Acknowledgement

Acknowledgement is given to Lyndal Spencer for her comments on drafts of this second edition chapter, and to Greg Price for his comments and assistance in preparing the first edition version of this chapter.

References

ACIL Consulting—Crowley P & Cutbush G (ACIL) 1999, *Ageing Gracefully: An Overview of the Economic Implications of Australia's Ageing Population Profile*, Occasional Papers: New Series No. 10, Commonwealth Department of Health and Ageing: Canberra.

Aged Care Act 1997, Commonwealth Parliament, AGPS: Canberra.

Aged Care Standards and Accreditation Agency 1998, *The Agency Update*, Aged Care Standards and Accreditation Agency: Parramatta. Online: www.accreditation.aust.com

Australian Bureau of Statistics (ABS) 1999, *Australian Social Trends*, AGPS: Canberra.

Australian Bureau of Statistics (ABS) 2003, *Population Projections Australia*, Cat. No. 3222.0, AGPS: Canberra.

Australian Institute of Health and Welfare (AIHW) 1997c, *Older Australia at a Glance, Fact Sheet No. 35, Health Expenditure on Older People*, AIHW: Canberra.

Australian Institute of Health and Welfare (AIHW) 1999, *Older Australia at a Glance, Fact Sheet No. 31, Fitting the Pieces Together*, 2nd edn, AIHW: Canberra. Online: http://www.aihw.gov.au/publications/welfare/oag02/oag02.pdf, accessed 15 July 2003.

Australian Institute of Health and Welfare (AIHW) 2002a, *Older Australia at a Glance, Fact Sheet No. 35, Health Expenditure on Older People*, AIHW: Canberra.

Australian Institute of Health and Welfare (AIHW) 2002b, *Older Australia at a Glance, Fact Sheet No. 29, Hostels*, AIHW: Canberra.

Australian Institute of Health and Welfare (AIHW) 2002c, *Ageing in Place: Before and After the 1997 Aged Care Reforms*, Bulletin, Issue 1, June, AIHW Cat. No. AUS 26, Canberra.

Australian National Audit Office (ANAO) 2003, *Managing Residential Aged Care*, The Aged Care Standards and Accreditation Agency Ltd, Audit Report No. 42 2002-03, ANAO: Canberra.

Barker J 2001, The centenarians are coming: are we ready?, *Australasian Journal of Ageing*, 20(3), Suppl 2, pp 66–8.

Braithwaite J 2001, The challenge of regulating care for older people in Australia, *British Medical Journal*, 323(7310), International Edition, pp 443–6.

Commonwealth Department of Community Services and Health (CS&H) 1986, (Chair: G. Rees), *Nursing Homes and Hostels Review*, AGPS: Canberra.

Commonwealth Department of Health and Aged Care 1999a, *The National Strategy for an Ageing Australia: Background Paper*, AusInfo: Canberra.

Commonwealth Department of Health and Aged Care (DH&AC) 1999b, *Aged Care Principles*, AusInfo: Canberra.

Commonwealth Department of Health and Ageing (DOHA) 2000, *National Strategy for an Ageing Australia*, Healthy Ageing Discussion Paper, Highlights Sheet. Online: http://www.ageing.health.gov.au/ofoa/posageing/hahilite.htm, accessed 12 July 2003.

Commonwealth Department of Health and Ageing (DOHA) 2002, *Ageing in Place: A Guide for Providers of Residential Aged Care*, DOHA: Canberra.

Commonwealth Department of Health and Ageing (DOHA) 2003, *Resident Classification Scale Review: a Report Prepared by Aged Care Evaluation and Management Advisors*, Aged and Community Care Service Development and Evaluation Reports, No. 43, DOHA: Canberra. Online: www.health.gov.au/acc/rcspage/rcsrev/rcsrprog.htm

Commonwealth Department of Health and Family Services (DH&FS) 1997a, *The Documentation and Accountability Manual*, DH&FS: Canberra.

Commonwealth Department of Health and Family Services (DH&FS) 1997b, *Standards and Accreditation Training Seminar Participants Workbook*, DH&FS/Australian Healthcare Associates: Canberra.

Commonwealth Department of Health, Housing and Community Services (HH&CS) 1991, *Aged Care Reform Strategy Mid-Term Review 1990–91*, AGPS: Canberra.

Commonwealth Department of Health, Housing, Local Government and Community Services (HHLG&CS) 1993, *Aged Care Reform Strategy Mid-Term Review Stage 2*, Australian Government Publishing Service: Canberra.

Commonwealth Treasury 2002, *Intergenerational Report 2002–03*, 2002–03 Budget Paper No. 5, Treasury: Canberra.

Craik DRS 1981, *Report of the Auditor-General on an Efficiency Audit of Commonwealth Administration of Nursing Home Programs*, AGPS: Canberra.

Curtis K 2002, Nursing crisis in aged care, *Healthcare*, August, pp 14–16.

Dowrick S & McDonald P 2002, *Comments on Intergenerational Report 2002–03*, Australian National University. Online: http://www.acpr.edu.au/Publications/IntergenReport.pdf, accessed 20 July 2003.

Duckett S 1995, *Keynote Address to the Aged Care Australia 8th National Conference*, Canberra, 9 November 1995: Office of the Secretary, Department of Human Services and Health: Canberra.

Duckett SJ 2000, *The Australian Healthcare System*, Oxford University Press: Melbourne.

Gibson D 1998, *Aged Care: Old Policies, New Problems*, Cambridge University Press: Melbourne.

Gray L 2001a, *Two Year Review of Aged Care Reforms*, Commonwealth Department of Health and Aged Care: Canberra.

Gray L 2001b, Beyond the two-year review: the new generation of issues in aged care? *Australasian Journal of Ageing*, 20(3), pp 123–6.

Grenade L & Boldy D 2002, The accreditation experience: views of residential care providers, *Geriaction*, 20(1), pp 5–9.

Hogan W 2002, Pricing review, *Healthcare*, November, pp 14–16.

Howe A 1992, Participation in policy making: the case of aged care. In: Gardner H (ed), *Health Policy: Development, Implementation and Evaluation in Australia*, Churchill Livingstone: Melbourne.

Ireland J 2002, The future assured, *Healthcare*, November, pp 31–2.

Jones D 1997–98, Nursing home policy reverse, *Australian Nursing Journal*, 5(6), p 10.

Legge K 2003, No helping hand, *The Australian*, Tuesday 6 May, p 13.

Lippert N 1998, Aged care reforms: policy implications for rural and remote Australia, *Australian Journal of Rural Health*, 6, pp 161–4.

McCallum J, Calder R, Walsh J, Moy S, Adamzcuk S, Bye R & Nakamura T 2001, Australian aged care and the new international paradigm, *Australasian Journal of Ageing*, 20(3), Suppl 2, pp 5–14.

Mitchell M 2002, Gazing into the fiscal crystal ball: the first intergenerational report, on-line opinion. Online: http://www.onlineopinion.com.au/2002/Jun02/Mitchell.htm, posted 15 June 2002, accessed 10 June 2003.

National Aged Care Alliance 2002, *Options for Financing Long-Term Care for Older People in Australia.*

Palmer GR & Short SD 1989, *Health Care and Public Policy: An Australian Analysis*, Macmillan: Melbourne.

Palmer GR & Short SD 2000, *Health Care and Public Policy: An Australian Analysis* (3rd edn), Macmillan: Melbourne.

Rowland DT 1991, *Ageing in Australia*, Longman and Cheshire: Melbourne.

Sax S 1990, *Health Care Choices and the Public Purse*, Allen & Unwin: Sydney.

Sax S 1993, *Ageing and Public Policy in Australia*, Allen & Unwin: Sydney.

Working Group of the National Aged Care Forum 2002, *Report of the Lessons Learned from Accreditation*, Commonwealth Department of Health and Ageing: Canberra.

Young R 2003, Reporting on the RCS Review, *Healthcare*, May, p 19.

CHAPTER 2

Do the elderly cost more?
Casemix funding in acute settings

STEPHEN DUCKETT AND TERRI JACKSON

INTRODUCTION

Promoting efficiency of health care is a perennial concern of health policy makers and analysts. Allowing inefficiency to continue means that money is wasted that could have been used for other purposes such as—in the face of long waiting times for care—treating more patients. A number of State governments and private health insurance organisations now use 'casemix' measures to standardise funding for acute hospitals. Under casemix funding, hospitals are paid on the basis of the number of patients they treat, with the payment per patient varying according to the relative costs of treating those types of patients. All hospitals get paid the same for treating the same type of patient. Efficient hospitals can keep any surplus, and inefficient hospitals are put under financial pressure to find savings.

Elderly patients are significant consumers of health-care resources: hospital admission rates increase with age, and people aged over 65 occupy more than half the beds in acute hospitals. The introduction of casemix funding in Victoria (and now in other States) led to fears that the elderly would be discriminated against because they were not 'profitable'. The evidence presented in this chapter, drawn from a sizeable sample of Victorian hospital admissions, indicates that although elderly patients may have a longer than average length of stay, this does not translate into higher than average costs.

CASEMIX FUNDING

Casemix funding relies on a system for accurately describing patients and their relative costs. Such a classification system was developed in the United States by Fetter and associates in the late 1970s (Fetter et al 1980) and has been subsequently modified in Australia (Reid et al 1992). This classification system, known as *diagnosis-related groups* (DRGs), is based on three important attributes.

- There are a limited number of categories (the Australian version has around 660 groups).
- Each category is clinically meaningful.
- The treatment costs for patients in each category are roughly the same (resource homogenous).

Essentially, the development of DRGs involved analysing the resource use of patients treated in hospitals and grouping the 10,000 or so diagnosis and procedure codes—which are assigned to each patient on discharge—into a more manageable number of groups. The data used for defining DRGs are routinely collected and recorded in hospital computerised discharge abstracts.

Australia began developing its own version of DRGs in the late 1980s and the first version of *Australian National Diagnosis Related Groups* was released in 1992. The contemporary version (Version 4) was released in 1998. The Australian classification system was built using length of stay as the principal measure of resource use, although it would now be possible to develop classification systems using the full resource cost rather than a surrogate such as length of stay.

If the design of the classification system is not appropriate, or the payment rate by the funder is set too low, hospitals and patients can be disadvantaged. Both these concerns were articulated when casemix funding was first introduced in Australia, in Victoria in 1993. A particular concern at the time, and continuing today, is that the Australian DRG classification system may leave more complex patients underfunded and hospitals at risk financially when they admit complex patients.

The introduction of casemix funding in Victoria was not without controversy, as a 15% cut in hospital budgets was implemented simultaneously, and this led to a substantial reduction in staffing (Lin & Duckett 1997). Despite the bad press associated with casemix funding and budget cuts in Victoria, this new ability to compare the efficiency of hospitals was seen by policy makers as a valuable tool, and all Australian States except New South Wales now use casemix funding to pay for hospital care.

The move to casemix funding in Victoria was welcomed by most hospitals, although the potential adverse impact of casemix funding was also highlighted in public debate. The fear among many in the Australian community, including some professionals, was that the elderly would be discriminated against under the Australian casemix funding arrangements (Hanson & O'Dea 1994; Joseph 1994; Nelson 1994). It was reasoned that discrimination would occur because 'everybody knows that the elderly cost more'. Certainly, older patients stay on average longer than younger patients and, to the extent that costs reflect length of stay, the conventional wisdom is true. One of the most common of the criticisms was the risk that patients would be discharged 'quicker and sicker', as had happened following the introduction of casemix funding for the US Medicare system, the national funding scheme for the elderly and the disabled (Berenson & Pawlson 1984; Kosecoff et al 1990). Casemix funding in the United States is known as the Prospective Payment System because payments are determined prospectively based on characteristics of the patient. It replaced the retrospective payment scheme, whereby payments were based on incurred costs. The US Senate held an inquiry into the effect of the Prospective Payment System two years after its implementation. This inquiry was in response to reports of difficulties for elderly patients in getting access to care. The Chairman of the US Senate Special Committee on Aging (Senator Heinz) said in his opening remarks to the inquiry:

Seriously ill Medicare patients are being denied admissions to hospitals or have been catapulted out of hospital wards prematurely as a result of inflexible, inaccurate pricing and packages of illnesses. And patients are judged 'DRG winners or losers', depending on the profit potential that they represent under this current payment system.

US Senate 1985

The assignment of DRGs relies principally on the diagnosis and procedures performed. An underlying assumption is that any additional resource use is due to multiple diagnoses or other diseases the person may be suffering from (termed *co-morbidities* in the DRG system), rather than the person's age *per se*. Where splits in the DRG classifications are required because of the resource implications of these co-morbidities or complications, the split categories are identified as 'catastrophic' or 'severe'. These designations are used in Australia. For example, there are two DRGs for heart failure and shock: F62A for those cases with catastrophic co-morbidity and complications, and F62B for those without.

Although DRGs are defined on the basis that patients in each DRG consume similar amounts of resources, there will still be variations within a DRG, with some patients costing more and some less than the average. Even if this variation is systematic and the average older person does cost more than the average younger person, discriminating between patients on this basis, aside from being unethical, may not be a feasible financial strategy. This is because of the practical difficulty of controlling emergency presentations. In addition, because of the high proportion of hospital admissions from elderly patients, there may be an adverse effect on economies of scale in clinical areas where admissions might be discouraged. Furthermore, every older patient will not necessarily cost more than every younger patient, as older patients (as with younger patients) vary in their physical fitness, case complexity and co-morbidities. In addition, as hospital information systems are still fairly rudimentary, most hospitals are unable to predict with any degree of accuracy or certainty the profitability of each patient. Picking 'winners' may be neither possible nor sensible from the hospital's point of view.

The operation of the casemix funding system means that if an older patient has complications or co-morbidities that are likely to increase resource use, they will generally be assigned to a more complex DRG and will attract an additional payment. Together with the individual variability for older patients this means that it is very difficult to predict at admission whether a particular older patient will cost more than a younger patient. It would thus be difficult for hospitals to predict whether they will make a 'profit or loss' (surplus or deficit) on each individual patient in advance. Even if hospitals do not discriminate against the elderly, they may feel that casemix payment for the elderly is inadequate, a view reinforced in a questionnaire circulated to hospitals as part of the Victorian Auditor-General's evaluation of casemix funding in Victoria, which asked hospitals about the adequacy of funding for 'higher cost patients such as ... the elderly', implicitly assuming that the elderly do indeed cost more (Auditor-General of Victoria 1998, pp 175–6).

THE ELDERLY IN ACUTE CARE

The assumption that 'the elderly cost more' may have arisen from confusion of a number of different elements. The first element of the 'elderly cost more' argument is unrelated to the health sector: older people require higher levels of income support than younger people. The second assumption does relate to the health sector—on average, older people have more hospital admissions and consume more hospital days. However, there have been no Australian studies demonstrating that the cost of each of those hospital admissions and each of those hospital days is more than for younger patients.

Figure 2.1 shows hospital utilisation rates (in terms of admission, termed 'separations' and 'patient-days' or bed-days) for males and females by age. The graph shows a dramatic escalation in utilisation rates in later years, with separation rates per 1000 population for people over 65 being more than double those of people aged 25 to 45. (A 'separation' is a discharge, transfer or death.) Patient-days per 1000 population for the over-65 population are more than ten times higher than those of younger age groups. For most age groups, patient days *per 100* population (as shown in Figure 2.1) is about one-third of the separation rate *per 1000* population, suggesting an average length of stay of about three days. However, for the over-75 age group, the relativity between bed-days and separations begins to vary. In the 85+ age group, patient days per 100 population is about equal to separation rates per 1000 population, reflecting the much longer average length of stay for this age group.

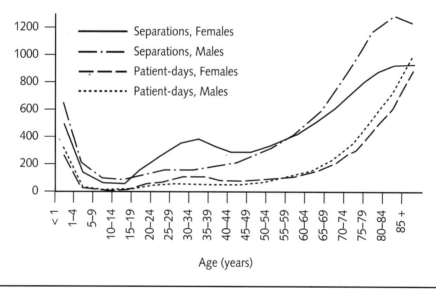

Fig 2.1: Hospital utilisation rate (separations per 1000 population; patient-days per 100 population) by age group and gender 2001–02

Source: AIHW 2003, Australian Hospital Statistics 2001–02.

More importantly, even though the elderly are a relatively small proportion of the population, these very high rates of utilisation also translate into high proportions of hospital activity. Figure 2.2 shows the proportion of separations and bed-days by age group and gender in Australia.

It can be seen that the over-65 population represents about one-third of all hospital separations but one-half of bed-days (56% of all bed-days). These very high proportions emphasise the critical role of care of the elderly in hospital planning and management. Indeed, given that people over 65 occupy more than half of all acute beds, there is a strong case for ensuring that all nurses have skills in gerontic nursing. However, these data do not show that elderly persons' use is 'disproportionately large', as McKie et al (1996 p 50) suggest. Although the elderly have higher per capita utilisation rates, as shown in Figure 2.1, their use may indeed be proportionate to need.

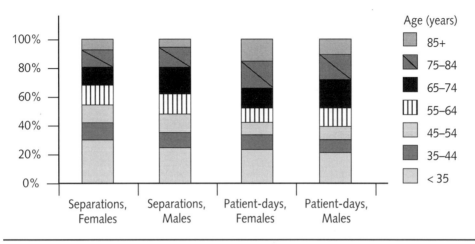

Fig 2.2: Proportion of separations and patient days by age group and gender, 2001–02

The combination of increased use of services by the elderly and increased income support for the elderly has led to scaremongering about the implications of an ageing Australian population (Clare & Tulpulé, 1994). The assumption is that the ageing population will bankrupt Australia unless draconian action is taken. Schulz (1997) has referred to the basis of this argument as 'voodoo demographics', as it rarely takes into account the effects of economic growth. Furthermore, the elderly in Australia make up a smaller proportion of the population than in many European countries that provide similar levels of social support to those provided in Australia and that have coped well with this higher proportion of the elderly (Gibson 1998; Richardson & Robertson 1999).

DO THE ELDERLY IN ACUTE CARE COST MORE?

The previous section has shown that the elderly consume a very high proportion of hospital separations and bed-days. As outlined earlier, the conventional wisdom is that each admission of an elderly patient is more costly than for non-elderly patients. Under casemix funding systems, the critical issue is whether this cost difference remains *after* standardising for casemix—that is, whether older patients *within a given DRG* cost more than younger patients. This chapter sets out to test this hypothesis.

The analysis uses information on patient-level costs from a data set of over 0.5 million recorded patient admissions to nineteen Victorian acute-care hospitals from 1 July 2000 to 30 June 2001. Because most major tertiary hospitals are included in the sample, these cases represent over 50% of total Victorian admissions to acute-care hospitals in the period. Coded clinical information and demographic information is matched to each costing record, making it possible to analyse the relationship between costs and patient age within DRGs.

In Victoria, the public hospital unit of payment is a Weighted Inlier Equivalent Separation (WIES). The terminology reflects the derivation of the payment unit. The basic unit is a *separation* (discharge, transfer or death) that is *weighted* by a set of payment relativities (or cost weights) which are DRG-specific. (For example, an appendicectomy is weighted lower than an open-heart operation, reflecting relative costliness.) The DRG system distinguishes very-long-stay patients (called *outliers*) from patients who stay for an average amount of time (called *inliers*). The WIES calculation transforms the very-long-stay outliers into their *inlier equivalents* by multiplying up the inlier payment to take account of the extra days of stay. The WIES calculation thus yields for every inpatient episode a payment relativity which summarises how costly the episode is expected to be, given the inlier and outlier days consumed by the patient. In the Victorian casemix funding system this relativity is multiplied by a standard payment rate to yield the payment to a public hospital for treating that patient.

In order to test whether a hospital might be disadvantaged by treating more older patients than another hospital, we created a new measure of 'cost per WIES' by dividing the total cost of a patient's care by the WIES value. A higher value therefore indicates that a patient costs relatively more than the payment rate.

Our aim was to determine whether age could be used to predict the value of this new variable. We used linear regression with cost per WIES as the dependent variable and patient age, hospital and emergency admissions as independent variables and to take account of known sources of within-DRG variation. In all, this model explained only 4.5% of the variation in cost per WIES. Eighty per cent of this explained variation was attributable to eleven of the hospital variables and the emergency status variable, with patient age explaining almost none of the variation in cost per WIES.

WHY ARE THERE DIFFERENCES IN COST?

The conventional wisdom that the elderly cost more is belied by the above analysis. Why do nurses and other health professionals hold strongly to the belief that elderly patients cost more? The answer relates in part to staff perceptions of costs and the extent to which the costs incurred are visible to all staff.

Two DRGs, one medical and one surgical, will be examined in this chapter to explore why there may not be a relationship between increasing age and increasing cost.

AR-DRG E65B

The 2390 cases in AR-DRG E65B (chronic obstructive airways disease without catastrophic or severe co-morbidities or complications) in the database had an average cost of $2760 (median = $2043) and an average length of stay of 4.1 days (median = 3 days.). Persons aged 65 and over stayed longer on average than persons under 65 (4.41 days versus 3.51 days, $t = 4.92$, $p < 0.001$), although the total cost of their stay (on average $2747) was lower but not statistically significantly different than the cost for people under 65 ($2783).

The composition of these total costs, however, was strikingly different between the two age groups, as Table 2.1 shows.

Table 2.1: Average cost for AR-DRG E65B (chronic obstructive airways disease without catastrophic or severe co-morbidities or complications) by cost component for patients aged under 65, and 65 and over, in 19 Victorian hospitals, 2000–01

Cost component	Under 65 years $	65 years and over $	Total population $
Allied health	112	141	130
Critical care (ICU + CCU)	127	21	59
Emergency department	471	470	470
Imaging	96	101	100
Medical	528	383	434
Nursing	1003	1063	1041
Pathology	96	113	107
Pharmacy	185	173	177
Prostheses	0	0	0
Theatre	49	19	30
Other	0	2	1
Total cost	**2783**	**2747**	**2760**
Average length of stay (days)	3.51	4.41	4.10

Source: authors' analysis.

Despite the differences in length of stay, nursing costs for patients aged 65 and over are not statistically significantly different from those for patients under 65. This is also the case for most other cost components. Only three cost components reveal statistically significant cost differences. Pathology costs in the elderly are $16 more than in people under 65 ($t = 3.00$, $p < 0.005$), medical costs are $145 less in people 65 and over ($t = 4.9$, $p < 0.005$), and critical care costs are $106 higher in people under 65 ($t = 4.93$, $p < 0.001$).

Although AR-DRG E65B is a 'medical' DRG, certain incidental procedures can be undertaken on patients without changing the DRG assignment, hence the recording of operating theatre costs. In all, only 173 patients had surgical procedures; there was no statistically significant difference in the incidence of surgical operations in the under-65 population compared to the 65-and-over population ($\chi^2 = 1.387$, $p = 0.248$). However, for those patients having surgery, theatre costs were higher in the under-65 population relative to the 65-and-over population ($1522 versus $602; $t = 1.963$, $p = 0.05$).

The overall pattern of costs in this DRG reflects slightly more intensive treatment for patients under 65: more incidental surgical intervention, more medical (as opposed to nursing) care and more frequent use of critical care. The additional costs incurred in these areas for younger patients offset any savings resulting from their shorter length of stay and savings in other cost components. The clinical reasoning behind the differences in costs cannot be discerned from these data.

AR-DRG I03C

The database includes 752 cases in AR-DRG I03C (hip replacement without catastrophic or severe co-morbidities or complications). The average length of stay for all patients is 9.2 days (median = 8 days) with patients under 65 staying on average 7.9 days, and patients 65 and over staying 9.7 days (the difference of nearly two days is statistically significant, $t = 4.13$, $p < 0.001$). The mean cost for all patients in this DRG is \$12,088 (median = \$11,727), with older patients (65 and over) costing an average of \$11,669 and those under 65 costing almost \$1600 more at \$13,255. This difference is statistically significant ($t = 3.9$, $p < 0.001$).

Table 2.2 shows the average cost for each of the major cost components for patients under 65 contrasted with those for patients 65 and over.

Table 2.2: Average cost for AR-DRG I03C (hip replacement without catastrophic or severe co-morbidities or complications) by cost component for patients aged under 65, and 65 and over, in 15 Victorian hospitals, 1996–97

Cost component	Under 65 years $	65 years and over $	Total population $
Allied health	531	516	518
Critical care (ICU + CCU)	28	40	36
Emergency department	14	119	87
Imaging	142	225	199
Medical	1,805	1,779	1,777
Nursing	2,731	3,427	3,198
Pathology	137	189	172
Pharmacy	391	348	359
Prostheses	3,596	1,998	2,472
Theatre	7,415	4,823	5,583
Other	0	0	0
Total cost	**13,255**	**11,669**	**12,088**
Average length of stay (days)	7.93	9.78	9.20

Source: authors' analysis.

Costs of elderly patients for emergency department care (t = 6.4), imaging (t = 4.9), nursing (t = 4.9), and pathology (t = 2.6) are generally higher than for younger patients. All these differences are statistically significant (p < 0.01). The two largest sources of the difference between the costs of the elderly and of patients under 65, however, relate to costs incurred in the operating theatre, a difference of almost $2600 per admission (t = 8.5, p < 0.001) and the costs of prostheses where, on average, patients under 65 have prostheses costing almost $1600 more than patients over 65, a statistically significant difference (t = 6.74, p < 0.001).

CONCLUSION

There are differences in other aspects of care that overwhelm the cost differences associated with the longer than average length of stay for the elderly, differences that have also been found in other countries (Bond et al 2003). It may be that the analyses of the two DRGs reported in this paper simply reveal other aspects of discrimination against the elderly. For AR-DRG E65B, is it clinically reasonable that patients aged under 65 are managed slightly more intensively? Do the differences revealed here in the COAD DRG reflect an implicit policy of lower expectations of what should be done for elderly patients? For the hip replacement DRG, is it fair that the elderly should be provided with cheaper prostheses? Are decisions about prostheses based on reasonable expectations regarding the life of the patient and the life of the prosthesis, or on other less relevant criteria?

These data show that the perception and the realities of cost profiles can be quite different. Most large hospitals either have now, or will have in the near future, databases similar to that used to analyse costs in this chapter. The analyses in this chapter have focused on differences between the cost patterns for patients in different age groups. Similar analyses comparing hospital cost profiles, or different medical (or surgical) units within a hospital, could be done. Analyses of these kinds will become more common over the next few years and lead to more informed debates about health care priorities. It is important that nurses learn to use and interpret cost data to understand the real costs of care and budget implications of treatment decisions, in order to advocate for their patients' quality of care. Reliance on hunch, guesswork or perceived wisdom may distort priorities or lead to lower average quality of care.

References

Auditor-General of Victoria 1998, *Acute Health Services under Casemix: A Case of Mixed Priorities, Special Report No. 56*, Victorian Government Printer: Melbourne.

Berenson RA & Pawlson LG 1984, The Medicare prospective payment system and the care of the frail elderly, *Journal of the American Geriatrics Society*, 32(11), pp 843–8.

Bond M, Bowling A, McKee D, Kennelly M, Banning AP, Dudley N, Elder A & Martin A 2003, Does ageism affect the management of ischaemic heart disease? *Journal of Health Services Research and Policy*, 8(1), pp 40–7.

Clare R & Tulpulé A 1994, *Australia's Ageing Society*, Economic Planning Advisory Council: Canberra.

Fetter RB, Shin Y, Freeman JL & Averill RF 1980, Case mix definition by diagnosis related groups, *Medical Care*, 18, pp 1–53.

Gibson D 1998, *Aged Care: Old Policies, New Problems*, Cambridge University Press: Cambridge.

Hanson R & O'Dea J 1994, The casemix conundrum—trick or treat?, *Medical Journal of Australia*, 161, pp S2–S3.

Joseph K 1994, Ethical problems in the use of diagnosis-related groups (DRGs), *New Doctor*, Summer, pp 8–11.

Kosecoff J, Kahn KL, Rogers WH, Reinisch EJ, Sherwood MJ, Rubenstein LV, Draper D, Roth CP, Chew C & Brook RH 1990, Prospective payment system and impairment at discharge. The 'quicker-and-sicker' story revisited, *Journal of the American Medical Association*, 264, pp 1995–6.

Lin V & Duckett SJ 1997, Structural interests and organisational dimensions of health system reform. In: Gardner H (ed), *Health Policy in Australia*, Oxford University Press: Melbourne, pp 64–80.

McKie J, Kuhse H, Richardson J & Singer P 1996, Allocating healthcare by QALYs: the relevance of age, *Cambridge Quarterly of Healthcare Ethics*, 5, pp 534–45.

Nelson B 1994, Casemix—an AMA perspective, *Medical Journal of Australia*, 161, pp S4–S6.

Reid B, Aisbett C, Ng L-M, Lohmann J & Palmer G 1992, *Evaluation of the Performance of the Australian National DRG Grouper. Report to the Commonwealth Department of Health, Housing and Community Services*, Centre for Hospital Management and Information Systems Research, University of New South Wales.

Richardson J & Robertson I 1999, *Ageing and the Cost of Health Services*, Working Paper No. 90, Health Economics Unit, Monash University: Melbourne.

Schulz JH 1997, The Economics and financing of long-term care, *Australian Journal on Ageing*, Supplement, 17, pp 82–4.

United States Senate Special Committee on Aging 1985, *Quality of Care Under Medicare's Prospective Payment System*, US Government Printing Office: Washington.

CHAPTER 3

Clinical safety and quality in residential aged care

ELIZABETH PERCIVAL

INTRODUCTION

The following account is adapted from a case study prepared by concerned family members who wanted to bring attention to the need for quality health care in residential aged-care facilities. It provides a background for this chapter and highlights the potential for error resulting in clinical adverse events. The case illustrates the need for professionals working in residential facilities to have highly developed clinical assessment skills and for effective organisational systems to support safety and quality of care.

A resident who had suffered a cerebrovascular accident had lived in a residential facility for a number of years. Over a period of time the resident complained of severe pain in the back and called out in pain. The staff labelled the resident a 'behaviour problem'; in his relatives' view he was not given appropriate care to alleviate his pain and discomfort. The family observed that the resident had gained considerable weight in a relatively short time (approximately six weeks). They noted that he had pitting oedema of his legs and a swollen and distended abdomen. On questioning staff about their father's condition, they were told that the resident had swollen legs because he would not keep them elevated. However, the man's pain was made worse by keeping his legs elevated.

The relatives recognised that their father was ill, and requested that he be seen by a medical practitioner. They were told to contact the doctor and to speak directly to him about their father. The relatives believed that the resident was not given a comprehensive assessment by the doctor at that time.

In the residential facility a medication error occurred with the resident, and as a result he was transferred to an acute hospital for care. On admission to the hospital, the resident was diagnosed with a lung tumour. He died a few days after admission. Medical staff at the hospital also diagnosed pneumonia, urinary tract infection and congestive cardiac failure.

This resident experienced unnecessary pain and discomfort during the last months of his life. His relatives and loved ones also experienced additional anguish and concern during a very emotionally distressing time. Much of this pain, suffering and anguish was preventable.

Improving safety and quality of health care for older people accommodated in residential aged care is of concern to professionals, clients and their families, and the community. It is also of particular concern to the Australian Government. Against a backdrop of providing suitable accommodation as well as high-quality clinical care, this chapter highlights the essential principles of clinical safety and quality in health care, and canvasses the issue of ensuring a systematic approach to clinical safety and quality care in residential aged care. Although residential aged care has its own specific issues, the general principles and framework of the prevailing safety and quality agenda in acute health care in Australia can be applied to residential aged-care facilities.

This chapter also discusses an initiative currently being conducted by the Commonwealth Government—a pilot project of different models and approaches to Quality of Care Committees (QCC) in residential facilities. The aim of this pilot project is to support the leadership required to facilitate a culture of safety and continuous quality improvement in health care in residential facilities. According to Ramadge (2002) health care as it applies to older people should be interpreted as care that affects an older person's need for the prevention of disease states or disability arising from illness. Quality health care for older people also includes clinical intervention for illness and disease, rehabilitation to maximise physical, cognitive, social, emotional and mental functioning, management of the dying process, and safe and enjoyable accommodation (Ramadge 2002).

DEVELOPING A SAFETY AND QUALITY APPROACH

Substantial work to improve safety and quality in the acute-care context has been undertaken by the Australian Council for Safety and Quality in Health Care (the Council). Although providing health care in a residential setting presents different clinical issues and involves less medical intervention, the research and work undertaken by the Council in the acute setting can be applied to residential aged care. The Australian framework for safety and quality in health care is underpinned by the work of the American Institute of Medicine (Institute of Medicine 2000) and Australian research undertaken in the acute-care setting into the level of adverse events. The seminal Australian research, the Quality in Australian Health Care Study into patient safety, documented the extent of adverse events and the subsequent degree of patient harm in the New South Wales public health system. The results of this study were extrapolated to a national level to obtain an understanding of the extent of the issue across Australia. In New South Wales, 16.6% of admissions involved an adverse event and 51% of adverse events were found to be highly preventable (Wilson et al 1995). It is now generally acknowledged that much of the unintentional and unforeseen harm caused to patients may be due to preventable human error and/or systems failure. The Harvard Medical Practice study found that two-thirds of adverse events involving hospitalised patients were preventable (Rothschild, Bates & Leape 2000). Other research in America has found that the majority of adverse events in the acute-care context are the result of system failures within health-care delivery organisations (Leape 1994). In addition, it has been suggested that some systems are more vulnerable than others due to basic organisational disorder. In these circumstances the tendency is often to blame the staff delivering the care rather than examining the errors in the health-care delivery system and implementing risk management and improvement strategies (Australian Council for Safety and Quality in Health Care 2001a, p 26; Reason et al 2001).

According to experts in the area, the contemporary approach to safety and quality in health care is to agree that human error is inevitable and that the systems, processes and culture within organisations bring about or contribute to clinical errors. Accepting this approach to safety and quality requires a cultural change, as the general view in health-care settings and in professional education is frequently not to acknowledge the actuality of human error. The data extracted for identifying errors and adverse events can be very sensitive for patients/residents, relatives, staff and health-care facilities. It is essential therefore that proper protective measures be implemented to ensure that the processes involved do not compromise the privacy or rights of any party (Australian Patient Safety Foundation 2001).

Similar Australian research into clinical safety and quality has not been undertaken in the context of residential aged care. It has been suggested (Ramadge 2002) that one reason for this lack of research is that, in the past, residential aged-care facilities have been seen as only an accommodation option for older people, rather than a health-care service. One American study involving older people in acute-care settings reports that due to the clinical complexity of care, preventable adverse events were more common among elderly patients (Thomas & Brennan 2000). Another American author (Kapp 2003) reports that the acuity and complexity of illness and disability among nursing-home residents has risen over the past decade. He suggests that safety concerns in residential facilities include adverse drug events, injurious falls, pressure ulcers, problems with tube feeding, breakdowns in communication during transfers to and from acute facilities, and equipment failures. Initial feedback from the Australian Government's pilot project to establish Quality of Care Committees shows that similar safety matters are of concern in Australian facilities.

The demographic transition in Australia will continue to put pressure on aged-care services, and on health responses within those services. Between 2001 and 2031 the number of people over 65 years of age will more than double (from 2.4 to 5.05 million). Over that period the proportion aged 70 and over will almost double (from 8.9 to 15.9% of Australia's population), while the number and proportion of those aged over 80 will also double (to 1.3 million, or 5.8% of the population). As people age they are more likely to develop disabling and multiple illnesses, and currently 21% of people aged 70 and over use aged-care services, and of these 7.9% are in residential aged care. A person aged 70 has a 36% chance of needing high-level residential care. About 64% of high-level care residents enter from hospital, 26% from low-level care, and 10% directly from the community. The delivery of aged health care in residential facilities has become progressively more complex, and will continue to present ongoing challenges for staff who work in these facilities. The safety of clinical care for older people has therefore become increasingly important (data in this paragraph from Commonwealth Department of Health and Ageing 2002a, p 28).

THE CURRENT SAFETY AND QUALITY FRAMEWORK IN AUSTRALIA

Over the past decade, clinical care in the acute health-care sector has been recognised as not being risk-free, and efforts have been made to make the health sector as safe as possible. The Australian Council for Safety and Quality, which was established in 2001, has provided national leadership to improve the safety of patient care in the acute-care sector. The Council proposes a vision for a safer health-care system that:

- is customer centred;
- has open and honest communication;
- is accountable and supports multidisciplinary approaches;
- has a culture of learning for quality improvement; and
- constantly strives to maximise safety, eliminate error and improve systems design (Australian Council for Safety and Quality 2001b, p 34).

Building on this work, in 2002 the Council revised its strategic plan to focus on achieving outcomes in its priority areas. The areas identified for improvement in patient safety were:

- the development of national standards for open disclosure;
- reducing preventable patient harm associated with medication use;
- reducing patient harm as a result of infection associated with health care; and
- coordinating national action to learn from serious adverse events (Australian Council for Safety and Quality 2002).

The Council (2001a, pp 33–6) has developed and published definitions related to the area of safety and quality in health care which have national application. Several terms referred to in this chapter have been defined by the Council as follows:

- An *adverse event* is an incident in which harm resulted to a person receiving health care.
- *Risk management* is the culture, processes and structures that are directed towards effective management of risk.
- An *error* is the failure to complete an action as intended, or the wrong use of a wrong plan to achieve an aim. Errors may occur by doing the wrong thing (commission) or by failing to do the right thing (omission).

Another international expert in the area, Lucien Leape, suggests that the human and organisational factors affecting the safety of health-care provision can be considered at two levels. He clarifies and expands on the elements in these factors as follows:

- At the immediate human–system or practitioner–patient interface, common features include dynamic environments, multiple sources of concurrent information, shifting and often ill-defined goals, reliance on indirect or inferred indications, actions having immediate and multiple consequences, moments of intense time stress interspersed with long periods of routine activity, advanced technologies with many redundancies, complex and often confusing human–machine interfaces, and multiple players with differing priorities and high stakes.
- At the organisational level, these activities are carried on within complex institutional settings and entail multiple interactions between different

professional groups. This is extremely important for understanding not only the character and aetiology of mishaps but also for devising more effective remedial measures (Leape 1994, pp 1851–7).

To improve safety and reduce clinical risk it is necessary to minimise error by identifying and analysing fundamental system problems, correcting faulty systems, evaluating and providing evidence of what works, and educating staff to deliver clinical and technical expertise.

As identified above, many factors influence clinical practice. The most important and obvious include:

- *institutional context*—regulations, economics, systems;
- *organisational and management factors*—resources, structure, policies, cultures;
- *work environment*—staffing levels, skill mix, workloads, shift patterns, management support;
- *team factors*—communication, supervision, team structures;
- *individual staff factors*—knowledge and skill levels, motivation, attitudes and health;
- *task factors*—availability and use of protocols and guidelines; and
- *patient/resident characteristics*—medical condition, language and communication, personality and social factors (Vincent et al 1998).

IMPROVING QUALITY AND SAFETY IN RESIDENTIAL AGED-CARE FACILITIES

It is generally accepted that the framework and principles that guide the work and strategies of the Australian Council for Safety and Quality in Health Care can equally be applied to the aged-care sector. At a Clinical Safety and Quality in Aged Care Workshop hosted by the Department of Health and Ageing (DOHA) in September 2002 Professor Bruce Barraclough, Chair of the Council, strongly suggested that there was an opportunity to apply 'lessons already learned' by the Council to the residential aged-care setting.

Older people have the same legal rights as younger people, including the right to quality health care which is appropriate to their needs. Nurses working in aged care will be aware that the right to quality care is set down in the *Aged Care Act 1997* and its subordinate legislation, and is underpinned by the law relating to negligence. Focus on clinical safety has become more important as research has been conducted into the level of iatrogenic harm caused through incidents, errors and adverse events to consumers of health-care systems. Some of these events result in death, permanent disability and other personal loss. Through setting standards, monitoring compliance and providing support for workers in various ways, the DOHA plays a direct leadership role in promoting safety and quality of care for people in residential facilities. One of the objects of the *Aged Care Act 1997* (section 2-1(1)(b)) is to promote a high quality of care and accommodation for the recipients of aged-care services. Furthermore, the Code of Ethics and Guide to Ethical Conduct for Residential Aged Care (Commonwealth Department of Health and Ageing 2001) sets out the ethical obligations of the partners (providers, employed and contract staff, attending professionals, volunteers, and residents and their families/representative) in residential aged care. Value 5 of the Code relates to the resident's right to an appropriate standard of care to meet their individual needs. Providers, staff and attending professionals are obliged to administer care that is in line with best practice, and to participate in risk-reduction programs where mistakes and adverse events are identified, reported without blame, discussed and corrected.

An argument has been articulated above that safety and quality of clinical care delivered to residents may be jeopardised by a variety of systematic errors. Improving safety and quality of care in residential facilities therefore involves identifying, understanding and managing risks across the many and complex systems within a facility. The principles of continuous quality improvement, including interdisciplinary approaches and systems analysis, are important for preventing errors in the care of elderly people. Their safety is an essential component of the concepts of quality improvement, risk management and clinical governance.

Rothschild et al (2000) found that injuries associated with hospitalisation and residential care are more common in older (65 and over) people than in younger patients (under 65), and they may be more severe and more often preventable. In addition, under-diagnosis and delayed diagnosis of illnesses are more common in elderly patients, and under-diagnosis in older patients appears more likely to occur when a non-geriatric physician cares for the patient (Rothschild et al 2000). According to these authors, the main cause of increased risks to older people appears to be the diminished physiological reserve of elderly patients; however, age alone is a less important predictor of adverse events than co-morbidities and functional status. These findings are of great importance to nurses working in residential facilities when assessing the risks of adverse events for residents in their care.

IMPLEMENTING QUALITY OF CARE COMMITTEES IN RESIDENTIAL AGED-CARE FACILITIES

The Department of Veterans' Affairs (DVA) and the Department of Health and Ageing (DOHA) have each been considering appropriate methods of supporting continuous quality improvement in residential aged care. Both departments are interested in exploring the potential role of Quality Care Committees (QCCs) in assisting aged-care facilities to meet this agenda. However, each department prefers a slightly different approach to the role of a QCC.

In March 2001, the DVA and the Aged and Community Care Division (ACCD) of the DOHA agreed to jointly fund a consultant to research and give advice on an appropriate strategy for piloting quality committees in aged-care facilities. They also agreed to jointly implement a pilot project following receipt of advice from the consultant. In addition, the General Practitioner Branch (GPB) of DOHA also indicated its willingness to participate and to contribute to the pilot project.

The scoping study, undertaken in 2001, established that monitoring quality and safety in residential aged care is still in a developmental stage. It also suggested that few Australian aged-care facilities have established multidisciplinary structures to monitor safety and quality. The DVA identified the need to focus on communication and interaction between a facility and the community. The DOHA saw that the role of a quality committee would be primarily focused on monitoring, implementing and evaluating the provision of care, and recommending changes to systems that affect the provision of safe, quality care.

The consultant appointed to undertake the scoping study did so with the guidance of an Interdepartmental Reference Group (IDRG) comprising representatives of DVA, ACCD and GPB. The issues were researched and consultation occurred with a range of stakeholders. The resulting reports identified possible broad options, discussed the potential problems of having committees in place, addressed issues related to the different DVA and DOHA approaches to the committees, and suggested how pilot facilities might be recruited (Bollen 2002).

To enable both the DVA and DOHA approaches to be incorporated, it was recommended that three separate models of QCC be piloted:

- Divisions of general practice to establish and coordinate committees with representatives from facilities, the community and providers. The committees would focus on generic quality-of-care issues relevant to each of the participating facilities.

- Individual facilities to establish a committee with representatives from facility management, residents, GPs/Divisions, and community nominees. The committees would focus on quality care at the individual facility and would review quality care information collected by the facility.

- Individual veterans' facilities to establish committees with representatives from facility management, residents, GPs and community nominee(s). These committees would focus on communication and interaction between the facility and the community.

During the consultant phase, some sites were identified that either already had a quality committee operating or would like to trial such a committee.

Following review of the consultant's report by the IDRG, the DVA and the DOHA agreed to establish a pilot project which would aim to:

- implement only two models of QCCs—a clinical care model (with several components) and a community participation model;

- evaluate how well these committees function and whether they can meet their objectives;

- identify what processes and incentives are required;

- identify problems, difficulties and/or barriers preventing them from achieving good outcomes and how these might be overcome; and

- evaluate the outcomes directly related to quality care issues.

Specific objectives for the individual committees would be determined by each facility.

THE PILOT PROJECT

Building on the outcomes of the DVA scoping study, in April 2002 the DOHA commissioned a pilot study to establish and evaluate models of Quality of Care

Committees in selected residential aged-care facilities. At that point it was determined that the models should include a *community participation model* and a *clinical care model* with three components. Further explanation of these models and the various components is provided below.

An important feature of the pilot project is the partnership arrangements between the DOHA and the DVA, and with the Aged Care Division of DOHA and the General Practice Branch of the DOHA. The two departments acknowledged that the principles of continuous quality improvement and resident-centred care, including interdisciplinary approaches and systems analysis, are as important for preventing errors in the care of elderly people as they are in the care of people in acute health-care facilities.

The joint project was undertaken as a pilot to identify appropriate models of QCCs, to identify strengths, weaknesses and barriers in the development and sustainability of QCCs, to identify the required support for QCCs, and to identify further research.

Quality of Care Committees

The committees were convened to act in an advisory capacity in order to assist residential aged-care facilities to improve the safety and quality of care by minimising the risk of adverse events. The purpose of the committees was to:

- improve safety and quality of care by minimising the risk of adverse events, incidents and error;
- assist in developing a culture of continuous improvement and resident-centred care in facilities;
- promote best practice;
- promote an integrated, multidisciplinary approach to improving care through committee membership; and
- establish support mechanisms for staff who work in the facility to practise safely.

Committee models

The two models of QCCs are a clinical care model and a community participation model.

Clinical care model

The clinical care model has been established in two facilities as well as a project currently being conducted at a Division of General Practice. The model has three components:

- *Facility-based component*—This component is established in two facilities: a high-care dementia-specific charitable facility in a large regional centre in New South Wales (withdrawn September 2002); a high-care private facility in the Australian Capital Territory; and a high-care charitable facility in regional New South Wales (since December 2002).

- *Division of general practice-based component*—A division of general practice in Victoria is the pilot site for a regional QCC. This project involves three residential aged-care facilities in rural towns in western Victoria.

- *Existing committee evaluation*—This component is based in two facilities: a high-care charitable facility in metropolitan Sydney; and a high-care private facility in rural Victoria. It should be noted that both these facilities had established a model of a QCC; the original IDRG considered that it would be useful to include these existing models in the pilot.

Community participation model

The community participation model is based in two DVA facilities, in Queensland and Western Australia. This model emphasises community participation in resident lifestyle, with a subcommittee that focuses on clinical care matters. It was agreed that the pilot project would have three stages.

- **Stage 1, Development and implementation**, includes:
  - formulating a detailed work plan;
  - establishing a project advisory committee;
  - liaising with stakeholders, the DVA and the DOHA;
  - developing guidelines and definitions, draft terms of reference for both models, fact sheets and reference material;
  - assisting pilot facilities to establish and implement agreed committee models;
  - designing a framework for evaluation; and
  - establishing acceptable support systems between the project coordinator and participating facilities.

- **Stage 2, Ongoing monitoring and support**, involves:
  - communicating regularly with participating facilities and other stakeholders;
  - monitoring the implementation of the QCCs;
  - providing advice and support when required; and
  - maintaining records and reporting to the project officer and other DOHA personnel as required.

- **Stage 3, Evaluation and reporting**, is ongoing, as issues emerge throughout the pilot. Prior to commencing the project it was important to communicate the evaluation framework, agree to the ground rules about evaluation with the stakeholders, and manage expectations. The process of evaluation of the QCC models is essential in order to acquire, analyse and use information to assess the effectiveness of the project and assist with a comparison of different models. The information may also be used in decision-making associated with planning, programming and implementation of components of the project.

The evaluation processes involved in this pilot project will require a specific evaluation method for each committee model and will identify the individual approaches within each facility and model. At the time of writing this chapter, the evaluation process had just commenced and was scheduled for completion early in 2004, and the report of the project was to be finalised shortly after this.

Implementation progress

Originally the pilot project was to be completed in twelve months. This timeframe has been extended because of difficulties with staffing resources and other commitments and priorities, such as accreditation and commissioning new buildings. Such delays can be common in projects of this type and should be factored into any implementation plan. Start-up issues and implementation difficulties are an important component of the project evaluation.

At the time of writing this chapter (2003), the pilot has been running for twelve months. One QCC is ready for evaluation, and the other committees will complete the twelve-month timeframe in early 2004. The Existing Committee Evaluation in two facilities has been documented. The following vignette provides an illustration of an effective improvement action implemented by one pilot facility as a direct result of implementing a QCC.

VIGNETTE

Applying quality improvement principles to wound care

Suzanne Sawyer

Through the work of our Quality of Care Committee, skin tears were identified as an adverse event because of the potential to negatively affect residents' quality of life.

Anecdotal evidence of prolonged wound healing times prompted the need for an investigation. This was carried out in line with quality improvement principles to establish the cause of prolonged healing times.

Problem

The following wound management issues were identified via audit:

- a number of wounds taking an extended time to heal;
- wound management protocols not being followed and treatments constantly being changed;
- expenditure on medical items running over budget; and
- residents' quality of life being reduced by wound pain and discomfort, and interruption of daily routine by wound dressings.

Solution

Contemporary wound management by a dedicated wound management nurse was introduced to the facility of 106 residents after the following steps:

- Education and training in best practice wound management undertaken by an enrolled nurse and a senior registered nurse.

- New arrangements discussed with all stakeholders including residents, registered nurses and care managers.
- Close liaison with the ACT Wound Management Association.

Results

At the end of the first two weeks of trialling contemporary wound management by a dedicated wound management nurse, the number of wounds had been reduced from twenty to six.

The average time of healing for skin tears is now ten days and the number of nursing interventions per wound has been reduced to two. The Wound Management Nurse derived great personal satisfaction from the results, which has led to increased self-esteem and job satisfaction.

Other goals that have been achieved include the following:

- All residents with wounds have documented assessments, wound plans and evaluations in place.
- Evidence-based wound management protocols which are evidence based are being followed.
- Staff education is ongoing.
- Costs, including those of wound dressings and staff time, have been reduced.
- Disruption of residents' lifestyles due to prolonged treatments has been reduced.

Similar outcomes have been achieved for more complex wounds, as outlined in the following case study.

Case study

This case study outlines the treatment of two wounds sustained by the same resident at different times.

The resident is a frail 81-year-old who has severe rheumatoid arthritis, peripheral vascular disease and anaemia, and has received prolonged steroid medication.

Episode 1—The resident sustained a haematoma measuring approximately 5 cm by 2 cm on his lower leg. Three weeks later the area was surgically debrided and treated with a daily dressing of saline, Vaseline gauze and dry dressing. One month later, daily saline cleansing and application of an absorbent dressing was introduced. Antibiotics were prescribed to treat an infection. Daily dressings continued and the wound finally healed after more than four months of daily treatment.

Episode 2—The resident fell in the courtyard and sustained two extensive skin tears on his lower leg. The larger measured approximately 15 cm in length. The skin was rolled back and preserved apart from an area measuring approximately 5 cm by 1 cm. After administration of first aid the resident was transferred to hospital for assessment. He returned with a wound plan consisting of daily saline cleansing followed by the application of Vaseline gauze and a dry dressing. Healing remained static for ten days.

On the eleventh day our wound management nurse took on the management and after reassessment introduced dressings to maximise healing, manage wound debris and exudate and help prevent infection. Warm water was used to cleanse. Dressing times were extended to third daily and then rapidly to weekly. After six weeks of uninterrupted progress the wounds were completely healed.

Conclusion

Prior to the introduction of a dedicated wound management nurse with education and skills training in contemporary wound management, there were great fluctuations in healing times, use of wound cleansing and dressing agents, and frequency and number of interventions. In addition, there was incomplete documentation of wound assessment, planning and evaluation. This resulted in costly outcomes for residents and staff.

The quality improvement process was applied to the problem, with outstanding results for residents and staff—costs were reduced, and the quality of life of residents and job satisfaction of nursing staff were enhanced.

EMERGING ISSUES

To date the pilot has provided an opportunity to determine any emerging issues and problems. There will be more opportunity to examine these matters in detail during the evaluation process. Some of the emerging issues and problems are described here.

Getting started

Establishing the committees proved to be more challenging than originally anticipated. Because of competing priorities there was an underestimation of the time required for setting up. It took much longer than expected to work through some logistical matters, such as gaining approval, finding suitable committee members, lack of available human resources, and the ability of facilities to take action on implementation.

Leadership

Ongoing and committed leadership at various levels is seen as critical to the implementation of QCCs. Strong commitment to safety and quality at a senior level is essential. In one pilot facility, the QCC is a committee of the Board of Management. Experience gained during this project has shown that, to ensure the ongoing effectiveness of committees, it is necessary to get the commitment of leaders at different levels within the facility. For example, it is essential that leadership be given at executive level, at a divisional or service area level, at a multidisciplinary level, and at an education and training level. A most noticeable reason for failure in establishing a QCC is reliance on one person providing leadership for safety and quality.

Ownership and individual approaches

A feature of the pilot project has been the encouragement of facilities to implement a QCC that is suitable to the specific facility. Reference materials such as guidelines, fact sheets and draft terms of reference were provided for the participating facilities as a draft framework for the structure and operations of the committees. It is seen that the participating facilities must develop a QCC that is relevant to the context of the facility and that the staff must have ownership of safety and quality outcomes.

Conflicting priorities

Demands on the time of staff in addressing other priorities emerged as a major factor delaying the implementation of QCCs. Actual and important matters, such as preparing for accreditation processes, recruiting new and critical staff, coordinating capital programs including monitoring building renovations and extensions, and implementing other service programs took priority for staff time. Under these circumstances, implementing another committee was a daunting task for staff, who felt they were already over-stretched.

Confidentiality and misinterpretations

Privacy, confidentiality, misinterpretations and leakage of information were issues of concern. Staff at some facilities were concerned that the government would require details about adverse incidents and that this data could have negative repercussions for the facility during the accreditation process. Reassurance and clarification was given to the facilities that specific data on adverse events was not required by the government, and that its interest was in the structures, processes and outcomes involved in thoroughly examining adverse events, incidents and errors, as well as the issues involved in making the QCC operational.

Available staff expertise

Some key staff involved in providing leadership for safety and quality in facilities indicated that staff members working at the coalface have limited knowledge and confidence in the concepts of continuous quality improvement. Critical analysis and high levels of problem solving in safety and quality matters are more difficult for staff who have limited training and experience. Staff training and continuing education are integral to safety and quality outcomes for residents. The two vignettes in this chapter illustrate the relationship between staff training and education, and quality outcomes.

In addition, in some facilities staff members have English as a second language or have limited literacy skills, which makes it difficult for them to contribute fully to continuous quality improvement processes. Staff training in these matters is required, although if staff members do not have some elementary knowledge of safety and quality, it can be beyond the capacity of the facility to provide the basics through training.

A broader perspective on safety and quality

At facilities where a new or expanded multidisciplinary committee was established, feedback suggests that there is now a broader perspective on safety and quality matters. As well as having registered nurses as committee members, two committees have included a community member, a carer, a GP, a pharmacist and other health professionals as members of the QCC. This multidisciplinary approach to membership has been seen in an overwhelmingly positive light at those facilities where the membership has deliberately been formed on a multidisciplinary basis.

Networking and links

Staff members in participating facilities have developed networks and links with other individuals and organisations that have an interest in safety and quality. They have created opportunities to share knowledge and lessons learned, and to gain support from like-minded people. Feedback given by staff working in facilities participating in the project suggests that they have gained more confidence in dealing openly with adverse events and errors, and in their approaches to safety and quality.

Correlation to accreditation

Several Directors of Nursing employed by the participating facilities believe that the work of the QCC assists with the accreditation process. They have stated that the QCC is the quality pivot of the facility—if the committee works effectively, the pathway for gaining accreditation is put in place. The links between the work of a QCC and facility accreditation is viewed as a positive and helpful outcome by facility staff. The vignette below presents an example of education provided by the accreditation agency that supports a systematic approach to improving safety and quality in residential aged care.

CONCLUSION

The results reported in this chapter do not detail improvements in quality, but rather focus on processes and emerging issues. The aged-care system operates within a broader system of health-care delivery, and thus the type of care provided in residential aged-care facilities has changed significantly over the past decade. People accommodated in these facilities have higher levels of dependence and more complex clinical needs. As a result of these changes, residents require not only long-term accommodation but also skilled health care. The potential for preventable adverse events in clinical care increases in frail older people who suffer from disabling and multiple illnesses, and therefore clinical safety and quality in residential aged care has emerged as an important issue.

International and Australian research has found that clinical adverse events occur at an alarming rate in the acute-care health sector. It has also been found that many adverse events are preventable. This chapter has raised the issue of clinical safety and quality in the residential aged-care setting, which has not been researched. Leaders in safety and quality in health care believe that the research and principles established in the acute-care sector can generally be applied to the residential aged-care environment, although aged care requires its own specific application of these principles. The first stage of the Australian Government's pilot project to implement and evaluate models of QCC in residential facilities has been reported in this chapter. The final stage of project evaluation commenced in August 2003, and at the time of writing was scheduled for completion in early 2004. It is hoped that the report and outcomes of this important project to emphasise clinical safety and quality in residential aged care will have positive and lasting results which will enhance the quality of care and quality of life for people living in residential facilities.

VIGNETTE

Achieving quality care: shifting from a blame culture to a learning culture

Elizabeth Pringle

The Aged Care Standards and Accreditation Agency conducted an accreditation audit on a high-care facility, and rated it non-compliant on eight outcomes, with serious risk reported in 2.7 (medication management).

The Agency worked with the facility to achieve a timetable for improvement and increased its monitoring of the facility. It became evident that many of the staff viewed 'quality systems' as a hurdle to be overcome at every audit—a superficial overlay to operations, rather than part of everyone's daily practice, underpinning all delivery of care and services.

The facility's management and Director of Nursing realised the need for a better approach and, together with key staff, analysed the Agency Site Audit Report and support contact records, and conducted an internal audit. They identified the following problems in their organisation:

- lack of leadership and ambiguous lines of authority;
- lack of understanding of quality principles at all levels of the organisation;
- poor internal communication systems;
- inadequate processes for dealing with complaints from residents and a 'blame and cover up' culture in relation to errors and incidents;
- low staff morale—high turnover of staff, high absentee rates and high OH&S claims, including stress claims;
- ad hoc, superficial and unfocused training and education;
- virtually non-existent skills assessment;
- inadequate measurement and monitoring of processes and outcomes; and
- almost non-existent performance management systems.

  The service responded in a number of ways.
- The existing systems were reviewed with key staff from each area within the facility.
- An organisation structure with clear position descriptions, responsibilities and lines of accountability was developed.
- Policies and practices were established to change the closed culture to an open and inclusive learning culture.
- Systems were established to measure, monitor and report on performance and outcomes.
- Staff training and education was aligned to organisation goals, identified gaps in competency, and achieving quality improvement objectives.
- A rejuvenated Medication Advisory Committee (MAC) collectively analysed the possible causes and effects of problems and advised on solutions.

One of the recommendations of the MAC was the importance of developing a comprehensive plan to equip staff with skills and knowledge. All staff were provided with education on quality principles and their application to their specific work within the wider organisation. A formal staff education and training program was established for registered nurses in the safe management of medication, including topics such as medication interactions, reactions, dosage, storage, and accountability and administration.

Training was also provided in the implementation of policies and procedures, staff performance expectations and the importance of measuring and monitoring performance. Staff were also regularly assessed on their skills in providing clinical care and undertaking specific procedures. The result was that, with a strong commitment from management and staff and the implementation of a sound quality system, there was a marked reduction in medication incidents. Errors found were relatively minor, quickly identified and used as learning experiences for wider application and dissemination.

There was a fundamental shift from a blame culture to a learning culture. As staff felt better equipped to perform their roles, morale improved dramatically, resulting in lower turnover, improved absentee rates and fewer OH&S claims.

The outcome for residents was a dramatic increase in the quality of medication management. On the vast majority of occasions, the right resident receives the right medication and dosage at the right time, the right way. The residents are also more aware of the importance of correct medication management.

The organisation's capacity to harness the learning that overcame these problems enabled it to apply the learning across other processes within the organisation, with similar results.

References

Australian Council for Safety and Quality in Health Care 2001a, *First National Report on Patient Safety*, Safety and Quality Council: Canberra, www.safetyandquality.org

Australian Council for Safety and Quality in Health Care 2001b, *National Action Plan 2001*, Safety and Quality Council: Canberra.

Australian Council for Safety and Quality in Health Care 2002, *National Action Plan 2002*, Safety and Quality Council: Canberra, www.safetyandquality.org

Australian Patient Safety Foundation (APSF) 2001, *Iatrogenic Injury in Australia*, ACHS, www.apsf.net.au

Bollen M 2002, *Scoping Report*, Department of Veterans' Affairs: Canberra.

Commonwealth Department of Health and Ageing 2001, *Code of Ethics and Guide to Ethical Conduct for Residential Aged Care*, CDHA: Canberra.

Commonwealth Department of Health and Ageing 2002a, *Aged Care in Australia*, CDHA: Canberra p 28.

Commonwealth Department of Health and Ageing. 2002b, *Aged Care in Australia*, Section 1. Online: www.health.gov.au/acc.ofoa/ageing_policy/nsaa/nsaabk8.htm

Commonwealth Department of Health and Ageing 2002c, *Aged Care Act 1997*. Online: www.scaletext.law.gov.au/html/pasteact/2/3051/0/PA000100.htm

Commonwealth Department of Health and Ageing, Office for an Ageing Australia 2002, *National Strategy for an Ageing Australia*, www.health.gov.au/acc/ofoa/ageing_policy/nsaa/nsaabk8.htm

Institute of Medicine 2000, *To Err is Human*, National Academy of Sciences: Washington.

Kapp MB 2003, 'At least Mom will be safe there': The role of resident safety in nursing home quality, *Quality and Safety Health Care*, 12, pp 201–4.

Leape LL 1994, Error in medicine, *Journal of the American Medical Association*, 272, pp 1851–7.

Ramadge J 2002, *Clinical Safety in Aged Health Care*, unpublished discussion paper.

Reason JT 2001, Understanding adverse events: the human factor. In: Vincent C (ed), *Clinical Risk Management*, pp 9–29, BMJ Publishing Group: London.

Rothschild JM, Bates DW & Leape LL 2000, Preventable medical injuries in older patients, *Archives of Internal Medicine*, 160(18), pp 2717–28.

Thomas E & Brennan T 2000, Incidents and types of preventable adverse events in elderly patients: population based reviews of medical records, *British Medical Journal*, 18 March, pp 741–53.

Vincent C, Taylor-Adams S & Stanhope N 1998, Framework for analysing risk and safety in clinical medicine, *British Medical Journal*, 316, pp 1154–7.

Wilson R, Runciman WB, Gibberd RW, Harrison BT, Newby L & Hamilton JD, 1995, The Quality in Australian Health Care Study, *Medical Journal of Australia*, 163, pp 458–71.

Further reading

Australian Council for Safety and Quality in Health Care 2001, *Safety in Practice: Making Health Care Safer*, Safety and Quality Council: Canberra.

Australian Council for Safety and Quality in Health Care 2001, *Safety in Numbers: A Technical Options Paper for a National Approach to the Use of Data for Safer Health Care*, Safety and Quality Council: Canberra, www.safetyandquality.org

Brennan TA, Leape LL, Laird NM, Herbert L, Localio R, Lawthers AG, Newhouse JP, Weiler PC & Hiatt HH 1991, Incidence of adverse events and negligence in hospitalized patients, *New England Journal of Medicine*, 325(3), p 210.

Leape LL 1999, Editorial: adverse drug events, *Journal of Quality in Clinical Practice*, 19(1), p 3.

Runciman WB 1999, Editorial: incidents and accidents in health care: it's time! *Journal of Quality in Clinical Practice*, 19(2), pp 1–2.

Vincent C 2001 (ed), *Clinical Risk Management: Enhancing Patient Safety*, BMJ Publishing Group: London.

CHAPTER 4

Nursing workforce issues in aged care

INTRODUCTION

You would have to have been asleep for the past fifteen years not to have noticed how much the world has changed around us. Indeed, one of the things nurses complain most about is the constant change that confronts them. And yet, too many seem to think we can continue to organise and deliver nursing in the way we 'always have'. Any suggestion that we think about nursing and its delivery differently is bound to meet resistance. This chapter argues that if we are to address the current 'crisis' in nursing we must be prepared to let go of old traditions and role boundaries and keep apace with the changing demands in the health-care system. It draws upon Australian research undertaken for projects where I was either the lead author or co-author:

- Recruitment and Retention of Qualified Nurses in Aged Care 1999
- Australian Aged Care Nursing: a critical review of education, training, recruitment and retention in residential and community settings 2002
- Recruitment and Retention of Nurses in Residential Aged Care 2002
- Review of Aged Care Nursing Component of the Undergraduate Nursing Program 2002
- Aged Care Enrolled Nursing Working Party (ACENWP) Report to the Minister for Ageing 2003

and contextualises these using other Australian research and the international literature.

THE CHANGING CONTEXT

Perhaps the most significant change that has affected health care, and society generally, is the ageing population. World population statistics show that the median age increased by barely three years between 1950 and 2000, from 23.6 to 26.4 years. However, over the next 50 years, the world's median age is predicted to increase by more than 10 years to 37 years (United Nations Populations Division 2003). In 1976, 9% of the Australian population was aged 65 years or older; in 2001 this had grown to 12% and is predicted to increase to 16% by 2016 and over 25%

by 2051 (Access Economics 2001). The fastest-growing cohort is the over-85s. Between 2011 and 2020 the over-85s age cohort is expected to grow by 50%, compared with an increase of 28% for those aged 65–74 (Australian Institute of Health and Welfare [AIHW] 2002). Although the majority of older Australians are independent and contributing in numerous important ways to family, through voluntary work, to the economy and society generally, it is the case that disease and disability increase with age and thus older people are the single largest users of the health-care system (AIHW 2002). The highest disease burden is related to dementia (AIHW 2002), with depression prevalence growing rapidly. Concomitant with an ageing society has been the increasing emphasis on managing complex, chronic illness and disabilities. A combination of economics and consumer demand has resulted in a shift away from acute care in hospitals toward shorter hospital stays and more community care. For older people and their families, the desire to avoid nursing home entry at all costs has been supported by government policies aimed at keeping people in the community for as long as possible (Angus & Nay 2003). Numerous programs and services have been introduced with the purpose of reducing hospital admission, discharging patients in the shortest possible time, avoiding re-admission and preventing admission to aged-care facilities (Australian Health Care Agreement [AHCA] 2002). While care in the community is on the face of it immediately appealing to most people, it comes at a cost to older people and their families (Rogers & Barusch 2000; Williams et al 1997). Many older people could not remain in the community if they did not have a spouse, adult child or other carer to meet most of their care needs, sometimes supplemented by formal services (see Chapter 7).

The level and extent of support that older people and governments can rely on is changing, however, and can be expected to change even more over the next ten to twenty years. The challenges to traditional family support are many. For example, what constitutes a family has changed. Families now include same-sex couples, couples without children, 'blended' families with several sets of parents but no parental set as such, single parents and the usual nuclear family. These changed families may reduce feelings of filial duty. Geographical mobility more often means that children and parents are not closely located, making direct support impossible. Increased life expectancy also means that spouses are often frail and unable to provide support to each other, while 'children' may also be in their seventies and/or have responsibilities already caring for spouse or grandchildren. Many more women are working in paid employment and may not be able, or willing, to give up work to provide care. In Western countries, this transition is well progressed. The effect is just beginning to be felt in Asian countries. As a consequence we are seeing more governments exploring educational opportunities in care of older people for nurses and paid carers. Compounding the situation is the very low birth rate in Australia. It is estimated that fewer people will enter employment in the whole decade from 2020 to 2030 than the number that currently enter in one year (Access Economics 2001, p xvii). The policy implications are that every effort and incentive will be introduced to keep people in the workforce, reducing further availability of informal carers. As a result, I predict (although few agree with me yet) that we will see a swing back to residential care. Community care is cheaper for the government while informal carers carry a significant proportion of the hidden cost and/or when care needs are not too great. When carer support is minimal or unavailable and care needs are complex and frequent, servicing many individuals across numerous sites and even suburbs will require more staff time and become more expensive than meeting those same needs in one care facility (Chiu et al 2000).

Other changes affecting the health-care system include the information and technological explosions, the increasing expectations of individuals and their understanding of their 'rights', alongside an increasing expectation that users will pay. All of the former encourage litigation when people feel that the service they paid for, and have read about on the internet, does not meet their expectations. So health-care professionals are expected to continuously improve the quality of care provided and be able to justify any care decisions made. Evidence-based practice (EBP) attempts to address these expectations. That is, by basing practice on the best available evidence, care decisions can be justified and quality improved. (Evidence-based practice is discussed in detail in Chapter 19.) Technology has affected all aspects of society and has resulted in unprecedented employment re-engineering, redeployments, redundancies and entirely new workplaces and practices.

No doubt there are many other changes that could be listed, but the purpose here is to underscore the fact that the context and demands of the health-care system are changing rapidly. If nursing is to remain relevant it cannot ignore these changes.

NURSING OLDER PEOPLE

Governments across Australia have recognised that broad policy initiatives are required to respond to the ageing of the population and specifically that there are insufficient nurses entering and remaining in the system to meet current and predicted needs. The nursing workforce itself is ageing and it is anticipated that many nurses will soon retire, making recruitment and retention issues even more pressing. Governments around the world are struggling with increasing demands and a decreasing nursing workforce. The Australian Government instigated two broad reviews which were reported in 2002: The Senate Inquiry into Nursing—*The Patient Profession: Time For Action* and the National Review of Nursing Education—*Our Duty of Care*. A number of State reports into nursing have also been published (for example, The Australian Institute of Health and Welfare Labour Force Study 1998; New South Wales Government Nursing Workforce—The Way Forward Study 2000). In addition, a number of projects have looked specifically at issues related to aged care (Cheek et al 2003; Nay & Closs 1999; Nay et al 2002, 2003; Pearson et al 2002a,b). Common themes identified in these reports are discussed here, relating them to international literature where appropriate. The common themes can be organised under the following headings:

- image of nursing
- education
- workplace conditions
- relationship and personal issues.

Professional issues have also been identified but range across all of these areas and will be covered accordingly.

IMAGE OF NURSING

All recent reports into nursing in Australia have identified image as a hindrance in attracting school-leavers into nursing. Nursing continues to be seen as the poor cousin of the health professions and essentially the forced choice of females who are unable to get into a higher-status course. Reasons suggested include entry qualifications, university experience, workplace experience and the association of nursing with females.

Students, their parents and career advisors tend to judge course status on the basis of how difficult it is to enter any course. The relatively low ENTER score required to enter nursing courses supports the traditional view that medicine (and now speech pathology, physiotherapy and so on) are for the brighter students and nursing is for the least qualified. In fact the entry score is determined more by supply and demand than difficulty of the course, but the public perception is proving hard to change. This disparity between health profession entry qualifications can also affect the image of nursing within universities, with nursing students seen by staff and peers as less able than the high ENTER-scoring students in other disciplines. It is not surprising that this hierarchy continues in the workplace, with nurses often complaining that they experience a lack of respect from other disciplines.

Nursing as a natural female role

Nursing and caring have traditionally been seen as extensions of the female/mothering role. Probably since Nightingale established nursing as fit work for moral middle-class women, this view has prevailed. Despite many historically male professions, including medicine, now attracting higher percentages of women, nursing has remained predominantly female. This affects not only its image, but also its overall recruitment opportunities. In the past, young women seeking a career had few options and thus many chose nursing. Now there are more opportunities for women and nursing must compete with higher-status professions. It is illogical to argue that other (previously male) professions need a gender balance to better serve the population and ignore the gender imbalance in nursing. The image and recruitment potential of nursing can only improve by promoting nursing as a discipline that is learned—not acquired by gender—and can be learned by either sex of sufficient intellect. Men are also more likely to work full-time, and thus fewer are required to boost effective full-time numbers.

Geronic nursing

If nursing is the poor cousin of the health professions, geronic nursing has been seen as the untouchable illegitimate of nursing! The devalued status of elderly people and the associated ageism in society generally and among health professionals specifically is recognised as largely contributing to the low status of geronic nursing. Aged care competes poorly against highly valued, high-tech acute care (Levin 1988; Newbern et al 1994; Stevens 2002; Stevens & Herbert 1997). Old people, chronic illness, slow-stream care and being female (which most older people are) all attract low status relative to young people, acute illness, curing and being male (Nay 1993). Nursing elderly people has been portrayed as easy and requiring little, if any, more knowledge and skills than those with which women are equipped through their mothering experiences and general experiences of being female (Nay 1993). It is still not uncommon to hear of nurses being placed in aged-care wards as 'punishment' for poor care practices. New graduates who undertake their graduate year in extended/ aged-care hospitals are still experiencing pity from peers, academics and Registered Nurses in the workplace and being encouraged to 'get experience in real nursing' as soon as possible. Nursing homes, especially, are associated with stigma. There is also evidence that younger staff may be afraid of frail older people and that working with older people in nursing homes forces nurses to confront the realities of disease, disability and death, which tend to be denied and avoided in broader society (Nay & Closs 1999). A further problem issue concerning image and gerontic nursing was identified in recent reports, and relates to the gerontic nursing component of the undergraduate curriculum. To summarise concerns, nursing older people is seen to be associated with basic tasks in the initial clinical placement and undertaken in nursing homes. The fact that the majority of nursing experience across the health-care continuum is with older people is often lost as students are taught higher-level skills and knowledge in later years by non-gerontic experts and with little attention to the specific needs of older people. The emphasis on basic tasks and inattention to good role models and positive clinical environments in which care of older people is valued, innovative and challenging leaves graduates with a negative view of older people and gerontic nursing.

The image of nursing, and particularly gerontic nursing, is further tarnished by constant negative media. Genuine efforts to improve nurses' salaries and working conditions, and media attraction to sensationalist reporting, have resulted in numerous stories of poor conditions, workplace bullying and violence against nurses. This is exacerbated in relation to gerontic nursing by 'revelations' of 'appalling conditions' in aged-care facilities and 'granny dumping' in hospitals.

The need to improve the image of nursing generally and gerontic nursing specifically has featured in all Australian reports and in the international literature. Importantly it has also been noted that any efforts to change the image will only succeed if the image reflects reality. In other words, changing the image may attract more students and staff but retention relies on real-world experiences being positive.

EDUCATIONAL EXPERIENCES

Recent Australian reports into nursing and nurse education have recommended that the minimum entry education for registered nurses remain at a three-year Bachelor degree (Heath 2002; Senate Community Affairs References Committee 2002). I believe this support for the maintenance of the status quo lacks vision, ignores changes in the health-care system and leaves nursing in a disadvantaged position relative to other health professions. The 1994 National Review of Nursing Education (Reid 1994) noted strong support for four years as entry preparation to nursing. Since that time it has been argued that there is insufficient clinical experience and that the curriculum needs to include more mental health, gerontic nursing, community and palliative care, complementary health care, evidence-based practice, information technology … and the list could go on. Role expectations are changing as health-care demands, responses and systems change. To expect those students who have achieved less well at school to be able to prepare adequately for practice in less time than the higher-achieving students in other disciplines devalues nursing knowledge and skills and reinforces the lower status of nurses and the discipline of nursing. It also suggests that the much-lauded support for reflective practice is little more than rhetoric. More importantly, it could be expected that a four-year program would give students more time to develop their skills and knowledge, improve the transition-to-practice experience (as new graduates' own and their workplaces' expectations could be better aligned), and facilitate confident collaboration with other disciplines.

I have argued for some years for an articulated educational program that recognises and includes Assistants in Nursing (AINs)[1], Enrolled Nurses (ENs) and Registered Nurses (RNs). Such a model would acknowledge changing health-care demands, the ageing population and associated need in many cases for a level of care that could be provided by a less-qualified carer or EN, the relative shortage of nurses, and the need for different entry and exit points if we are to maximise workforce potential. It would support a larger EN workforce with an extended scope of practice, and a relatively smaller, better-educated professional RN workforce. Given the reduced recruitment pool of eager high-achieving nursing students and the increasing demand for care—much of which does not require an RN to deliver—it seems sensible to take a team approach to care and vary the skills mix according to the complexity of care needs. Registered Nurses would be more involved in planning, monitoring, evaluating, teaching and policy development and implementation. The emphasis of the RN's role would be on ensuring that older people receive high-quality evidence-based care and that staff skills are appropriate to care needs rather than repeatedly undertaking tasks that leave no time for thinking. Registered Nurses would deliver care in situations where the assessment indicates that high-level skills and knowledge are required.

In this model, initial entry for students either not meeting university entry requirements or not wishing to commit to a professional career in nursing could be at the Certificate II/III/IV or Diploma level. Clear articulation and RPL/RCC would facilitate ENs who demonstrated academic ability to enter the third year of the four-year Bachelor of Nursing (BN). Entry requirements for the BN would be aligned with other health professions, to reflect the expectations of the course and improve the perceived status of nursing. The university degree could equip undergraduates with the Enrolled Nurse competencies within the first two years and thus permit them to work as ENs outside semester time. This would add to nurse availability while also providing additional clinical experience for the students. Some students may choose to exit at this point and remain ENs. Others may choose to exit for a time to gain experience and/or engage in childbearing/rearing and then return and complete the degree at a later stage.

Such an approach could: improve the status of professional nursing; improve the university experience for students; graduate more confident nurses who would have entered, experienced and graduated from university on a par with other health professionals; improve the articulation and reduce the costs of an educational pathway; educate a workforce that better reflects changing demands and provides a replacement workforce more rapidly. As it seems likely that nursing will remain predominantly female, at least for some time, and that women will continue to leave the workforce to have and care for children, nurse workforce planning should predict and allow for this level of non-participation in overall numbers.

[1]AINs is used throughout this chapter to define unlicensed, third-level carers undertaking nursing work.

Gerontic nursing in the curriculum

Studies have pointed to problems associated with the teaching of gerontic nursing in the undergraduate curriculum. A recent study undertaken for the Nurses Board of Victoria (Nay et al 2002) reflects many of the issues raised in other literature. It established a need to emphasise and make more explicit aged care in undergraduate nursing. Specifically, the following issues were identified:

- lack of emphasis on aged-care nursing generally;
- the linking of aged-care nursing to learning basic tasks in the first clinical experience;
- lack of opportunity to develop aged-care nursing competencies as a senior student;
- insufficient quality clinical experience;
- lack of evidence that staff teaching aged-care nursing have qualifications in the field and/or have continuing relevant competence and credibility;
- too few appropriate role models in clinical practice;
- insufficient educational development of clinical preceptors/teachers;
- lack of sound university/industry partnerships;
- lack of processes to select quality clinical placements; and
- insufficient evidence of specific aged-care nursing content.

Recommendations included using gerontic nursing experts, improving partnerships between universities and clinical agencies, teaching gerontic nursing at all levels of the course, offering gerontic nursing as a specific subject in the senior year of the course and offering an elective subject in gerontic nursing. The plight of undergraduate education in aged care in Australia was also highlighted in the recent *National Nursing Review of Education* and the *Senate Inquiry into Nursing*. Recommendations of these inquiries included urging universities to review the content and quality of clinical placements and experiences of student nurses, and that clinical placements should include a range of aged-care settings (Heath 2002; Senate Community Affairs References Committee 2002, p 158). The Commonwealth Government has recently commissioned Queensland University of Technology to conduct a national review in response to these recommendations.

Postgraduate education and re-entry/refresher programs

Postgraduate gerontic nursing has not, for all the reasons already mentioned, been a popular choice for many nurses. Some argue that there is a perception that 'anyone' can do gerontic nursing (no skills required) and that the effort and cost involved are not rewarded sufficiently in the workplace. Others say that as they are working to improve the financial situation of their family, it makes little sense for them to then spend that money on their own education (Nay & Closs 1999; Pearson et al 2002a). Numerous recommendations have emanated from recent reports in relation to government providing scholarships, refresher and re-entry programs to encourage and support more nurses to improve their knowledge and skills and ultimately develop a career in aged care. Governments have responded and the current public focus on care of older people is at least providing some much-needed good press. Whether that translates into more qualified nurses participating in the care of older people remains to be seen.

Clearly there are many opportunities and initiatives related to education that can encourage nurses to consider working with older people as a more positive option. But that is just the beginning—once staff are recruited they will only be retained if the workplace meets their needs.

WORKPLACE ISSUES

All nursing and aged-care studies have reported dissatisfaction with the current workplace environment for nurses—both in hospital settings and in aged care. Common areas of concern include the need for:

- greater support for the transition from study to work;
- wages and wage parity for aged-care nurses with their public-sector peers;
- improved staffing levels;
- appropriate skills mix;
- career pathways;
- improved staff development;
- reduced documentation requirements;
- appreciation and recognition of nurses;
- better relationships with management, peers, other health professionals and families;
- a safe, supportive work environment; and
- a stronger research base

(c.f. Bennett 2001; Heath 2002; Nay & Closs 1999; Pearson et al 2002a,b; Senate Community Affairs References Committee 2002).

The transition from study to work

The Australian and international literature report negative student experiences as they enter the workplace as neophyte nurses. New graduates report feeling incompetent, lacking support and shocked by reality. It appears to take around six months for them to feel organised, competent and accepted. In a US study, Boychuk Duchsher (2001) found that new graduates experienced tension between what they had learned and how they were expected to practise; they were confronted by their own infallibility and desired more support. Time management can also be a problem as the new organisation and its policies, practices and pan-rooms have to be negotiated. Boychuk Duchsher (2001), Greene & Puetzer (2002) and Cordeniz (2002) suggest that older nurses adopt preceptor and mentor roles to support the transition. This may also be a strategic way to keep older nurses in the workforce by reducing the physical demands of direct care, while capitalising on their knowledge and experience (Buchan 2002).

Wages, staffing levels and skills mix

In Australia, the wages of nurses working in aged care can be up to 20% less than those received by nurses with similar qualifications and experience in the public hospital sector. While the international literature suggests that money is not the top priority for nurses (Duffield & O'Brien-Pallas 2002; Upenieks 2003), there is no doubt that wage disparity reduces the attractiveness of working with older people and reinforces the devalued image of gerontic nursing. Until and unless this situation is rectified, recruitment into aged care will remain a major challenge. Similarly, inadequate staffing levels and skills mix leaves nurses feeling burned out and unable to provide quality care. A recent study by Stechmiller (2002) notes UK nurses' perceptions that care quality has drastically changed—citing falls, medication errors and nosocomial infections as indicators. Australian nurses in aged-care environments report frustration and fear of litigation related to working with AINs and poor overall staffing levels (Heath 2002; Nay & Closs 1999; Pearson et al 2002a; Senate Community Affairs References Committee 2002). The increased pressure they face in a short-staffed environment leaves no time for supervision, planning and evaluation of care. In addition, workplace injury, sick leave and staff turnover are less likely in workplaces that have sufficient appropriately qualified staff.

Two conflicting arguments are presented to explain the lack of qualified nurses in aged care: one is that aged-care managers want to replace qualified nurses with AINs because the latter are cheaper; the other is that managers in aged care are desperately trying to attract qualified nurses but are forced to employ lesser-qualified staff because they cannot attract nurses. My guess, in the absence of hard evidence, is that both are true. However, the facilities that are substituting qualified nurses to save money are ill-informed. Ample evidence now shows that the employment of sufficient qualified nurses can indeed save money while improving care quality (Duffield & O'Brien-Pallas 2002; Romano 2002). On the other hand, well-considered, evidence-based substitution is required if health-care demands are to be met. Nursing cannot logically remain static in a changing context. Delegation decisions must be related to educational preparation, demonstrated competence and context.

The Queensland Nursing Council (QNC) developed a scope of nursing practice decision-making framework to 'provide guidance to individual nurses, the nursing profession, other health care personnel, service providers and consumers in decision-making about issues of nursing practice' (QNC 1998, p 2). This framework has been adopted in Western Australia and is gaining support by nursing authorities for national implementation (Minister for Ageing Meeting 2003) to assist decisions regarding scope of practice and delegation.

The role of gerontic nurse practitioner offers exciting possibilities for RN career development, a positive response to the increasing need for expertise at this level across the health-care system, and another avenue for attracting and retaining well-qualified nurses. Nurses have supported RNs advancing their practice and have been very critical of doctors who have resisted this. Yet those same RNs often seem reluctant to support ENs in extending their scope of practice! Decisions about substitution should derive from consideration of health-care demand, required and available skills and cost effectiveness—not territory protection. Doctors cannot complain that they are overworked yet refuse to share that work with nurse practitioners; similarly, RNs cannot complain about the time required to document care and administer medications and then resist ENs taking up some of these responsibilities. Current Australian inconsistencies in EN education and scope of practice result in the unjustifiable situation where an EN moving from Western Australia to Victoria is unable to use the full extent of his or her knowledge and skills despite the stated nursing 'crisis', because Victoria prescribes a more limited scope of practice for ENs than does Western Australia. More importantly, the safety of older people is compromised due to the shortage of staff qualified in medication administration.

Leadership, career pathways and staff development

Research into Magnet Hospitals (Shobbrook & Fenton 2002) illustrates the critical link between good nursing leadership, staff development, and recruitment and retention. For years, studies have reported that nurses are more satisfied in their job—and thus likely to stay—where they have opportunities to be involved in decision-making, greater autonomy, flexible rostering and career development. The Magnet Hospital concept has capitalised on this and apparently reaped the benefits. Nurses remain on average 8.6 years, compared to a national average of 3.5 years. Ten per cent of nurses nationally report giving good to excellent care, whereas in Magnet Hospitals the figure is 89%, indicating that nurses are satisfied and quality improved. The major characteristics of Magnet Hospitals are as follows:

- A nurse executive is a formal member of the governing body in the hospital.
- Nursing services are organised in a flat organisational structure rather than a pyramid.
- Decision-making is decentralised to the unit level for staffing and patient care.
- Administrative structures are supporting nurses and physicians.
- Investments are in the education and expertise of nurses.
- BSN RN staffing is increasing.
- RN-to-patient ratios are increasing.
- RN salaried status is implemented.
- Flexible and varied nursing care delivery is designed to meet patient and staff needs (Stechmiller 2002, p 580).

Australian reports reveal similar principles as influencing a nurse's decision to remain in or leave a workplace. Excellent nursing leadership, that has a clear vision and is prepared to take risks and to support nursing staff where required, appears to increase nurse retention (Romano 2002). The need for nurse leaders to be educated for their positions and not just expected to move from clinical nursing to management has been noted and recommendations for leadership training are included in all recent reviews. 'Good' nurse leaders can reduce workplace conflict and generally smooth relationships.

Documentation

The issue of documentation is of sufficient significance to nurses to be addressed separately. All recent reports strongly recommend a reduction in documentation. In aged care specifically, the linking of funding to care has attracted enormous concern, mountains of apparently unnecessary documentation, and complaints that nurses are being prevented from providing and supervising direct care because of the time involved in meeting documentation requirements. There appear to be three issues involved: the use of paper-based systems, the linking of funding to individual care requirements, and the vested interests of consultants! Anecdotal evidence indicates that where nurses undertake comprehensive nursing assessments and develop care plans based on these assessments, the documentation for funding is less onerous. Indeed, the information required to validate funding is already available in the care documents. Nevertheless, a review of funding requirements and current associated research should make this more explicit and reduce duplication of information (RCS Review 2003). Lack of understanding of the documentation required and inconsistency in feedback to aged-care facilities from government, coupled with subsequent loss of funding, encouraged many providers to bring in consultants to assist them. There are widespread reports of such consultancies resulting in duplication—with nurses' documentation being driven by the funding requirements and then supplemented where necessary for care. This approach, apart from increasing workload, moves the focus from client care needs to facility funding requirements. Finally, much of the duplication could be avoided by using computerised information and care-planning systems. (The benefits of moving with the times in this way are detailed in Chapter 18.) Furthermore, if younger recruits are to be attracted, attention must be given to their expectations. Recent research into the expectations of Generation X-ers (Gen X) gives some indication of how management and workplaces will need to change.

Cordeniz (2002) reported that Gen X nurses' expectations and work values included: work that aligned with values and demands; training; liberal vacations; day-care centres; workout rooms; on-site dry-cleaning; flexibility; and emails/website information rather than lengthy meetings. It is unlikely that out-of-date paper-based systems will be valued by this generation!

RELATIONSHIP AND PERSONAL ISSUES

Good relationships are reported in most, if not all, studies as highly influential in job satisfaction for nurses and their decision to remain in or leave a workplace. Relationships with management, doctors, peers, administrators and families have received significant comment. Relationships with management have been commented on already and will not be laboured here except to note that Gen X-ers want their managers to: be good communicators, work with them, stand up for them, know them, be with them (e.g. have a cuppa), help them grow and make them laugh. A quick review of contemporary leadership books suggests that the authors have already been surveying Gen X!

As good leadership is integral to recruiting and retaining staff, good leaders must also be retained. A study by Singh & Schwab (2000) reported a 40% turnover of nursing home administrators each year in the United States. They surveyed 1035 nursing home administrators in Michigan and Indiana and found that most left their posts voluntarily, and of these 81% left because they were promoted. Factors involved in the retention of administrators included:

- consistency between their own philosophy and that of the organisation;
- a high level of trust in the organisation;
- enthusiasm;
- loyalty to the organisation;
- realised expectations;
- career opportunities and rewards;
- autonomy in decision-making;
- support; and
- a good match between their desired lifestyle and the community.

These factors overlap considerably with factors identified by other nurses as important to them. Relationships with doctors seem to be particularly important to job satisfaction (Boychuk Duchsher 2001; Duffield & O'Brien-Pallas 2002; Nay & Closs 1999; Shobbrook & Fenton 2002; Upenieks 2003). Rosenstein (2002) identified a number of strategies aimed at improving nurse–physician relationships. These included 'greater opportunities for collaboration and communication ... education and training of nurses and physicians through programs designed to improve working relationships ... more open forums and group discussions ... and greater accountability among nurses and physicians for their actions' (p 32). Further strategies suggested were better organisational processes to reduce the potential for confrontation, zero-tolerance for disruptive behaviour, a code of conduct, improving nurse competencies and having physicians on nurse recruitment panels. It was interesting to note that no suggestion was made regarding nurses being on medical selection panels!

Horizontal violence has long been recognised as a cause for low job satisfaction (Nay 1993; Roberts 1983). Numerous papers have also referred to nurses 'eating their young'. More recently the term 'workplace bullying' has become popular (e.g. Lewis 2001; Quine 1999). In essence, some nurses report that personal attacks, undermining and other workplace relationship problems influence their decision to leave a position (Stevens 2002; Strawbridge 2001). These behaviours seem to occur less frequently in organisations with fewer hierarchical structures and more participative management styles.

Relationships with families are inescapable in the care of older people and nurses value relationships that are constructive and in which families express appreciation for the work the nurses do. This is more likely to occur in environments where families feel valued and can determine their role in the ongoing care of the older person (Bauer & Nay 2003; Nay & Closs 1999; Pearson et al 2002a). In summary, relationships are far from marginal in care contexts; where leadership, processes and policies support respectful collaborative relationships, job satisfaction is higher.

Finally, perhaps because the workforce is predominantly female, personal issues are often central to a nurse's decision to commence or remain in employment. The most frequently cited issue is that of accommodating family responsibilities.

Workplaces that can offer flexible rostering, school vacations, child-care assistance and, increasingly, elder-care assistance, are more likely to retain staff pressured by informal caring responsibilities. As noted previously, Gen X have their own expectations; Cordeniz (2002) reported that they ranked their priorities in this order: family, health, time, friends, religion, living comfortably, career and money. Facilities that recognise and support the personal desires of staff are likely to win in recruitment competitions in the future.

A STRONGER RESEARCH BASE

Being required to practise evidence-based nursing in the absence of a strong research base was identified as a concern for participants in the Nurse Returners study (Pearson et al 2002a). Funding for nursing research is very limited and much of the research that has been conducted to date has been fragmented, with a substantial amount remaining unpublished. Practitioners often do not know how to access or implement research findings. The need for research is considered sufficiently important that it is addressed in detail in three chapters of this book (Chs 19, 20 and 21) and the issues will not be laboured here.

CONCLUSION

The ageing of the population demands an expanded health-care workforce. This requires all stakeholders to think and act more creatively. Although some effort has been expended to improve the image of ageing, nursing and aged care, an increased and sustained strategy is required to overturn entrenched ageist societal views. If nursing is to remain relevant to the care of older people it must be prepared to anticipate and respond to changes in flexible and constructive ways. Changes are needed in what education is offered and how it is delivered. Partnerships between governments, education providers and clinical facilities are essential to success. Workplace cultures, structures and practices will need to change to reflect workforce needs and staff expectations. Staff will not stay if they do not feel valued. A commitment to undertake and support lifelong learning and recognise staff development as an investment, rather than a cost, will give organisations the competitive edge. Many organisations and individuals are already providing examples of innovation in recruitment and retention, as is demonstrated by June Heinrich in the following vignette.

VIGNETTE

Innovations in the recruitment and retention of staff

June Heinrich

There have been a number of innovations in the recruitment and retention of all levels of staff in community and residential aged care. While some innovations such as increased remuneration and self-rostering relate to the quality of working life, the high-impact innovations are in the area of staff professional development. Significant among these are education opportunities in both the vocational and tertiary areas. Innovations include:

- articulation of programs so that any education given to employees can lead to academically recognised professional qualifications;
- scholarship provision for employees enrolled in workplace-related studies;
- vocational education opportunities, including employer support to complete the Certificate III and IV in Aged Care Work. These programs provide a career pathway for direct-care workers and ensure greater job satisfaction through an enhanced scope of practice. This provides employees with the opportunity to become workplace champions in clinical areas of practice interest.
- provision of a new graduate program in aged care through the Aged Care Career Pathways (ACCP) Consortium.

The ACCP Consortium was established in 1999 to provide a relevant graduate transition program in aged care. In 2002 the ACCP introduced a similar program for registered nurses returning to the aged-care sector. The aims of the ACCP are to attract and retain newly registered nurses into the aged-care workforce and to provide an industry-relevant refresher program for registered nurses returning to the workforce who wish to work in the aged-care sector. The current provider members of the ACCP Consortium operate a diverse range of aged-care facilities and services, and are drawn from all sectors of aged care.

The professional members of ACCP provide support and advice in the management of the program. Professional members are the Australian Nursing Homes and Extended Care Association (NSW), the Aged and Community Services Association (NSW), Geri-action (NSW), The NSW Nurses Association, and the School of Nursing and Midwifery at the University of Newcastle. The program is also supported by the Commonwealth Department of Health and Ageing.

The program focuses on the consolidation of a cross-section of clinical abilities and the development of leadership and management skills in aged care. The outcomes have been extremely positive and have addressed educational and clinical needs.

Acknowledgement

Acknowledgement is given to Bernie Closs for her assistance in preparing the first edition version of this chapter.

References

Access Economics 2001, *Population Ageing and the Economy*, Commonwealth of Australia: Canberra.

Angus J & Nay R 2003, The paradox of the Aged Care Act 1997: the marginalisation of nursing discourse, *Nursing Inquiry*, 10(2), pp 130–8.

Australian Health Care Agreement (AHCA) 2002, Commonwealth Department of Health and Ageing. Online: http://www.health.gov.au/haf/ahca.htm

Australian Institute of Health and Welfare (AIHW) 1998, *Nursing Labour Force 1998*, AIHW: Canberra.

Australian Institute of Health and Welfare (AIHW) 2002, *Older Australia at a Glance*, Commonwealth of Australia: Canberra.

Bauer M & Nay R 2003, Family and staff partnerships in long term care: a review of the literature, *International Journal of Gerontological Nursing*, 29(10), pp 46–53.

Bennett M (Chair) 2001, *Nurse Recruitment and Retention Committee Final Report*, Department of Human Services, Victoria.

Boychuk Duchsher JB 2001, Out in the real world: newly graduated nurses in acute care speak out, *Journal Of Nursing Administration*, 31(9), pp 426–39.

Buchan J 2000, Planning for change: developing a policy framework for nursing labour markets, *International Nursing Review*, 47, pp 199–206.

Buchan J 2002, Nursing shortages and evidence-based interventions: a case study from Scotland, *International Nursing Review*, 49, pp 209–18.

Cheek J, Ballantyne A, Jones J, Roder-Allen G & Kitto S 2003, Ensuring excellence: an investigation of the issues that impact on the registered nurse providing residential care to older Australians, *International Journal of Nursing Practice*, 9(2), pp 103–11.

Chiu L, Tang K, Shyru W, Huang C & Wang S 2000, Cost analysis of home care and nursing home services in the Southern Taiwan area, *Public Health Nursing*, 17(5), pp 325–35.

Cordeniz J 2002, Recruitment, retention, and management of Generation X: a focus on nursing professionals, *Journal of Health Care Management*, Jul/Aug, pp 237–49.

Duffield C & O'Brien-Pallas L 2002, The nursing workforce in Canada and Australia: two sides of the same coin, *Australian Health Review*, 25(2), pp 136–44.

Greene M & Puetzer M 2002, The value of mentoring: a strategic approach to retention and recruitment, *Journal of Nursing Care Quality*, 17(1), pp 63–70.

Heath P (Chair) 2002, *National Review of Nursing Education 2002 Our Duty of Care*, Commonwealth of Australia: Canberra.

Levin WC 1988, Age stereotyping—college student evaluations, *Research on Aging*, 10(1), pp 134–48.

Lewis M 2001, Bullying in nursing, *Nursing Standard*, 15(45), pp 39–42.

Minister for Ageing Meeting 2003, with Australian nurse regulatory authorities and other stakeholders to discuss implementation of ACENWP report, Canberra, 18 June.

Nay R 1993, *Benevolent Oppression*, unpublished doctoral thesis, University of NSW.

Nay R & Closs B 1999, *Recruitment and Retention of Qualified Nurses in Aged Care*, unpublished report, Department of Human Services, Victoria.

Nay R (Chair) 2002, Review of the Aged Care Component of the Undergraduate Curriculum, Nurses Board of Victoria: Melbourne.

Nay R (Chair) 2003, Aged Care Enrolled Nurse Working Party Report to the Minister for Ageing, Commonwealth of Australia: Canberra.

New South Wales Department of Health 2000, *NSW Nursing Workforce: The Way Forward*.

New South Wales Nurses Association (NSWNA) 2000, *Nursing Home and Hostel Workforce, Third Survey Report*, NSWNA: Sydney.

Newbern VB, Barba BE, Courts NF & Kennedy-Malone L 1994, Required clinical course in gerontology: the key to providing competent nurse caregivers for the elderly, *Nursing Outlook*, 42(4), pp 170–4.

Pearson A, Nay R, Koch S & Rosewarne R 2002a, *Recruitment and Retention of Nurses in Residential Aged Care Final Report*, Commonwealth Department of Health and Aged Care: Canberra.

Pearson A, Nay R, Koch S & Ward C 2002b, *Australian Aged Care Nursing: A Critical Review of Education, Training, Recruitment and Retention in Residential and Community Settings*, National Review of Nursing Education 2002, Department of Education, Science and Training, and Department of Health and Ageing, pp 1–97.

Queensland Nursing Council (QNC) 1998, *Scope of Practice Decision Making Framework*, QNC: Brisbane.

Quine L 1999, Workplace bullying in NHS community trust: staff questionnaire survey, *British Medical Journal*, 318, pp 228–32.

Reid J 1994, *Nursing Education in Australian Universities*, Resident Classification Scale (RCS) Review, February 2003, Commonwealth Department of Health and Ageing, No. 43, AGPS: Canberra.

Roberts SJ 1983, Oppressed group behaviour: implications for nursing, *Advances in Nursing Science*, July, pp 21–30.

Rogers A & Barusch A 2000, Mental health service utilisation among frail, low-income elders: perceptions of home service providers and elders in the community, *Journal of Gerontological Social Work*, 34(2), pp 23–38.

Romano M 2002, A strong attraction, *Modern Healthcare*, 32(50), pp 28–34.

Rosenstein A 2002, Nurse–physician relationships: impact on nurse satisfaction and retention, *Australian Journal of Nursing*, 102(6), pp 26–34.

Senate Community Affairs References Committee 2002, *The Patient Profession: Time for Action. Report on Enquiry into Nursing*, Commonwealth of Australia, Canberra.

Shobbrook P & Fenton K 2002, A strategy for improving nurse retention and recruitment levels, *Professional Nurse*, 17(9), pp 534–7.

Singh D & Schwab R 2000, Predicting turnover and retention in nursing home administrators: management and policy implications, *The Gerontologist*, 40(3), pp 310–19.

Stechmiller J 2002, The nursing shortage in acute and critical care settings, *AACN Clinical Issues* 13(4), pp 577–84.

Stevens S 2002, Nursing workforce retention: challenging a bullying culture, *Health Affairs*, 21(5), pp 189–93.

Stevens JA & Herbert J 1997, *Ageism and Nursing Practice in Australia*, Discussion Paper No 3, Royal College of Nursing, Australia.

Strawbridge Y 2001, Bullying: a soul shattering experience, *Australian Nursing Journal*, 9(2), p 40.

United Nations Populations Division 2003, *World Prospects: The 2002 Revision, Highlights*.

Upenieks V 2003, Recruitment and retention strategies: a magnet hospital prevention model, *Nursing Economics*, 21(1), pp 7–13.

Williams J, Lyons B & Rowland D 1997, Unmet long-term care need of elderly people in the community: a review of the literature, *Home Health Care Services Quarterly*, 16(1/2), pp 93–119.

CHAPTER 5

Rights, regulation and aged-care practice

JOHN FIELD AND SALLY GARRATT

INTRODUCTION

The focus on health-related law that currently exists in Australia parallels developments in other developed Western nations, but is unprecedented in our legal history. There is considerable evidence of an explosion in health-related law. One has only to look at the range and scope of books on law for various health disciplines. Nursing is a good example, with most Australian books that deal with nursing and the law having been published in the past decade. The fact that many Australian law schools now include a unit on health law in their curriculum should send a very clear message to all health-care practitioners. Litigation will become an increasingly common aspect of practice.

It is not possible in one chapter to address every aspect of the law relating to the nursing care of older people. However, depending upon the area of aged care in which one is engaged, nurses need an understanding of the law, not merely with respect to clinical practice, but also with respect to funding and policy. A recurrent theme in Australian law is an emphasis on rights, so it is this that will form the organising framework for this chapter. Much of the law relating to the nursing care of older people—whether it be in residential facilities or hospitals—can be understood from this perspective. The implications of a rights-based approach to nursing practice raises issues for nurses that previously they have not had to address so rigorously. The aged-care reform process has raised many issues for nurses who endeavour to deliver personalised, individual care within a collective living environment. Meeting the needs of all parties when the rights agenda is driving practice is not easy. This chapter explains the legal aspects of rights, and briefly explores issues that may arise when endeavouring to give effect to rights in practice.

THE CONCEPT OF RIGHTS

It is important, as a preamble to this discussion, to clarify the sense in which the term 'right' is to be used. The term 'right' is used here to denote anything that is allowed, or claimed as due, where that claim is recognised in law. Thus, a distinction is drawn here between legal rights and rights which have only moral force. Nevertheless, in practice, moral rights also have some legal suasion for nurses because of the relationships among the *Code of Ethics for Nurses in Australia* (Australian Nursing Council [ANC]

Inc 2002), the *Code of Professional Conduct for Nurses in Australia* (ANC 2003) and the disciplinary powers of the nurse registering authorities.

A further concept related to legal rights is that of 'remedies'. There is little point to a right that has no available remedy. Thus, as each right is identified in this chapter, the possible legal remedies for its breach are canvassed.

In recent times, considerable attention has been paid to the individual's rights in Australia, and this is a vital component of social development. Less attention is paid to the corollary of rights. Where one person has a right, the existence of that right imposes obligations on another. For example, since a person has a right to expect quality health care, the providers of health care have an obligation to deliver their services with reasonable care and skill. However, a right will only be a right in the sense used here where there is a mechanism for its enforcement, and it will only be a legal right where that mechanism is the law. Thus, taking as an example the right to quality health care, the mechanism for its enforcement—or, put another way, the remedy for its breach—lies in the law in the form of a legal action in negligence.

Legal rights may arise in a number of ways. The most straightforward way is for Parliament to pass an Act which spells out a right. Unfortunately this is an infrequent occurrence. Sometimes a right will come into existence through what is referred to as delegated legislation. For instance, in New South Wales, the Department of Health issued guidelines on the management of dying patients (Health Department of New South Wales 1993). These guidelines reinforce the patient's right to make decisions regarding their own care and, although they do not carry statutory force, they would be taken into consideration by a court or tribunal. It is important to note, however, that guidelines need to be updated periodically to take account of developments in law and social expectations, among other things. For instance, the NSW guidelines are in the final stages of revision for a second edition to be published this year after a protracted period of consultation and review.

Another way in which a right may come into existence is through the development of case law; that is, where a court determines the status of a right. An example of this can be found in relation to informed consent in Australia. In 1992, in the case of *Rogers v Whitaker*, the High Court said that patients had a right to be informed of the material risks of any treatment they were being offered. Since there is no higher court in the Australian legal system, and leaving aside the option for the High Court to change its view in a future case, the only way this right can now be taken away is by State governments passing legislation in their parliaments that destroys it.

LEGAL RIGHTS OF OLDER PEOPLE

People lose many things as they grow older. They lose their youthfulness. They often lose their agility. They may lose their vision. They lose some of their friends. They might even lose the ability to live independently. They do not lose their legal rights. Thus, older people have the same legal rights as younger adults. In some cases older people will have clearer evidence of their rights than those who are younger. As far back as 1990, the Commonwealth Government brought into law a *Charter of Residents' Rights and Responsibilities (Aged or Disabled Persons Care Act 1954)* for people living in nursing homes. Some of the rights expressly articulated in that Charter are not found so succinctly stated elsewhere. Some of the rights included in the

Charter derive their statutory force solely by being included in that publication. This means that those persons not subject to the legislation which includes the Charter, may not have such rights. The original Charter, which will be familiar to those nurses who work in nursing homes, was added in 1991 as a Schedule to the *Aged or Disabled Persons Care Act 1954* (as amended) and, until relatively recently, it applied to the residents of all nursing homes. The highly controversial *Aged Care Act 1997* (Cth) incorporates this Charter in a slightly amended form through s.23(14) of the User Rights Principles established under the Aged Care Act. The *Charter of Residents' Rights and Responsibilities* identifies the rights of residents in nursing homes as being:

- a right to full and effective use of his or her personal, civil, legal and consumer rights;
- a right to quality care which is appropriate to his or her needs;
- a right to full information about his or her own state of health and about available treatments;
- a right to be treated with dignity and respect, and to live without exploitation, abuse or neglect;
- a right to live without discrimination or victimisation;
- a right to personal privacy;
- a right to live in a safe, secure, homelike environment, and to move freely, both within and outside the nursing home, without undue restriction;
- a right to be treated and accepted as an individual;
- a right to continue one's own cultural and religious practices and to retain the language of one's own choice, without discrimination;
- a right to select and maintain social and personal relationships with any other person without fear, criticism or restriction;
- a right to freedom of speech;
- a right to maintain one's personal independence—which includes a recognition of personal responsibility for one's own actions and choices;
- a right to maintain control over, and to continue making decisions about, the personal aspects of one's daily life, financial affairs and possessions;
- a right to be involved in the activities, associations and friendships of one's own choice, both within and outside the nursing home;
- a right to access services and activities available generally in the community;
- a right to be consulted on, and to choose to have input into, decisions about the living arrangements of the nursing home;
- a right to access information about one's rights, care, accommodation and any other information that relates to one personally;
- a right to complain and to take action to resolve disputes; and
- a right to have access to advocates and other avenues of redress.

The Commonwealth Government's intent with respect to nursing home residents is evident from this reduction to writing of their rights: there should be no diminution of rights merely by reason of admission to a nursing home. As foreshadowed above, a corollary of this is that there should be no diminution of one's legal rights merely by reason of growing older. Hence, the rights of older people should be precisely those of any adult citizen of our society. This is as true of rights relating to health care as of any other rights. Since the *Charter of Residents' Rights and Responsibilities* forms the broadest array of rights enshrined in legislation for the benefit of aged persons, an analysis of these rights provides very useful guidance for those charged with responsibility for the nursing care of aged persons. The mechanism contained in the *Aged or Disabled Persons Care Act 1954* to assure the rights contained in the Charter was a specified agreement that was to be entered into between the resident and the service provider. Note that the *Aged Care Act 1997*, because of perceived difficulties in enforcing the rights contained within the Charter by way of the agreement, has adopted a different approach in an attempt to guarantee the rights of residents of non-government nursing homes.

REMEDIES FOR WRONGS: CONSEQUENCES OF THE BREACH OF RIGHTS

In this context, the most useful form of analysis is a consideration of remedies available to aged persons in the event of a breach of any of the rights in the Charter. This can shed considerable light on the ways in which nurses can adjust their practice in aged care to ensure the observance of the consumer's rights. Note the language here, because these are effectively consumer rights that are being considered.

A right to quality care which is appropriate to his or her needs

The right to quality care is underpinned by the law on negligence. Every nurse is familiar with the common-law mantra of the elements of negligence—duty of care, breach of duty, damage and foreseeability. A consumer who believes that their treatment has been substandard can commence an action in negligence against the provider(s) of that treatment. The law of negligence is not reviewed here, but it is important to recognise that this generic right is being increasingly exercised in Australia.

What is required of nurses in order to observe this right of the consumer is the exercise of reasonable care and skill in the conduct of their practice. What this means in practice is dependent upon all of the circumstances prevailing at the time, but requires that the nurse do what a reasonable, competent nurse of similar education and experience would do in those same circumstances.

Although this right derives from common-law principles, in the case of care of the aged it also finds a statutory basis in the Commonwealth Aged Care legislation, and some of the States also have legislative provisions reinforcing the common law. There is a trend towards the use of codes and charters of health rights that is likely to add further weight to this and other health-related rights.

A right to full information about his or her own state of health and about available treatments

This right is expressly articulated in the Charter. However, since *Rogers v Whitaker* (1992) was determined by the High Court of Australia, all persons have a common-law right to be informed at least of the material risks associated with any proposed treatment. A failure to inform a patient of a material risk may form the basis for an action in negligence, where that failure results in harm. As well, the mechanisms of the *Aged Care Act 1997*, together with emerging State-based codes or charters of health rights, are likely to strengthen this right.

Practice issue

Situations often arise where the nurse cannot give information regarding their care to the older person because of that person's cognitive impairment. In Australia, the matter of guardianship is not yet clearly understood by the community. The older person is often admitted to a facility without clear definition of who is responsible for care decisions. There may be several family members involved in the care of the older person and in such cases they may present staff with different and often conflicting information and expectations. In such circumstances it is imperative that one person be identified by the family as the person with authority to present the family perspective and liaise with staff in the decision-making process. Deciding who takes this responsibility is a family matter, but if it cannot be resolved, the staff of the facility may need to get independent assistance. The practice constraints of deciding who to deal with on matters of care when family members disagree can become a strain on the decision-making capacity of the staff. Such tensions can potentially lead to judgemental outcomes that polarise the care team. The core of the decision-making process must always be the 'best interests' of the older person receiving the care. However, determining what constitutes the 'best interests' of a cognitively impaired individual is a major challenge and it is very likely—if not inevitable—that there will be competing views about this. In practice, it will be at times such as this that nurses should draw most heavily on the guidance contained within the principles of the *Code of Ethics for Nurses in Australia* (ANC 2002).

A right to be treated with dignity and respect, and to live without exploitation, abuse or neglect

Although those persons who live in government-operated nursing homes have these requirements enshrined in legislation, and although abuse and neglect are addressed through various mechanisms (such as the law of negligence), dignity, respect and exploitation in relation to nursing practice have largely been within the province of professional regulation. Thus, conduct that may be regarded as unprofessional has been most commonly dealt with by the disciplinary processes of nurse registering authorities—but only where a complaint has been made in relation to that conduct. Every nurse needs to be conversant with the legislation that regulates his or her practice. As well, the additional complaints processes that have been put in place (described later in this chapter), ensure that many more breaches of rights result in formal complaints being lodged. Here again, the *Aged Care Act 1997*, together with the codes of conduct and ethics for Australian nurses, have given further substance to these rights for residents of non-government nursing homes. The complaints mechanisms for aged care, which now parallel those for health care generally, have given considerable access to those who wish to complain about the care provided to a person in an aged-care facility.

Practice issue

Notwithstanding the changing nature of the aged-care workforce and the increasing numbers of staff who are not registered or controlled by any authority except civil law, the registered nurse in charge at any time is accountable and responsible for care delivery. Delegation of direct care provision to a minimally skilled workforce is an increasing part of the manager role, as is supervision of that workforce. Nurses traditionally have not had this level of managerial responsibility in aged care. There is a need to educate clinical management staff about specific aspects of care and how they can be managed on a daily basis without the registered nurse becoming part of a culture of blame, overwork and negativity. Ethical behaviour concerning dignity and respect and the fostering of self-esteem for an older person begins with a foundation of knowledge built on professional care values. These values are part of the education process that all professionals are taught in their practice preparation. Values that other workers bring to the workplace are often based on prevailing norms in society, where there is still an element of ageism and undervaluing of the old. Unless these attitudes and values are constantly challenged by health-care professionals they will permeate the care-delivery system.

A right to live without discrimination or victimisation

Antidiscrimination legislation is now well established in Australia—at both Commonwealth and State levels. The effect of this legislation is to make unlawful discrimination against a person on the basis of such characteristics as sex, marital status, race, disability and—most importantly in the present context—age, with respect to employment, accommodation, education and the provision of goods and services. Health care falls within this last category.

Practice issue

This right is clearly addressing the needs of the older person who receives care in a communal living situation. In communal living in a multicultural society there will be people from different backgrounds and cultures. Staff must constantly juggle the needs of each resident in an aged-care facility that may not have the space to separate groups with different interests. Older people can exhibit their own form of discrimination and reject those of different colour or creed. By the age of 80 plus, a person's outlook on life may be somewhat set, making them less tolerant of those with different beliefs. This presents a challenge for staff who have to treat each person with the same respect and tolerance, recognising the needs of each person, without acting on their expressed wishes. An example of this dilemma is when an older person whose past history has not been positive because of involvement in war cannot tolerate another person from a country that was 'the enemy' during the war, and demands that the other person be removed from the premises. Should the staff isolate the other person, keep the complaining person away, or try to mediate with them, knowing that their values are set and not likely to change? These situations—which are not uncommon—are often not easily resolved.

A right to personal privacy

This is one of those rights that used to derive its legal force solely from its inclusion in the *Charter of Residents' Rights and Responsibilities*. As such, the remedy for its breach lay in the provisions of the *Aged or Disabled Persons Care Act 1954* and subsequently in the *Aged Care Act 1997*. However, further redress can be found in the complaints processes that now exist in the *Code of Ethics for Nurses in Australia* (ANC 2002) and in the *Code of Professional Conduct for Nurses in Australia* (ANC 2003).

Practice issue

The development of new building codes and the need for single rooms with either shared or ensuite bathroom accommodation has removed the problem of insufficient toilet space or traversing long corridors to shower rooms and so on. It has not changed the concept of personal space within the building. Human lifestyle improves when there is a sense of control over one's life, including the use of space around their person. Bedroom space is the only area that is really non-public in residential care environments. However, when staff treat this space as public, the older person has very little redress. Knocking on the door and seeking permission to enter is one act of respect for privacy, but how the room is used is quite another. It is often very difficult for staff to accept that personal use can be as varied as the personality of the residents themselves. The use of personal furnishing, colour, hoarding of objects, cleanliness, smells, positioning of items and so on all make for a distinctive personal stamp on the space. To deprive a person of this 'branding' because of environmental clashes is to reduce the nature of personal ownership and remove privacy.

A right to live in a safe, secure, homelike environment, and to move freely within and outside the nursing home without undue restriction

This provision actually encompasses two distinct rights, each having a different legal remedy when breached.

First, the right to live in a secure, homelike environment is another of the rights that derives its legal force solely from its inclusion in the *Charter of Residents' Rights and Responsibilities*. Thus, the remedy for any breach of this right is to be found in the *Aged Care Act 1997* or the *Aged or Disabled Persons Care Act 1954*.

The second right—to move about freely without undue restriction—derives its legal force not only from its inclusion in the Charter but also from the common law. Depending on the nature of the breach, it may be actionable in tort as assault and battery or as false imprisonment.

Practice issue

Safety is a major concern for all care staff. The accepted practice of key-coded doors to provide controlled entry and exit points seems well accepted in aged-care facilities. Further, surveillance technology is becoming prevalent. For example, the use of video cameras in public spaces, sensor tracking in bedrooms, bracelet tracking devices worn on the wrist, clothing tags that raise an alarm when taken through a sensor device at exit points, and alarm sensors at doorways are now commonly used. Just how much surveillance is required to promote safety is debatable. If the environment is secure and the space friendly for older people, personal tagging should not be necessary. The difference between homelike and institutional environments relies on the ability of the person living in the space to be free to move within it, to undertake personal decisions as to when to open windows, close doors and so on. A controlled environment—to the extent that personal choice is restricted—is very institutional. The ability to obtain food and fluid at will, rearrange the furniture, change the environmental stimulus and go outside at will constitutes 'home'. The challenge for care staff is to manage the environment so that maximum freedom of choice is achieved without compromising safety. It is much easier to control the environment and the people who live in it under the guise of safety and duty of care than it is to provide the closest possible conditions to the ideal of home, and choice.

A right to be treated and accepted as an individual

This is another right that derives its authority solely from its inclusion in the Charter. Most people in our society take it for granted that they will be treated and accepted as individuals. However, in institutions that provide services to vulnerable populations—whether residential or otherwise—individuality can be overlooked in the need to achieve efficiency. Many aged persons are obviously vulnerable in this sense, but institutions are now generally aware of the need to take steps to preserve individuality. Note, however, that this problem is not confined to institutions—as the many reported cases of domestic elder-abuse demonstrate.

Practice issue

The notion of 'individual' is one that nursing has adopted for some time. As Leonard (1989) suggests, 'individual' is merely one of something—a tree or a chair can be an individual chair or tree. Only when the concept of 'person' is understood can differences to care be made. *Person* implies more than 'one of'; it represents a uniqueness that is solely that of this person, not any other. Person-centred care is the approach aged-care nurses are slowly adopting for dementia care and this has ramifications for all nursing practice. When the term 'person' is applied it means that the care is tailored to meet the unique needs of this human being, that knowing the person is the only way this type of care can be delivered. Without knowledge of the person, their life and the meaning they create for themselves, care cannot be made purposeful. Care planning should therefore reflect the day-to-day nuances that make a difference for this particular person. This approach is time consuming; it requires knowledge of the person's life and should not be problem oriented. Current care-planning and assessment strategies tend to be based on problem-solving approaches that seek the negative rather than the positive.

A right to continue one's own cultural and religious practices and to retain the language of one's own choice, without discrimination

This right is clearly subsumed by the discussion relating to discrimination generally, but a breach of this right is also subject to the provisions of the *Aged Care Act 1997* or the *Aged or Disabled Persons Care Act 1954*.

Practice issue

An aged-care facility admitted eight Japanese residents who continued to practise their daily prayer ritual, which required a Shinto shrine. The manager organised a specific room that was arranged in the proper manner with incense and a space for prayer. At other times the room was used for activity, mostly by the Japanese elders. Over time the remaining residents became annoyed at the perceived 'extra care' that these residents were receiving. The matter was raised at a resident meeting and family members became involved. After much debate, management faced two options: remove the shrine or make more space available for a chapel for other denominations. The compromise was to create a purposeful space that became the chapel for all, with designated areas within for altars, shrines and any other religious icons required. During the heated debate over the matter, the staff were in danger of being polarised and 'taking sides'. Tension is created when these issues are being resolved and recourse to the *Aged Care Act 1997* is necessary to defuse this tension before the care of residents is affected.

A right to complain and to take action to resolve disputes

The Commonwealth's Charter of Residents' Rights and Responsibilities clearly articulates the right to complain about the services received by aged persons in residential care. In a general sense, this right has always existed, but traditionally it has only rarely been exercised by older persons. This has reflected a number of exigencies—such as the role models and power relationships between service providers and consumers, and the lack of any real mechanisms to facilitate complaints.

Times have changed, however, and as far as aged care is concerned, the Commonwealth has established a statutory body to address complaints relating to the provision of aged care. It constitutes a referee between facilities, individuals and their families. As well, where health care is concerned, a comprehensive complaints process has been put in place in all jurisdictions in Australia. Nurses engaged in the care of the aged need to be aware of the mechanisms available to their clients—both inside and outside the facility—for complaints relating to residential services and health.

Although health-care complaints legislation is a State responsibility—and thus there are differences between the various States' schemes—most schemes have followed a similar model. They all consist of a health-care complaints commission (or equivalent body), a broad jurisdiction to investigate complaints about health care (irrespective of the particular profession of the provider), a specified relationship with professional registration boards, and the ability to receive complaints from any person.

The *Aged Care Act 1997* reinforces this right by requiring approved providers of aged-care services to establish a complaints-resolution mechanism within the service, and to use it to address any complaint made by, or on behalf of, any recipient of care in that service.

THE CHARTER AND THE *AGED CARE ACT 1997*

All of the following rights contained in the *Charter of Residents' Rights* derive their legal authority solely from their inclusion in the Charter:

- a right to select and maintain social and personal relationships with any other person without fear, criticism or restriction;
- a right to freedom of speech;
- a right to maintain one's personal independence—which includes a recognition of personal responsibility for one's own actions and choices;
- a right to maintain control over, and to continue making decisions about, the personal aspects of one's daily life, financial affairs and possessions;

- a right to be involved in the activities, associations and friendships of one's own choice both within and outside the nursing home;
- a right to have access to services and activities which are available generally in the community;
- a right to be consulted on, and to choose to have input into, decisions about the living arrangements of the nursing home;
- a right to have access to information about one's rights, care, accommodation and any other information that relates to one personally; and
- a right to have access to advocates and other avenues of redress.

Before moving on to consider health-related rights specifically, some consideration of the effect of the *Aged Care Act 1997* is necessary because it is this legislation that is likely to preserve those nine rights that to date have had statutory authority only by virtue of their inclusion in the *Charter of Residents' Rights and Responsibilities.* So far in this chapter the major emphasis has been on the rights contained in the Charter of Residents' Rights. This emphasis has been adopted because, incorporated as it is in the provisions of the *Aged Care Act 1997*, the Charter spells out the rights that this legislation is seeking to preserve by more effective mechanisms for their enforcement than its precursor legislation. This later legislation is much more focused on principles. These principles include Accountability Principles, Quality of Care Principles, and User Rights Principles, to name but a few. They stipulate the standards required for the health, safety, personal care, environment and lifestyle of older people in residential, community and flexible care. The list of principles can be accessed on the website of the Commonwealth Department of Health and Aged Care (http://www.ageing.health.gov.au, select Legislation). The Charter is now incorporated in the *Aged Care Act 1997* through the User Rights Principles. The enhanced capacity of this legislation for enforcement suggests that it will be an effective means of assuring the rights of the older person.

This legislation created considerable consternation among the population generally, and among the elderly in particular, primarily because of its funding provisions for nursing-home care. The prime cause of concern was the introduction of accommodation bonds, but in the face of massive protestation by the community generally, and in particular by those affected, the legislation was amended to alter the funding arrangements. However, in this chapter, the significant issues relate not to funding but to the ways in which the *Aged Care Act 1997* approaches the rights of residents of nursing homes. This it does in a number of ways.

First, the Act details the responsibilities of 'approved providers' with respect to the quality of care provided and the rights of the recipients of that care. It does this by providing for 'quality-of-care principles' and 'user-rights principles'. In each case it is the Commonwealth Minister for Aged Care who can determine the actual nature of these principles.

The approved provider must then comply by providing the care and services specified in the quality-of-care principles. These stipulate standards that deal with the health, personal care and lifestyle of recipients of care. They also address issues of safety, environment and the management of nursing homes and hostels. Most importantly, approved providers are accountable for the care and services they provide, and failure to comply with the responsibilities may result in sanctions.

The 'user-rights principles' are intended to address the responsibilities of service providers with respect to such matters as fees, security of tenure, extra service agreements and complaints mechanisms.

LEGAL RIGHTS OF OLDER PEOPLE AND HEALTH CARE

Given that the rights of an older adult person are not different from the rights of younger adults, it is important in a discussion of the legal context of aged-care nursing to identify those rights that relate specifically to health care, and to examine how they may influence nursing practice in the care of the elderly. This is particularly appropriate at this time because of the emergence of codes or charters of health-care rights in some States and Territories. The rights contained in these codes or charters will apply to aged persons just as they would to any other adult. They are of more general application than the *Charter of Residents' Rights and Responsibilities*, but they are only operative within the specific State or Territory. Commonwealth legislation, on the other hand, applies throughout Australia. Remember too that the emphasis of the Commonwealth's *Charter of Residents' Rights and Responsibilities* is deliberately on residential rights—although it certainly contains some health-care rights too.

For nurses, the significant aspects of any health-related right are the nature of the right, the ways in which nursing care can be delivered that maximises compliance with the right, and the consequences of any breach of the right. Here, each of these aspects will be addressed with respect to those health-care rights not addressed in the analysis of the *Charter of Residents' Rights and Responsibilities*.

The first of these health rights is the right to consent. A legally competent person has the right to consent or refuse to consent to medical treatment. No health-care professional should administer treatment without a valid consent. An exception is the provision of emergency care. In some States there is legislative provision for the refusal of medical treatment. In Victoria, any adult of sound mind may refuse treatment under the *Medical Treatment Act 1988*. In South Australia, the *Consent to Medical Treatment and Palliative Care Act 1995* relates only to the terminally ill.

Note that this discussion has so far contemplated only those who are legally competent. However, in aged care, it is a common situation that the client is not competent. They may have dementia, or they may be legally incompetent for some other reason. Whatever the cause, the result is that the individual is unable to give a valid consent for any required treatment.

Until relatively recently, in the absence of a legally appointed guardian, there was no one who could give consent for such persons. However, all the States and Territories have now made legislative provision for such incompetent persons. In New South Wales, the relevant legislation is the *Guardianship Act 1987*. In South Australia, the relevant legislation is the *Guardianship and Administration Act 1993* and, in Tasmania, it is the *Guardianship and Administration Act 1995*. In Western Australia it is the *Guardianship and Administration Act 1990* and in Queensland, it is the *Guardianship and Administration Act 2000*. In the ACT it is the *Guardianship and Management of Property Act 1991* and in the Northern Territory, it is the *Adult Guardianship Act 1988*. This legislation is very important in aged-care nursing because of the prevalence of legal incompetency among the elderly. Nurses need to be aware of the specific provisions in their State. This is important in residential aged care but, because of the provisions relating to medical treatment, it is just as important in a hospital or any other medical setting.

Insofar as health care is concerned, a person has a right to confidentiality. This is not diminished merely by virtue of one's age. There are several bases to this right. There is, of course, the ethical obligation—but in this chapter the emphasis is on legal rights. There is a common law basis in contract. More importantly, however, every State has legislation that recognises this right—and provides penalties for its breach. It is also specifically recognised by both the *Code of Ethics for Nurses in Australia* (ANC 2002) and the *Code of Professional Conduct for Nurses in Australia* (ANC 2003). It is important to recognise that the right to confidentiality is not an absolute right. Thus, it is acceptable to communicate information about a patient's case to other health professionals where it is necessary to do so for the treatment of that person. There are a number of other exceptions—such as public interest—but these will generally be construed narrowly. With respect to aged-care services specifically, the *Aged Care Act 1997* obliges approved providers of aged-care services to respect the confidentiality of recipients of care of that service. Privacy legislation at the Commonwealth and State levels has now added to this right by making provision for the protection of personal information. The requirements are most extensive in Victoria, where the *Information Privacy Act 2000* has come into effect.

THE PRESERVATION OF RIGHTS IN PRACTICE

From this brief account of the rights of aged persons—and, in particular, the rights of aged persons with respect to health care—two things should be abundantly clear. The first is that aged persons have at least the same rights as any other legally competent adult. The second is that the legal basis of these rights is complex and diverse—and constantly developing through both legislation and case law.

The most salient advice offered here for nurses is this: although the discussion of rights has largely revolved around the *Charter of Residents' Rights and Responsibilities* (with its now more limited application), there is merit in using that Charter as a framework for nursing practice in general. This is because it is the broadest statutory articulation of specific rights of aged persons in Australian law. Thus, if a nurse conducts his or her practice within this framework, and in compliance with the various competency standards and codes that regulate the practice of nursing in their jurisdiction, they are likely to satisfy all prevailing standards with respect to the care of the elderly. Of course, it is also necessary to take account of those additional health-care rights identified in this chapter but not contained within the Charter. Close attention to both aspects should result in practice that respects all of the rights of the elderly person.

A number of strategies have been adopted by nurses as individuals, and by organisations, to protect the rights of the recipients of aged care. These includes the establishment of positions such as resident advocates and quality officers in residential facilities. Other organisational strategies have involved the education of nursing staff on the rights of residents and of patients.

ETHICAL DILEMMAS IN PRACTICE

Bioethics has evolved as an approach to health care. Johnstone (1999) discusses the term 'bioethics' and its origins and concludes that it has been medicocentric in its evolution (p 44). Ethical practice in nursing is described in the *Code of Professional Conduct for Nurses in Australia* (ANCI 2003), which has been developed by the profession itself to guide practice.

End-of-life decision-making is looming as the major ethical issue in aged care (Moody 1992). Traditionally, aged-care facilities did not have recourse to ethics committees for advice, nor did they have the use of the current technology to change care direction (Kane & Caplan 1990). Since the advent of life-sustaining technology such as percutaneous endoscopic gastrostomy (PEG) tube insertion, the problem of post-stroke dysphagia has largely been relieved. Nutrition delivered in this way can sustain life for long periods. However, when this technique is used for a person who has other disease processes, such as dementia or neurological disorders, the issue becomes one of quality of life rather than length of life. Australian society has generally not been educated sufficiently to consider end-of-life decision-making by way of enduring Medical Power of Attorney or Advanced Care Directives before the adverse event occurs. Such decision-making relieves the moral/ethical debate about end-of-life decisions and enables a legal approach to be adopted.

Often the staff of an aged-care facility are not able to contact the right relative in time to prevent hospitalisation and feeding tube insertion. Consider the case of BWV (2003) VCAT 121. A woman's husband requested the Guardianship board to appoint him as her legal guardian so he could make decisions about her continued PEG tube feeding. The case was contested by the Right to Life movement, who considered that the removal of the tube would be in breach of the law under the *Medical Treatment Act 1988*. The Tribunal found that artificial feeding in this case was palliative care and appointed the husband as guardian.

The outcome of this case was determined by legal means but the issues of concern to nurses were ethical in nature. To continue to care for a resident/patient who has a feeding tube in situ but not deliver hydration or food raises the issue of the code of conduct of professional nursing. Clearly the nurse 'must respect the dignity, culture, values and beliefs of an individual and any significant other person' (ANCI 2003, p 2). The ethical dilemma involved in, on the one hand, protecting the interests of the family and of the resident by not prolonging suffering, while on the other, withdrawing life support of feeding, is one that many aged-care nurses face. As the population ages in Australia these issues will need to be discussed openly and processes put in place to reconcile the ethical debates that will continue to surround end-of-life decisions. Legal developments will afford guidance for what can be done legally. The challenge will be for nurses to achieve ethically comfortable outcomes.

CONCLUSION

This account of the legal framework of aged care—and thus of the legal context in which the nursing care of older persons occurs—has focused almost exclusively on the legal rights of those persons, and the consequences of breaches of those rights. This reflects current approaches and developments in Australia's law, and in the attitudes of Australian society towards older persons and their care.

The many aspects that have not been discussed here include:

- the background to the developments in aged-care law;
- the obligations of nursing-home residents who are subject to the *Charter of Residents' Rights and Responsibilities*;
- the emerging role of trade-practices legislation as a mechanism for the enforcement of rights against providers of both health and accommodation services;
- the increasing use of practice guidelines; and
- the role of measures of quality of care.

Nor has there been any extensive consideration of how the recent Commonwealth legislation on aged care is working. However, there are differing views on its efficacy. This is shown by the public discomfort around the closure of nursing homes for failing to achieve satisfactory standards. Although the focus here is on the rights of the recipients of aged care, the objective is to enable nurses to practise in a way that respects their clients' rights—but also protects them legally and professionally. To respect clients' rights, nurses need to know what those rights are.

Remember, too, that the federal nature of the Australian system of government results in nine legal jurisdictions. Thus every nurse needs to be familiar with the legal provisions relating to both the rights of residents/patients and the practice of nursing of at least two jurisdictions. They need to be familiar with those of the Commonwealth and with those of the State in which they practise. The emphasis on rights in this discussion reflects a growing trend in Australian society. Increasingly, this emphasis will shape the practice of nursing in all its forms.

VIGNETTE

Managing unprepared families

Phillip Abbott

Mr X was admitted to a residential care unit from a busy teaching hospital for end-of-life palliative care management. He was not able to swallow and was clearly dying. The staff considered he should have gone to a hospice or palliative care unit. His wife realised he was close to death but could not contemplate that this was the end and that he could not feed without respiratory consequences. Both partners were of Jewish background, though non-practising. The staff began giving Mr X fluid through a subcutaneous infusion, as he was too ill for a PEG procedure and IV fluids were not appropriate. Mrs X was satisfied that something was being done for her husband, and although distressed thought the fluid replacement was appropriate.

Morphine (SC) and clonazepam (SL) were used for comfort and sedation and the resident comfortably progressed to terminal stage. As Mr X slowly went into systems failure, fluid began to build up in the tissues and was not being absorbed. The abdominal tissues were overloaded, and there were other signs of oedema in the lowest extremities, found as nursing staff changed his position regularly, in addition to early pulmonary signs of a wet chest, and the Nurse Unit Manager (NUM) decided to withdraw the subcutaneous line.

Despite education, support and counselling throughout this period, Mrs X was distraught at the thought of the cessation of treatment and believed it was not in her husband's best interests. Her grief obstructed good practice, as she demanded that the line be replaced, claiming that staff were 'killing' her husband. The NUM had spent considerable time with her prior to making his decision and eventually had to act on behalf of the resident and good nursing practice. The decision caused a rift in the relationship between the care staff and Mrs X and much unhappiness for the NUM and staff. Mr X died 24 hours later and the relationship between Mrs X and the NUM ended on a far less congenial note than either would have liked, with blame being levelled about the final doses of analgesia and sedation given.

In this case cultural influences and lack of appropriate preparation from the acute hospital for the family in transferring Mr X to residential care when he clearly required hospice care affected the outcome. It was not possible to provide the counselling time and resources normally available in residential care for prolonged family education and case management when Mr X was admitted in a moribund state and decisions had to be made quickly.

References

Australian Nursing Council (ANC) Inc 2002, *Code of Ethics for Nurses in Australia* Australian Nursing Council Inc: Canberra.

Australian Nursing Council (ANC) Inc 2003, *Code of Professional Conduct for Nurses in Australia*, Australian Nursing Council Inc: Canberra.

Department of Health, Housing and Community Services (nd), *Your Guide to Residents' Rights and Responsibilities*, DHHCS: Canberra.

Health Department of New South Wales 1993, *Dying with Dignity: Interim Guidelines on Management*, Health Department of New South Wales: Sydney.

Johnstone M-J 1999, *Bioethics: A Nursing Perspective*, 3rd edn, Harcourt Sanders: Sydney.

Kane RA & Caplan AL 1990, *Everyday Ethics: Resolving Dilemmas in Nursing Home Life*, Springer: New York.

Leonard VW 1989, A Heideggerian phenomenologic perspective on the concept of the person, *Advanced Nursing Science*, 11(4), pp 40–55.

Moody HR 1992, *Ethics in an Ageing Society*, Johns Hopkins University Press: Baltimore.

Table of legislation

Adult Guardianship Act 1988 (NT)
Aged or Disabled Persons Care Act 1954 (Cth)
Aged Care Act 1997 (Cth)
Consent to Medical Treatment and Palliative Care Act 1995 (SA)
Guardianship Act 1987 (NSW)
Guardianship and Administration Act 2000 (Qld)
Guardianship and Administration Act 1993 (SA)
Guardianship and Administration Act 1995 (Tas)
Guardianship and Administration Act 1990 (WA)
Guardianship and Management of Property Act 1991 (ACT)
Medical Treatment Act 1998 (Vic)

Cases

Rogers v Whitaker (1992) Australian Torts Reports 81-189 CCH Australia Limited: Sydney
Victorian Civil and Administrative Tribunal BWV 2003 VCAT 121 (28 Feb 2003)

CHAPTER 6

Care of people from Indigenous and culturally diverse backgrounds

IRENE STEIN

INTRODUCTION

Australia is rich in cultural diversity. With this diversity come issues related to health-care delivery for older people from Indigenous and Culturally and Linguistically Diverse (CALD) backgrounds. An Indigenous Australian is a person 'who is of Aboriginal descent, who identifies as being Aboriginal and who is recognised by his or her community as being an Aboriginal person' (Bourke 1998, p 175). This definition includes Indigenous people from the Torres Strait Islands. A person who is from a CALD background is born in a country other than Australia.

While there are significant differences between the care needs of older people from Indigenous and CALD backgrounds, there are also similarities, including:

- the need for appropriate communication support;
- the need for culturally sensitive assessment;
- the need for culturally appropriate care options;
- the need for care delivery by staff who are cognisant of ethno-cultural trends;
- the need for provision for culturally specific dietary requirements, recreation activities and spiritual expression; and
- the need for access to culturally appropriate advocacy services.

These care needs reflect and are embedded in an individual's culture. Older people from Indigenous and CALD backgrounds are not homogenous groups. There are, for example, significant cultural and linguistic differences between groups in terms of language and beliefs in the Indigenous population of Australia and among those from a CALD background.

Leninger (1991, p 47) asserts that culture is 'the learned, shared and transmitted values, beliefs, norms and lifeways of a particular group that guides their thinking, decisions and actions in patterned ways'. From this Leninger developed the concept of transcultural care, based on the premise that culturally sensitive and appropriate care should be provided for people from all cultures. Leninger defined *cultural care* as 'the subjectively and objectively learned and transmitted values, beliefs, and patterned lifeways that assist individuals or groups to maintain their well-being, health, improve their human condition and lifeway, or to deal with illness, handicap or death' (p 47). Inherent in this principle is the way individuals view their own ethnocentricity. The challenge this presents for those who work amongst Indigenous and culturally diverse older populations is to respect and enhance the care experience.

This creates tensions related to the care experience (Fig 6.1). These tensions affect the manner in which care is planned and delivered. The care planning cycle (Fig 6.2) that evolves from the recognition that these tensions exist is predicated on a non-judgemental approach to the person. From this a culturally sensitive and inclusive assessment can be carried out. The data collected from this process facilitates the development of a situationally relevant plan for care that is cognisant of ethno-cultural differences and needs. Congruent care application and outcomes are then identified. In this context relevant evaluation and further communication are enabled.

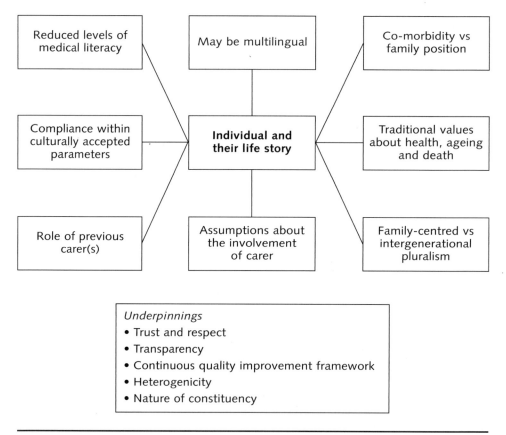

Fig 6.1: Tensions within a care paradigm for Indigenous and CALD older people

This chapter provides a demographic background to Indigenous and CALD older people in Australia, and identifies the major health concerns related to these people. It also provides examples of the health-care services available to meet their specific needs.

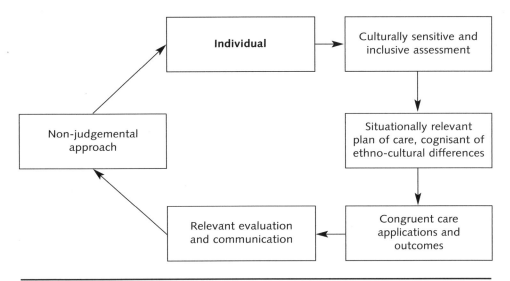

Fig 6.2: Care delivery planning cycle for Indigenous and CALD older people

CARE OF OLDER INDIGENOUS AUSTRALIANS

Profile

It is estimated that approximately 500,000 people in Australia identify as being Indigenous. Of this number, 18% are aged between 35 and 54 years. Only 7% are aged over 55 years. The Australian benchmark of 65 years as 'young old' is an inappropriate one in this cultural context. In response, the recognised age of 'young-old' for Indigenous people has been revised downward to 55 years. This allows for social security benefits normally available to non–Indigenous people aged over 65 years to be available to Indigenous people at age 55 years (Australian Indigenous Health*Info*Net 2003; Centrelink).

It is well documented that Indigenous people experience significant health disadvantage. This is characterised by:

- a reduced life expectancy by an average 20 years regardless of gender (ABS/AIHW 1999);
- higher rates of acute hospital admission; and
- higher levels of chronic disease.

Reduced life expectancy

The reduced life expectancy of Indigenous people is reflected in the fact that the death rate in the Indigenous population exceeded that in all groups across the Australian population. The 2002 Australian Census data identified that more than half of the deaths of Indigenous people occurred in those aged less than 50 years (www.healthinfonet.ecu.edu.au). Older Indigenous people are predominantly female and are from a range of intra-cultural backgrounds (ABS/AIHW 1991; Eckermann et al 1992).

Higher rates of acute hospital admission

Though under-reported, the age-standardised rate of acute hospitalisation amongst Indigenous people is estimated to be twice that of the Australian population as a whole. The most common causes of acute admissions amongst older Indigenous people are:

- cardiovascular incidents;
- renal disease or renal dialysis;
- cancer therapy;
- diabetes maintenance; and
- injury

(Cunningham & Beneforte 2000).

Higher levels of chronic disease

Indigenous people have higher levels of chronic disease. High levels of Types 1 and 2 diabetes mellitus and asthma are prevalent. Low levels of compliance with treatment modalities result in acute complications related to chronicity (ABS/AIHW 1999).

Underpinning these health disadvantages is poverty related to social situation, economic circumstances and learning. Indications of poverty are:

- poor or inadequate housing relative to the health needs of many Indigenous communities. Older Indigenous people live in overcrowded housing environments that have no hot running water, inadequate heating or cooling systems, no telephone services connected and no on-site health clinics (Australian Indigenous Health*Info*Net 2003; Tharawal Aboriginal Corporation 1994).
- high levels of unemployment and a dependence on social security payments for health maintenance. Conflicting family priorities can result in the use of these payments for items other than health-care needs (Eckermann et al 1992; Australian Indigenous Health*Info*Net 2003; Tharawal Aboriginal Corporation 1994).
- low education levels, which can result in a poor or limited understanding of issues such as compliance with treatment regimens, the progress patterns of a disease and patient education (Australian Indigenous Health*Info*Net 2003; Tharawal Aboriginal Corporation 1994)
- poor nutrition due to location and a restricted income limiting food choices. High prices for food in many rural and remote communities militates against a diet that would assist in some disease treatments such as cardiac disease and diabetes mellitus (Cunningham & Mackerras 1998).
- high levels of substance abuse. Older Indigenous people are twice as likely to smoke tobacco as the Australian population as a whole, and those who drink alcohol are more likely to consume unsafe levels (Brady 1998; Clelland 1996; Paterson et al 1999).

These conditions of poverty result in an over-representation amongst older Indigenous people of:

- cardiovascular disease;
- respiratory disease;
- cancer;
- Type 1 and Type 2 diabetes mellitus;
- renal failure; and
- trauma

(ABS/AIHW 1999; Cunningham & Beneforte 2000).

Implications for care delivery

The demographic profile of older Indigenous people has significant implications for care delivery. The prevailing patterns of morbidity and co-morbidity indicate a need for age-specific services at least twenty years earlier than for the Australian population as a whole. There are few culturally specific aged-care services for older Indigenous people. Initiatives directed towards this are through a mix of mainstream and culturally specific services (Woenne-Green 1995). These services include:

- housing for older Indigenous people;
- multipurpose services;
- Community Aged Care Packages (CACPs);
- Home and Community Care (HACC) services;
- Aboriginal Medical Service;
- Aboriginal health workers; and
- traditional healing practices.

Each of these services is discussed below.

Housing for older Indigenous people

Purpose-built housing for older Indigenous people has been developed across Australia. The various types of housing available include:

- independent living units;
- hostels offering low residential aged care;
- nursing homes offering high residential aged care; and
- bush camps for traditional elders

(Australian Indigenous Health*Info*Net 2003).

These care programs are staffed by Indigenous people and are managed by an elected community committee.

Multipurpose services

Multipurpose services are a joint Commonwealth and State/Territory health-care initiative in rural and remote areas of Australia. They aim to provide flexible and accessible health care to people living in those areas. In areas of high Indigenous population concentration, there is close liaison with the local Indigenous community. These services can be designed to meet specific community needs (Australian Department of Health and Ageing 2003).

Community aged-care packages

These are low-care packages for those Indigenous people able to remain at home. Packages for community aged care for Indigenous people are managed and funded by Home and Community Services (www.lm.net.au/~elders/packages/htm).

Home and Community Care services

Home and Community Care (HACC) services aim to support older Indigenous people in their own home and community. Strategies that improve independent activity and militate against premature admission to residential aged care are central to this aim. HACC services provide a flexible care model that facilitates:

- services such as home help, meal provision, home modification and transport;
- assessment processes;
- care coordination;
- carer support;
- community respite care; and
- consumer education and advocacy.

The application of these services in communities has been developed through a series of community consultations and advice (Tripp 1997).

The Aboriginal Medical Service

The Aboriginal Medical Service (AMS) is an Indigenous community-controlled organisation servicing the health needs of the local Indigenous community. Governed by an elected Board of Directors, the AMS provides a range of health-care services including:

- diabetes clinics;
- general practitioner services;
- dental clinics;
- immunisation clinics;
- transportation for health-related needs;
- pharmacy services; and
- podiatry

(Eckermann et al 1992; Tharawal Aboriginal Corporation 1994).

Aboriginal health workers

Aboriginal health workers (AHWs) provide in-hospital and home services to older Indigenous people. The role of the AHW includes:

- providing patient education concerning treatment modalities and compliance;
- providing medication management and ensuring compliance;
- providing dietary advice and meals; and
- providing transportation to health-related appointments and activities.

Aboriginal health workers understand the cultural milieu of older Indigenous people and are often the primary health-care professionals working in rural and remote communities of Australia (Tharawal Aboriginal Corporation 1994; Nganampa Health Council 2002; www.nfwrks.sa.gov.au/ab.health).

Traditional healing

There is a reliance on traditional healing methods within Indigenous communities. Traditional healers working in communities promote the use of naturally occurring substances and the power of cultural tradition to heal the ill person (Eckermann et al 1992; Pauling et al 1996).

While there are Indigenous health professionals caring for older Indigenous people, care is also provided by non-Indigenous people. Cultural education is required for these health professionals in areas such as:

- Indigenous history;
- cultural attitudes and beliefs concerning illness and death; and
- kinship patterns and obligations.

The education provides an initial framework for the practitioner in meeting the cultural needs and health needs of older Aboriginal and Torres Strait Islander populations (Cunningham & Wollin 1997; Eckermann 1992; Tsey et al 1999).

In rural and remote areas of Australia, mobile medical, renal dialysis and dental clinics have been established to service the needs of these areas. These clinics reach areas which older Indigenous people are reluctant to leave, for family and financial reasons. Based on a primary health care model, these clinics have the capacity for general practice, minor surgery and general dental services.

CARE OF CULTURALLY AND LINGUISTICALLY DIVERSE OLDER PEOPLE

Profile

It is estimated that approximately 25% of the Australian population aged over 65 years were born in other countries (Pillars 2001). The largest migrant groups are from the United Kingdom, Ireland, the Baltic States, Hungry, Italy, Greece and Asia. Of these, 82% came from English-speaking countries (Rowland 1999). Like the Indigenous aged, this population group is not homogenous. Predominantly resident in metropolitan areas, this rich cultural mix tends to age-in-place close to family members. Characteristically these people:

- have lower standardised mortality rates;
- are less likely to relocate to residential aged care; and
- have higher self-reported disability levels.

Seventy-five per cent of older CALD people rely on the means-tested aged pension for their income (AIHW 2002; Department of Health, Housing and Community Services 1993; Gibson et al 2001; Paterson 1999; www.centrelink.gov.au).

The health profile of CALD older people

Compared with the general aged population of Australia, CALD older people characteristically:

- have a lower standardised death rate;
- use less tobacco products and consume less alcohol;
- experience lower rates of respiratory disease, including asthma;
- experience higher rates of diabetes, circulatory disease, arthritis, kidney disease and some cancers; and
- have a higher usage of community-based HACC services

(AIHW 2002; Curtis 2002; Department of Health, Housing and Community Services 1993).

The health-care needs of CALD older people in Australia are met through a mixture of mainstream and culturally specific services. There is little national or State strategic planning for services to address the cultural sensitivities involved in the delivery of aged care (Barnett 1999). This inevitably leads to a mismatch between services and needs. The key issues related to this mismatch are:

- communication in an environment where there is scant language service availability;
- quality of care where diagnostic accuracy is compromised;
- compliance with treatment regimens; and
- gender, where women observe traditional cultural and religious practices, and are less likely to be English speaking

(Barnett 1999; Curtis 2002; Rowland 1999).

Implications for care delivery

To address these issues, a holistic model of culturally appropriate care delivery that can be used in a variety of care settings is required (Fig 6.3). Underpinning this model is the centrality of the CALD older person, effective communication, evidence-based care delivery and the recognition of cultural and spiritual dimensions. These factors are discussed below.

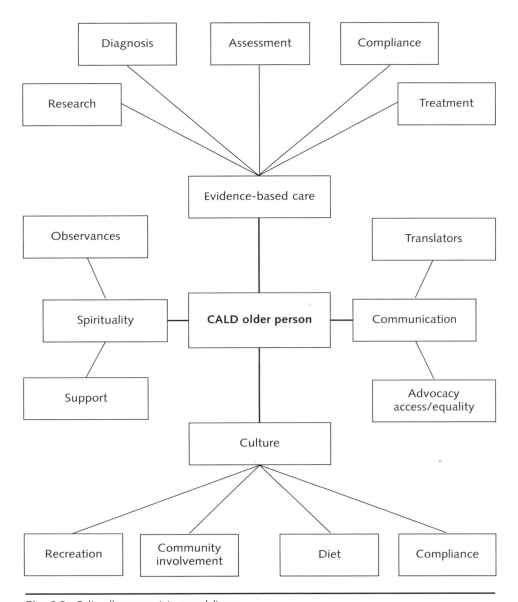

Fig 6.3: Culturally appropriate care delivery

Effective communication

While there has been an increase in the numbers of aged-care workers from CALD backgrounds and education programs for non-CALD aged-care workers (Barnett 1999), there remains a shortage of professional and accredited interpreters in the communication cycle. Competent translators interpret not only the spoken word, but the cultural context of the message being conveyed. Family and bilingual staff can be substituted, but it must be remembered that these people are not accredited translators.

Evidence-based care delivery

An evidence-based care-delivery cycle is the outcome of clinical and cultural research. It involves:

- thorough assessment;
- accurate diagnostics;
- appropriate clinical interventions;
- ongoing compliance with clinical interventions; and
- evaluation of the care-delivery cycle

(Daly et al 2000; Pillars 2001).

Cultural dimensions

Cultural isolation is a potential problem for CALD older people. Feelings of isolation can occur in all care-delivery settings. Strategies to minimise isolation include:

- relocation to residential aged care (RAC) that is ethno-specific;
- relocation to a RAC facility that operates cluster accommodation;
- attention to dietary preferences and requirements;
- CALD-specific community involvement in a program or facility;
- recreational activities that reflect the CALD background of participants; and
- participation in the Community Visitors Scheme

(Curtis 2002; Pillars 2001; Ray 2001).

Spiritual dimensions

Support for spiritual expression is integral to the well-being of CALD older people. It includes:

- attention to denominational dietary requirements;
- provision of multi-faith worship areas; and
- programming of care and activities around designated prayer and fasting times

(Carers Victoria 2003; Curtis 2002).

Some excellent examples of programs delivering culturally sensitive care to CALD older people are:

- ethno-specific low-care and high-care residential aged-care facilities;
- clustering in low- and high-care residential aged-care facilities;
- in-home meal provision; and
- community aged-care packages.

Ethno-specific low- and high-care residential aged-care facilities operate with bilingual staff and provide culturally specific meals, recreational programs and spiritual activities. Examples of these are the Saint Basil's Greek Homes operating nationally, and the Seaton Nursing Home in Port Adelaide, South Australia, which caters for older Ukrainian and Croatian people (www.members.iinet.au/~stbasils/basilsa.htm; Sniatynskj 1999).

Clustering in low-care and high-care residential aged-care facilitates cultural support for residents of the same cultural background. The identification of a discrete subgroup within the residential aged-care facility population means that food preferences, recreational and spiritual considerations can be recognised and accommodated.

The provision of culturally appropriate in-home meal services and Community Aged Care Packages reduces isolation and serves to maintain the individual in their home, avoiding premature admission to residential aged care.

CONCLUSION

As the Indigenous and CALD older populations grow in Australia, the need for more appropriate services will also increase, and this will provide many challenges to those who deliver care. The older Indigenous population will require more services at a community level which focus on their health needs, such as mobile renal dialysis and ophthalmology clinics, and education for compliance in areas such as Type 2 diabetes mellitus and cardiovascular disease. This service delivery will be through both Indigenous-specific health activities and mainstream care modalities.

The profile of CALD older people will alter—the predominance of older European people will be replaced by those from an Asian cultural background. A significant challenge associated with this change will be the provision of interventions that address the changing expectations and role of the extended family. Clustering in residential aged care and the provision of culturally appropriate community care will reduce isolation.

The challenges that providing care for older Indigenous and CALD older people present require sensitivity and an appreciation of the particular needs of each group.

VIGNETTE

Aged care fusion

Regina Barry

Mrs X was a 94-year-old Philippino woman who had nine children. All the family lived in Australia. Mrs X spoke very little English. She had been able to manage her affairs by relying on her family. She had lived with one of her daughters since her arrival from the Philippines.

Mrs X gradually became frail and exhibited dementia-type behaviours. At 92 years of age she was diagnosed with cancer of the breast. Treatment for this involved radiotherapy. Surgery was declined. At this stage support was required by her daughter. Initially the other siblings were supportive, but as Mrs X's condition deteriorated, the support of the other family members decreased, leaving the burden of care with the daughter she lived with.

An ACAT assessment was organised and as a result a Community Aged Care Package was implemented. As Mrs X's condition continued to deteriorate, her mobility decreased. She also suffered a series of transient ischaemic attacks, resulting in numerous falls and multiple soft-tissue damage. The family blamed their sister for neglecting their mother but still did not increase their level of involvement with her care. Family tension increased as they believed their sister was acting outside the Philippino tradition of caring for elders. The care package coordinator became aware of the carer's situation and arranged an ACAT reassessment. Admission to high-care residential aged care was recommended.

The daughter providing the care for her mother was relieved, but the rest of the family condemned her decision. No other family member was prepared to accept responsibility for care.

Mrs X was admitted to a high-care residential aged-care facility. The dysfunctional behaviours of the family became obvious to the facility staff, who had to intervene in disputes between family members. The family were reluctant to discuss issues with the staff, stating only that this was not the Philippino way of doing things.

The daughter who had been the primary carer explained that the family felt guilty about not being able to provide the care their mother needed.

Mrs X's condition deteriorated further. The family tension also increased. The staff of the facility found it harder to manage the family conflict and asked them to stagger their visiting times to minimise the general disruption caused to the other residents and their families, who had begun to complain about the situation. The family indicated that the facility had open visiting times and that they would come when they wanted to.

The staff then sought mediation through the facility's chaplain. The chaplain worked sensitively to identify the issues associated with the family's guilt and anger. Over a period of several weeks it became apparent that the issues required professional intervention. This was arranged and the outcomes were positive.

The family revoked their initial opposition to palliation for Mrs X and her death was pain-free, with her family present. Some weeks after her death, the family visited the facility. It was a good opportunity for the staff to talk to them about their experiences with their mother. In summary, they had felt unable to cope with the fact that their mother was dying and that they could not provide the care they believed she required. They admitted that previous family conflict had always been resolved by their mother and that they lacked the skills needed to manage their own inter-family conflict. Finally, they thanked the staff.

The staff asked them what the Philippino way of caring for the aged involved. Reluctantly the family described a changing culture, where in all probability their mother would have required care in her last years.

References

Australian Bureau of Statistics and Australian Institute of Health and Welfare (ABS/AIHW) 1999, *The Health and Welfare of Australian Aboriginal and Torres Strait Islander Peoples 1999*, ABS Cat. No. 4704.0, AIHW Cat. No. IHW 3, Canberra.

Australian Department of Health and Ageing 2003, Rural health. Online: www.ruralhealth.gov.au, last updated 30 October 2003.

Australian Indigenous Health*Info*Net 2003. Online: www.healthinfonet.ecu.edu.au

Australian Institute of Health and Welfare (AIHW) 2002, *Older Australians at a Glance*, 3rd edn, AIHW: Canberra.

Barnett K 1999, *Training as a Strategy for Meeting the Challenge of Cultural Diversity*, paper delivered to Diversity and Ageing Conference, Adelaide.

Bourke C 1998, Contemporary Australian Aboriginal identity. In: Day D (ed), *Australian Identities*, Australian Scholarly Publications: Melbourne.

Brady M 1998, *The Grog Book*, Commonwealth Department of Health and Family Services, Canberra.

Carers Victoria 2003, *Outside Looking in – Building Carer Friendly Practices*, Melbourne.

Centrelink, Department of Family and Community Services. Online: www.centrelink.gov.au

Clelland M 1996, *Keeping Company*, Centre for Indigenous Development Education and Research, University of Wollongong: Wollongong.

Cunningham J & Beneforte M 2000, *Hospital Statistics: Aboriginal and Torres Strait Islander Australians, 1997–1998*, Australian Bureau of Statistics Occasional Paper No. 4711-0, Canberra.

Cunningham J & Mackerras D 1998, *Overweight and Obesity, Indigenous Australians*, Australian Bureau of Statistics Occasional Paper No. 4702-0, Canberra.

Cunningham J & Wollin J 1998, The importance of clinical experience in Aboriginal communities, *Contemporary Nurse*, 7(3), pp 152–255.

Curtis K 2002, Ageing by diversity: multicultural Australia, *National Healthcare Journal*, February, pp 8–12.

Daly J, Elliott D & Chang E 2000. Research in nursing: concepts and processes. In: Daly J, Speedy S & Jackson D, *Contexts of Nursing*, pp 89–106, MacLellan & Petty: Sydney.

Department of Health, Housing and Community Services 1993, *Removing Cultural and Language Barriers To Health*, National Health Strategy Issues Paper No 6, Canberra.

Eckermann A, Dowd T, Martin M, Nixon L, Gray R & Chong E 1992, *Binan Goonj Bridging Cultures in Aboriginal Health*, University of New England: Armidale.

Gibson D, Bowler P, Benham C & Mason F 2001, *Projections of Older Immigrants, People from Culturally and Linguistically Diverse Backgrounds, 1996–2026*, Australia, Canberra, Australian Institute of Health and Welfare.

Leninger M 1991, *Culture Care Diversity and Universality: A Theory of Nursing*, National League for Nursing: New York.

Nganampa Health Council 2002, Nganampa health. Online: www.nganampahealth.com.au

Paterson K 1999, Keynote address to Diversity And Ageing—Resources For The Future Conference, Adelaide.

Paterson KM, Holman CDJ, English D, Hulse GF & Unwin E 1999, First-time hospital admissions with illicit drug problems in indigenous and non-indigenous Western Australians: an application of record linkage in public health surveillance, *Australian and New Zealand Journal of Public Health*, 23(5), pp 460–3.

Pauling C, Salisbury C & Bellear L 1996, *The Bugalwena Service: Our Story of a Partnership in Health*, Northern Rivers Area Health Service: Murwillumbah.

Pillars M 2001, Delivering culturally appropriate care within the context of continuous improvement, *Geriaction*, 19(2), pp 7–10.

Ray M 2001, Transcultural assessment. In: Koch S & Garratt S, *Assessing Older People: A Practical Guide for Health Professionals*, pp 35–47, MacLennan & Petty: Sydney.

Rowland DT 1999, The ethnic aged population and the likelihood of special needs, *Australasian Journal on Ageing*, 18(3), pp 50–4.

Sniatynskj J 1999, *Aged Care: A Ukrainian Perspective*, paper delivered at Diversity and Ageing Conference, Adelaide.

Tharawal Aboriginal Corporation 1994, *Aboriginal Health in South West Sydney*, Australian Institute of Aboriginal and Torres Strait Islander Studies and Research School of Social Sciences, The Australian National University: Canberra.

Tripp M 1997, Aboriginal and Torres Strait Islander aged care, *Aboriginal and Islander Health Worker Journal*, 21(5), pp 11–14.

Tsey K, Morrish S, Lucas A & Boffer J 1999, Training in aged care advocacy for primary health care workers in central Australia: An Evaluation, *Australasian Journal on Ageing*, 17(4), pp 167–71.

Woenne-Green S 1995, *'They might have to drag me like a bullock'*, Ngaanyatjarra Pitjantjatjara Yankunytjatjara Women's Council, Aboriginal Corporation: Alice Springs.

Websites

www.centrelink.gov.au

www.healthinfonet.ecu.edu.au

www.lm.net.au/~elders/package

www.members,iinet.au/~stbasils

ww.nfwrks.sc.gov.au/ab.health

www.nganampahealth.com.au

www.ruralhealth.gov.au

CHAPTER 7

Understanding community nursing for older individuals and carers

LIBBY BROOKE AND HAL KENDIG

INTRODUCTION

This chapter provides a social perspective on community nursing care for older people at the beginning of the twenty-first century. The focus is on clients in the context of their communities, thus extending nursing beyond its origins in technical and institutional care. While gerontic nursing is a speciality valued by the community, key challenges remain for nurses funded primarily for technical tasks in caring for older people at home. Advances in community nursing practice are required to meet increasing demands from governments as well as older people themselves.

The cornerstone of aged care has moved from hospitals and nursing homes to home care with its emphasis on older individuals and their daily lives, informal care-givers, and the home context. Older people overwhelmingly prefer to remain at home and most never enter residential care (Kendig & Duckett 2001). Governments support the redirection of care from institutions to the community in order to meet the preferences of older people and reduce public costs. Governments are also demanding more accountability for their money. Community nursing can be crucial in enabling frail older people to stay at home.

The notion of 'community' is often taken for granted in the world of the community nurse. A Queensland study (St John 1998) found that nurses' understandings of community were complex and fluid, involving: connections between people within geographical areas; pragmatic provision of resources; targeting subgroups in the older population; and working with relational networks (p 69). These concepts are significant influences on the sustainability of home care.

This chapter begins with a discussion of the substantial change and diversity in the older population, the orientations of older individuals, and caregiving relationships. The discussion then turns to the implications for practice, and case studies in community nursing. The chapter concludes by considering community nursing in the development of aged-care systems.

OLDER POPULATIONS AND CARE

The Commonwealth Government recognises that population ageing places substantial pressure on government spending (Commonwealth of Australia 2002).

However, two-thirds of the public costs of older people are in the area of income support, with costs being relatively less but also significant for hospitals (15%), medical services (6%), pharmaceuticals (3%), and residential (10%) and community care (3%) (Kendig & Duckett 2001). Health and welfare expenditure on older people as a percentage of GDP rose by a small amount over recent decades to reach 5% in the late 1990s. In 2002 the Commonwealth Budget allocated $5.5 billion to aged care including $674 million to the Home and Community Care Program, $265 million to Community Aged Care Packages, and $321 million for other non-residential areas including respite funding, dementia support, and support for carers (Kendig & Duckett 2001).

Numbers in the 80-years-and-older age group have been increasing relatively rapidly (5% per year) over recent decades. The very old population is expected to grow relatively less rapidly, however, until the babyboom cohort reaches advanced old age, late in the 2020s (Australian Institute of Health and Welfare [AIHW] 2002). The demand for aged care will increase over the next two decades, but it will be some time before the major impact of population ageing manifests in demand for aged care. While currently there are relatively higher concentrations of older people in rural areas and towns, the growth of older people is increasingly in post-war suburbs, where public transport is relatively poor, and in coastal areas where services can be relatively less developed and lag behind population growth (Kendig & Duckett 2001).

The proportion of people in the population likely to need care increases significantly with age. The proportion needing assistance with activities of daily living increases from 32% for those aged 65–74 years to 92% for those aged 85 years and over (Australian Bureau of Statistics [ABS] 1998). Similarly, the Victorian Aged Care Assessment Program Evaluation (July 2000–June 2001) shows that in 1999–2000 only 11% of clients were aged under 70 years, while 37% were aged 85 and over. It is in the advanced age groups where disabling diseases are concentrated. Dementia is the leading cause of non-fatal disease burden (17%), followed by adult hearing loss and stroke (8% respectively), vision disorders, and osteoarthritic and coronary disease (6% respectively) (AIHW 2002).

The vast majority of people live relatively independently and well for most of their later years. According to recent figures from the World Health Organization (WHO), Australian women at age 60 years can expect another 25 years of life, including only 4.5 years with disability, and men at 60 years can expect another 17 years with 4 years of disability (McCallum 2001). A Melbourne population survey of 1000 older people living in the community shows that the vast majority carry out at least some physical activity, and have wide-ranging social activities and hobbies (Kendig et al 1996).

More than 90% of those aged 65 years and over live in the community, in a variety of housing and household arrangements (Commonwealth of Australia 2001; AIHW 2002). The vast majority of disabled older people, even those in their eighties, continue to live in the community rather than in institutions. The major needs areas for older people with substantial disabilities, in order of their extensiveness, are property maintenance, housework, health care, transport, self-care and meals preparation (Bridge et al 2002). Three-quarters of these older people have informal support and half have both informal support and community services. Community care services aim to coordinate many variations of informal and formal support (Kendig & Brooke 1997).

There is increasing evidence that many of the functional limitations of old age can be prevented or postponed (Browning & Kendig 2003). For example, continuing physical activity, social activity and nutrition are important ways to maintain independence and well-being. The National Strategy for an Ageing Australia (Commonwealth of Australia 2001) highlights the need for positive individual and community attitudes to ageing to enable a greater number of older people to remain healthy and independent for as long as possible. This strategy is also consistent with the WHO strategy of maintaining functional capacity over the life course, through lifestyle and preventive interventions (WHO 2002).

The new cohort of baby boomers, now in their mid-fifties, may foreshadow very different orientations towards services (Kendig & Duckett 2001). The baby boomers now entering old age have benefited more from the post-war economic boom and are likely to have greater resources and expectations for their later years. Their lifelong perspectives contrast markedly with the stoicism that characterises older people who led their formative years during the Depression and World War II. The baby boom cohort, who are already influential as caregivers, may transform expectations and practice in aged care.

OLDER INDIVIDUALS

This section highlights critical issues for older people's identities in remaining at home when becoming frail. Quotations from interviews with four nurses, including direct care and case managers, illustrate how their understanding of individuals' perspectives has influenced nursing practice.

Policies are directed largely towards populations but *care* focuses on the preferences, resources and situation of each individual. Australian qualitative studies of older people emphasise independence rather than disabilities and impairments (Walker-Birckhead 1996). Older people have 'health identities' in which they seek continuity of meaningful activities, independence and well-being. Practitioners need to appreciate the health understandings and goals which arise out of each individual's lifelong experiences and personal interpretations.

Older people do not want to change who they are just because they have become frail. Walker-Birckhead (1996) shows how the 'old old' have developed robust constructions of the identities maintained in their life courses. Their survivorship attests to a strong sense of self in the face of changes that can threaten their identity. Even when people have major illnesses and experience chronic pain, their well-being can remain high as long as they can continue their activities and way of life (Kendig et al 2000). Brooke (1995) found that older people who were very frail and receiving community services held varying perspectives on dependence, and that independence developed over a lifetime. When confronted with decreasing physical capacities, in order to receive assistance, older people had to negotiate their care with nurses and informal caregivers.

Negotiations between an older person, caregiver and nurse commonly centre on the older person's sense of independence. A nurse interviewed for this paper expressed concern that nurses in the hospital medical system can predispose clients to depend on them rather than move away from dependency. She commented: 'We are hopeful and careful not to set up a dependency—we can't push clients to be more independent.'

Relationships with health professionals can be threatening for frail older people because they involve unequal power relationships and expose personal vulnerabilities. At the same time, nurses have great potential to enable the elderly to cope positively with age-related changes and to make informed decisions on care options. For people who are at sensitive and difficult points in their lives, nursing care can make a critical difference between supporting and eroding the older person's sense of self and identity.

Staying on in their own homes can be central to older people's sense of identity and control over their lives. Studies into the personal meaning of home indicate that older people's sense of self is symbolised by their homes, particularly their gardens, memorabilia, streetscapes and local neighbourhood. As Davison et al (1993) comment, 'there is a clear relationship between the physical environment they inhabit and their feeling of belonging' (p 63). When older people are on their own 'home turf' their individuality is revealed to service providers more so than in the hospital environment.

While older people may feel comfortable receiving care in their homes, informal carers can perceive the entry of formal carers into the home as intrusive. A UK study comparing and contrasting the role of family carers and nurses in domestic health care also indicated that professionals can threaten informal carers' control over care arrangements.

> Home is the centre of identity for many older people, and care-giving at home endows them with a certain measure of choice and control over the way they run their lives. However, professionals coming into the home can challenge the carer's perception of control in the home environment.
>
> Pickard & Glendinning 2002, p 149

Variation among older people

Nurses need to be responsive to diversity amongst older clients in their practice. Gender is a major social divide in the experience of ageing. Aged care is overwhelmingly directed towards women, who are much more likely than men to live to ages where they are widowed, disabled, on low income and living alone. Among those aged over 75 years and living in private dwellings, nearly half of women but only 22% of men live alone (ABS 2002). In 2011 there will be over twice as many women as men in the population aged 85 years and over (256,000 women to 133,100 men) (AIHW 2002). With the loss of age peers at older ages, 'old old' people can experience themselves as a vestige from a different time and place (Walker-Birckhead 1996).

Men and women can have very different interpretations of their ageing experiences. Older women, for example, can be reluctant to accept home help or delivered meals because these are perceived as replacing part of themselves (Russell & Oxley 1990). Women generally are more concerned than men to maintain close social relationships in the face of barriers imposed by limited mobility and poor transportation (Walker-Birckhead 1996).

Community care is heavily gender based. UK research based on the General Household Survey found that women aged 45–64 years caring for disabled husbands provided twice the number of hours of support that men did in caring for disabled wives (Arber & Ginn 1997, p 162). Pickard & Glendinning (2002) conducted a qualitative study into how lay and professional carers can work together effectively, by interviewing and observing carer/care recipient groups. They concluded that while female carers are viewed as a 'resource' in taking on complex and onerous tasks, at the same time they are 'not partners at all', in the sense that they are often not involved in decision-making about care (p 150).

Older men can be particularly reluctant to reveal their health or care needs and concern about declining physical performance. While they may have strong support when married, those who have never married are at high risk of isolation (Gardner et al 1998). The weaker social relationships of older men compared to women are also seen among residents of high-rise housing estates (Brooke et al 1998). Single men living in low-cost accommodation such as rooming houses are especially likely to have multiple problems of frailty, psychiatric disability, nutritional deficiencies and alcohol dependence (Hughes & Alexander 1995). Older men's lifelong approaches to social relationships can contrast sharply with those of women, who typically have been more socially engaged. Accordingly, older men may experience more social isolation and less support than women when they become frail. A nurse interviewed for this chapter commented on the influence of gender on assumptions underlying her practice:

> Understanding something about gender is important. Older men don't go out and socialise. Women have children and grandchildren. Men stay at home and get lonely. Once they get frail and have disability they don't access wonderful things out there … suffer grief and loss … starting with the job, with their garden, the loss of their spouse— it's cumulative grief over losses. The family is not what they aspire to. Women will get satisfaction more than men. They think 'Everyone around is dying. I've been here for too long'—they hate the loss of physical independence. The male has always been the provider—it's their responsibility to be strong. They went to war—strength is important; they do not cope with isolation. They are not social like women.

Increasing cultural and linguistic diversity also influences caregiving expectations. The proportion of the older population from culturally and linguistically diverse backgrounds is increasing, from 18% in 1996 to an expected 23% in 2011, a 66% growth rate, compared to only 23% for the Australian-born (AIHW 2001). The demographic basis for demand and access to appropriate services is increasing, whether it be for mainstream services or for ethno-specific groups.

Yet older people from culturally diverse backgrounds are under-represented as clients. They comprise just over 20% of the older population but only 16% of Home and Community Care clients (AIHW 2002, p 51). Older migrants can face many language and cultural barriers and there is great variation among groups in terms of their needs, informal support, and service use (Kendig & Russell 1998). Overall, they under-utilise formal community and residential care compared to other Australian older people (AIHW 2002). A small study of older Italian-Australians (Wells et al 2002) found that respondents preferred culture-specific service provision to mainstream services, but that there was poor awareness of Italian-specific and other services.

Cultural assumptions may also influence the assessment of older people for entry to aged-care systems. A nurse interviewed for this chapter considered that:

Cultural backgrounds affect the Mini Mental Test, which is not culturally specific. The test can say one thing but there is other evidence such as their ability to pay bills, shop, and medicate, be responsible nutritionally and be socially active. The Mini Mental—it's a tool and all tools are flawed.

Aboriginal people have life expectancies and disease patterns similar to those of people in developing countries (Harrison 1997). After years of neglect and inappropriate services, some attempts are now under way to provide aged care as envisaged and controlled by Aboriginal people themselves. An account by a community nurse interviewed for this chapter about working in a health centre with Pitjantjara people in central Australia indicated the value of a cross-cultural translator mediating understandings between the mainstream and Aboriginal health systems (Arch, verbal communication 2003).

Socioeconomic circumstances are a major influence on ageing and care needs. Arber & Ginn (1997), in an analysis of the United Kingdom General Household Survey data, assert that the social class of an elderly person is associated with becoming dependent and losing autonomy. Those with a less advantaged class background have a higher likelihood of experiencing chronic illness and impairment as well as fewer of the material, financial and cultural resources necessary to remain autonomous in their own homes. Whether or not older people own their homes has a crucial bearing on both their standard of living and the availability of wealth to buy into residential care (Howe 1992). Life expectancy and health are far worse for older Australians who have lower income and education (Mathers 1994). Less advantaged class background is also associated with higher risk of falls, depression and inappropriate use of medication (Kendig et al 1998).

Nurses working in the community are required to assess and respond to older people in widely diverse care situations. A nurse working in the community viewed client diversity as a professional resourcing issue:

Attention to diversity issues has to be one-on-one, which is not funded. That has to be done 'in house'. You go into those people (at home) rather than have them go out. *Every house you go into is going to be so different from the house before.* People are different, and their complexities—between men and women it's different. That's what makes it so enjoyable. It's their environment, their choices. That's not what happens in a hospital.

CARERS AND CAREGIVING

Caregiving and care receiving are widespread. According to the 1998 Survey of Disability, Ageing and Carers, there were 352,200 primary carers providing care for people with a profound or severe handicap who were living in the same household and a further 95,800 providing care to care recipients living elsewhere (ABS 1998). Having a co-resident carer increases the likelihood of an older person remaining in the community even in the face of their disabilities (Charlton et al 1996). Among older clients who leave community care for residential care, a major factor is a breakdown in the capacities of the caregivers (Wells & Kendig 1996; Wells et al 1999).

Care means different things to different people. Older people's perceptions of their care 'can only be understood in terms of the appreciation of the life histories of family members and of how present interdependencies are shaped by personal histories and environmental factors' (Wenger et al 1996, p 203).

The ability to care is affected by the carer's own resources, such as their mental health, social support and physical capabilities. Co-resident carers generally have higher levels of stress and are more likely to feel depressed or worried than non-co-resident carers (ABS 1998). Schofield et al (1994) report adverse effects of co-residency on emotional well-being, particularly for women carers. Their findings are based on a study of nearly 1000 carers of people with disabilities, half of whom were over 65 years.

Caregiving takes place within intimate relationships, which have accrued particular meanings over the lifespan. The tasks of care are set within these relationships and within the purposes of both the older person and the caregiver. Wells & Kendig (1997) show how positive aspects of spouse caregiving can outweigh the negative, providing a complex challenge which returns a sense of competence and satisfaction that may compensate for the losses. 'Caring' has been defined as 'only the continuation of normal relationships which becomes intensified in the face of unwanted, sometimes unexpected events which result in high levels of dependency' (Wenger et al 1996, p 203). When nurses assist older people they enter into these important pre-existing relationships and their meanings for the individuals concerned.

A nurse interviewed for this paper illustrates how attending to meanings within caregiving relationships is integral to nurses' practice:

> In case management you have to consider what is the ability of the carer to provide services that would be provided without putting the person at risk. There are environmental issues for families caring for a person with dementia—a carer may tolerate extreme behaviours, which another person does not tolerate. We have to *look at the relationship with the carer—within the carer's relationship with the patient.* We have to be acknowledging those things more. Or if the husband is mostly in control then when there is a change and the carer is, the carer may not cope with it. *It's very different for different individuals.* Similarly some carers have the ability to look after very disabled people—you have to be open to people's abilities—it's very easy to pass judgement on what people can or can't do without looking at the situation.

IMPLICATIONS FOR PRACTICE

Professional caring recognises that good care will vary according to the specific needs of each older person. Nurses need to be able to see what individuals want and how to make their practice congruent with the older people's perceptions. However, their relationships with clients also take place in a context of severely constrained resources and, desirably, in coordination with informal carers and other community-care professionals. Nurses need to negotiate work practices which reconcile the expectations of their clients with those of their organisations and the programs and policies behind them.

Community care is inherently different from the institutional context in which most nurses have been trained. First, care is no longer delivered at the workplace of the professional, under their (virtually) full control, but rather is delivered in the homes of clients. Secondly, care at home must make provision for the limited capacities to monitor and meet rapidly arising needs, and work out ways to provide care without the immediate availability of specialist staff and expensive technology. And thirdly, quality standards in community care cannot be implemented through senior staff located on site.

Nurses thus have extended responsibilities when they work in private homes. They need to carefully assess risk, and provide advice and reassurance to older people and carers. In addition to their technical nursing, 'nurses have become managers of environmental contexts so as to ensure hygiene, safety and comfort' (Kendig, Parker et al 1992, p 17). A recent Australian study of ageism in professional practice showed that nurses working in older people's homes exhibit more positive attitudes towards older people than those working in residential care facilities (Foreman et al 2002). Their positive and caring culture, so central to both older people and nursing principles, can be devalued if there is an imbalanced emphasis on technical, professional perspectives. Overall, older people perceive health professionals as displaying 'ageist' attitudes in which they are made to feel that they are 'old and dependent' rather than ageing normally (Minichiello et al 2000).

Requirements for practice have been identified in a report on community care for people with complex needs (Reynolds & Kendig 1997). Comprehensive and skilled assessment and care planning are required on an ongoing basis—not only when taking on a service. There is the need for an individual and flexible approach, collaboration with carers and families, and effective coordination between practitioners. Nursing is particularly important for people with complex needs, given that their needs and vulnerabilities are intense, multiple, varied and changeable.

A new development in practice is shifting the emphasis from solely a *care* strategy (responding after dependencies are entrenched) to also include a *preventative* strategy (which aims to maintain independence notwithstanding mounting vulnerabilities). As initially articulated in the National Healthy Ageing Strategy (Healthy Ageing Taskforce 1997), health and well-being can be enhanced through a holistic approach that incorporates physical, psychological, social and emotional well-being. Nurses can be proactive in supporting positive ageing in their practice.

Maintaining self-care requires early and timely interventions, often at critical points in people's lives such as widowhood, becoming a carer or relinquishing caregiving (Wells & Kendig 1997). It requires an emphasis on identifying and strengthening individuals' critical capacities as well as finding and meeting their functional deficits. New technologies, such as mobility aids, cooking facilities, monitoring devices and medical equipment formerly available only in institutional settings, can assist older people to stay in their homes. There is also increased awareness of the importance of the built environment, both within older people's homes and in their immediate surroundings and neighbourhoods, in both encouraging and reinforcing independent living (Bridge et al 2002).

Another feature of evolving practice is that nurses are operating in a multi-professional service system (Angus 1996). They are contributing to generic assessment and case management, and working with other professionals in addressing incontinence, dementia and rehabilitation. At the same time, governments are shifting some care responsibilities to less costly, less trained workers. Perceptions vary considerably about the appropriate boundaries between and potential of nurses, other health and community workers, and informal carers in the provision of community-based care (Kendig, McVicar et al 1992). Nurses need to demonstrate that their higher pay is more than matched by their increased effectiveness in meeting the needs of highly vulnerable people.

CASE STUDIES OF NURSING OLDER PEOPLE IN THE COMMUNITY

Of four nurses interviewed for this chapter, two worked in aged-care case management and two in front-line domiciliary nursing. The following case studies of nursing practice in the community illustrate how nurses employ notions of 'community' around which they construct care.

Case study 1

A man of Middle-Eastern background was discharged home from a hospital emergency department with a urinary condition requiring a catheter. His wife, also from the same background, had low skills in English literacy and had not been verbally informed of the procedures required to care for the catheter, or that it would have to be replaced. An operation had been booked for him to have a catheter inserted through an incision above his urethra.

A community nurse heard that this man had been discharged from a hospital emergency department with no arrangements for follow-up. She intervened by ringing the surgeon, and also the man's wife to explain the operation. The wife said that she did not know about the operation and that there was no way that they would accept 'a hole in his stomach'. The nurse commented that this case exemplifies situations in which 'cultural understanding is lacking'. The nurse commented: 'There are a lot of problems with discharge and a lot more with migrants. They think that the client or family member understands ... they get a new script and do not understand how to stop the old medication. *It's all to do with the way it's [nursing] fundamentally around tasks*'.

Lessons

Primary to this nurse's practice was her understanding that cultural assumptions and language problems could interfere with the clients' understandings of the potential operation. She also was able to connect the medical and hospital system to home care, knowing that the discharge system did not adequately provide information and prepare the informal carer for her care responsibilities at home. This could particularly disadvantage people from linguistically and culturally diverse backgrounds.

Case study 2

A woman in her early seventies had an intellectual disability and an underlying medical condition (pneumonia), which led to acute hospitalisation. She had been living in a Community Residential Unit (CRU) which provides for people with intellectual and psychiatric disabilities requiring support and monitoring in a shared community-based house. She had gone into an acute hospital bed for a medical problem and hospital staff had assessed her as requiring high-level care. The nurse was aware that this woman's dependency could be over-stated in the hospital. 'We assessed the lady—yes she can go back to the CRU. We also had her listed for a nearby nursing home in case her condition deteriorated.' The idea that she could remain in a CRU with support was maintained despite the fact that in hospital she was assessed as requiring high-level care.

Lessons

In this case the nurse's understanding of the extent of support offered to a woman in a community-based facility enabled discharge to a lower level of care than she had been assessed for. A primary aspect of the nurse's practice is that she had knowledge of community resources and specific understanding of the CRU as a supportive environment in the community. She was also able to bridge medical and community sectors through her knowledge and position at the interface between the medical and home contexts. Also important was the nurse's ability to act as an advocate for the older woman through her knowledge of facilities that would enable her to remain in the community.

Case study 3: negative case

In a negative case, a service was rejected by the client. The sister of the potential female client, aged in her late eighties, made the referral to the Aged Care Assessment Service, which recommended home care services. The potential client refused continence pads but also had mobility impairments and cardiac problems. The nurse believed that if supported by services this person could stay at home for longer than otherwise would have been the case; however, despite her sister's views, the potential client did not agree. The nurse expressed concern that this woman had rejected having a cognitive assessment, and felt that 'to get to the bottom of this is difficult'. The nurse commented that 'She really needs a Linkages [Community Options] place—there would be every advantage and it would defer hospitalisation'. The nurse commented that nevertheless 'The crux of this case is dealing with who people are … It's very important to understand … that they have a right to make decisions and you must respect whom they are. The term "noncompliant" should be taken out of nursing vocabulary'.

Lessons

The case illustrates the nurse's non-judgemental attitude and ability to understand the situation from the client's perspective. It also exemplifies a negative case of practice at the lower end of care, which enabled the nurse to maintain care at the minimal end of supervision and risk management—the nurse maintained contact with the sister and continued to monitor the woman by visiting regularly.

Common lessons from these case studies

These case studies illustrate how nurses' understandings of different manifestations of 'community' informs how they construct their care. One case illustrates a nurse's understanding of variations in cultural assumptions, while connecting the older person to both medical and community resource systems. In another case, a nurse uses her knowledge of community resources and the type of support required by an intellectually disabled person to maintain this person in the community rather than in residential care. At the level of informal relationships, these nurses demonstrated understanding of the older person's and carer's perspectives, which also included their disagreements.

NURSES' ROLES WITHIN COMMUNITY CARE SERVICE SYSTEMS

The context of community nursing for older people has been fundamentally changed by policy and funding developments since the mid-1980s. There is a need to work with more dependent people in their homes, given community demand and restricted access to residential care, and to meet the demands of post-acute care. Community care is increasingly based on the combined efforts of several services and professions, serving younger disabled people and those with mental illness as well as frail older people and their carers.

Nurses form part of multidisciplinary teams serving the community. They commonly share responsibilities and have blurred boundaries with other professionals, with these delineations heavily influenced by the availability of resources. Nurses may 'fill in' gaps in care, such as changing bed linen, when this is perceived to be necessary to hygiene, a task generally done by home carers. Nurses may by default act as interim case managers prior to assessments by Aged Care Assessment Services. They can stand in for other professionals, for example, by sharing common responsibilities such as helping to mobilise an older person in his or her home, thus crossing usual professional boundaries.

Complications in defining disciplinary boundaries in multidisciplinary teams were illustrated by nurses' difficulties in deciding whether bathing was professional nursing care or 'social care' in a UK study (Griffiths 1998, p 238). Griffiths comments: 'It is clear that if district nurses cannot decide amongst themselves how to define nursing care, the problem is likely to be amplified when health and social services, with their very different cultural backgrounds, attempt to reach a definition'. Brooke (1995) also found that clients could expect nurses to work longer than they are paid for, with the formal boundaries of care being crossed as a result.

Nurses practise in highly visible community care service systems, such as those coordinated by case management services and public and private providers of care. The informal care system may be more or less visible to nurses—for example, they may know that a neighbour monitors a frail older person—yet not know where this care begins and ends. Less visible care networks may also operate—for instance, a daughter may be the primary carer, but be in constant communication with a less visible network of the older person's friends, who support and supplement her care.

Nurses and other community care professionals are directing increasing attention to building service systems responsive to the diversity of clients' needs (Reynolds & Kendig 1997). Key service system capacities concern the range and adequacy of services, 24-hour and emergency coverage, and the ability to identify and address complex psychosocial circumstances. Much more needs to be done to develop effective quality assurance approaches at the system level as well as for individual services and practitioners. Well coordinated and collaborative approaches are essential for providing effective support.

Delivering client-centred assistance is facilitated by a shared vision and a collaborative and positive culture within local community service networks. Agreement is required on processes and protocols which share information about clients and facilitate cooperation with assessment, referrals and care planning. Equally important are common principles for targeting clients and ensuring continuity of care when people move from one service to another. Local approaches to service planning and service development assist in identifying gaps and problems in the local service network and strategies for addressing them.

Leading practitioners must be keenly aware of the management and policy context for delivering care. It is crucial that nurses understand the funding and program language, which so heavily influences the resources and scope for operations (Kendig 1995). Access to resources depends increasingly on the capacity to deliver good quality at a competitive price, and to work with and in innovative programs such as Community Aged Care Packages.

CHALLENGES FOR NURSES IN COMMUNITY CARE

A primary challenge for nurses in community care is that the nurse is required to look well beyond the immediate medical task in order to coordinate community resources around the client's needs. This demands a systemic approach to accessing community care systems, which transcends individual cases. Nurses' positions within both medical and community sectors enable them to act as advocates and brokers between medical and home contexts. Nurses' knowledge of what is available in the community enables them to mobilise medical and community care systems. A nurse commented:

> a good community nurse will be talking to a GP, hospital, family and firstly to the client. Hopefully it will all flow smoothly together ... You need to be tweaking those connections so that you work together.

Nurses need to have a strong understanding of case management processes and how to adapt these to suit each client (and carer). The growing demand for community care has increased pressure on assessment and case management capacities, which nurses commonly provide as interim measures. A nurse described how she was required to fill gaps in service coordination prior to the appointment of a case manager. As she commented:

> We are the first people through the door—the case manager can take six months to be appointed. They [nurses] can do feeding, washing, hanging clothes on the line—it's not in the job description but if there's dirty bed linen you'll start doing that before you get home help. Often it's combined nursing and home help.

A second challenge is that health-service provision in the community has been rationalised and rewards performance of tasks while not measuring or rewarding service coordination. Organisational tensions exist for nurses due to a lack of resources or mandate to go beyond standard nursing tasks, such as treating a wound, catheter care and supervising medication. As a nurse commented:

> Client advocacy is huge—nurses are often not doing it well as they are so interested in doing the [medical] task. They should be saying 'Where to next? What is the best for the client?' Often if we do it no one would know about it. *There is no measure for someone who goes beyond and advocates beyond his or her task.*

A third major challenge for nurses is to apply 'holistic' approaches which integrate medical and social perspectives in their care practice. These approaches include attention to present physical morbidities, co-morbidities, functional capacities and social relationships as well as biographical factors including previous employment, clubs attended, sporting, social and recreational activities and hobbies since retirement. A nurse articulated this approach:

> The non-clinical is very important—we look at people quite holistically. When you go in you need to understand the personal dynamics of the situation, what supports they have from family and friends, the dynamics of the situation, their education background and cultural background. These are real points to take into account. You are asking them what do they think they can or can't do, what are they doing and then whether they want to stay where they are. … [their needs] … and also the needs of healthy carers as well.

Finally, the overall context of rationalised resources means that nurses have to be smart managers of potential sources of social support for older people in their homes. This requires assessment of and responsiveness to the totality of support received within social relationships from carers and professionals. It also requires exploring the nature of community connections and how they can be activated and supported. This requires skills in discriminating between subtle, less visible forms of support as well as support from formal services. As one nurse commented:

> The issue is financial restraint. There's not enough dollars for carer respite. I do not believe that basic needs can be met due to unit cost [funding]. For social support you need to look at the family environment, monetary aspects, relationships and socialisation. Looking at ADLs without the intimacy relationship is difficult to understand and you need to know how their health is to be managed … It's exploring what people want, it's about respecting people's rights.

UNDERSTANDING 'COMMUNITY' IN PRACTICE

Nurses' academic education encourages a holistic understanding of community in their practice which goes beyond the technical tasks for which they are rewarded. But nurses are not financially reimbursed for what is integral to the practice of community care—that is, understanding the older person's need for support in their home in the context of their social relationships within the community.

Community nursing for older people is increasingly viewed as an interesting and valued field requiring specialised expertise. Task performance is under greater pressure now, as dependency is increasing together with directions from government for more throughputs of clients and demonstrated cost-effectiveness. There is an increasing expectation that nurses will do more with less—providing more individualised care without commensurate increases of resources.

Four approaches can be suggested for dealing with these issues. First, nurses can continue with innovations that coordinate practice to provide more with less. For some time nurses have in fact been developing coordination capacities, more multidisciplinary skills, and in some cases leading case management practices.

Second, nurses can work to improve their care provision through advocacy on behalf of older people across medical and community care systems, particularly for those who are most vulnerable and less able to speak for themselves. This can include advocacy on behalf of older individuals addressing home care issues. It can also extend to articulating problems at a systemic level and serving as a public spokesperson for older people and carers on care issues.

Third, holistic practice should recognise the various communities that can form complementary systems which support older people. At the relational level, older people's informal support may be easily visible or may consist of subtle arrangements which are not immediately obvious. Nurses need to be able to identify and evaluate social support and link these outcomes with their knowledge of available formal services.

Nurses can also encourage relationships within subgroups of older people based on their perspectives and characteristics. Possible communities could include social support groups based on geographic areas, affinity groups based on sharing common perspectives, and groups based on common cultural identities, in articulation with community resources, such as day centres, community activities and volunteer programs for social support. At the broadest level of community resources, they can link older people with formal services such as home and community care resources.

Fourth, nurses can play a major part in coalitions of professional bodies, consumer groups and industry groups in action to improve care provision. The 'Vision for Community Care', articulated by Aged and Community Services Australia (2002), aims to 'drive debate on the need for, and the shape of, reform required in community care' (p 1). The vision is that 'Community care of the future will support lifestyle choices to enable people who need support and their carers to live in the community'. The paper articulates the implications of this vision for philosophies of care, nature of service delivery, place of service delivery, and funding systems with clear budgeting for assessment, rehabilitation and other priority elements of care.

CONCLUSION

Nurses practice at the nexus of care for clients and carers, in health and welfare services, and across community and institutional settings. Their effective home care for older people requires interpreting and acting on the different meanings of 'community' in community nursing practice. This means that nurses make proactive and pragmatic connections between older people and the different communities to which they are, or could become, attached. It also involves advocating and bridging the medical/social hiatus separating community resources. And most fundamentally, it involves nurses recognising older people's closest connections with the caregivers who constitute their immediate and most intimate networks.

A strong practical understanding of 'community' within nursing practice is essential, as this provides substance to the terms 'community' and 'holistic' while affirming the identities of the older people who are cared for in their homes and communities.

References

Aged and Community Services Australia 2002, A Vision for Community Care. Online: www.agedcare.org.au

Angus J 1996 (ed), *Gerontology on the Move: Is Professional Education Keeping Pace?* Conference Proceedings of Lincoln Gerontology Centre for Education and Research 4th National Symposium 18–19 April 1996, Lincoln Gerontology Centre, La Trobe University: Melbourne.

Arber S & Ginn J 1997, Class, caring and the life course. In: Arber S & Ginn J (eds), *Ageing, Independence and the Life Course*, pp 149–67, Jessica Kingsley/British Society of Gerontology: London.

Australian Bureau of Statistics (ABS) 1995, *The Labour Force, Australia*, Cat. No. 6203, AGPS: Canberra.

Australian Bureau of Statistics (ABS) 1996, *Projections of the Population of Australia, States and Territories, 1995–2051*, Series A and B, Cat. No. 3222.0, AGPS: Canberra.

Australian Bureau of Statistics (ABS) 1998, *Disability, Ageing and Carers: Summary of Findings*, Cat. No. 4430.0, AGPS: Canberra.

Australian Bureau of Statistics (ABS) 2002, *Census of Population and Housing*.

Australian Institute of Health and Welfare (AIHW) 2001, *Projections of Older Immigrants— People from Culturally and Linguistically Diverse Backgrounds, 1996–2026*, Aged Care Series No. 6, AIHW: Canberra.

Australian Institute of Health and Welfare (AIHW) 2002, *Older Australia at a Glance*, AIHW and Office of the Aged, Commonwealth Department of Health and Family Services, Commonwealth of Australia: Canberra.

Bridge K, Kendig H, Quine S & Parsons A 2002, *Housing and Care for Younger and Older People with Disabilities*, Australian Housing and Urban Research Institute, Melbourne, 2001, p 136.

Brooke EM 1995, *Identity and Practice: Case Studies in Community Care in Australia*, unpublished PhD thesis, La Trobe University, Melbourne.

Brooke E, Davidson S & Kendig H 1998, *Support Needs of Older People in High Rise Public Housing*, Department of Human Services, Aged Care Division, Victorian Department of Human Services.

Browning C & Kendig H 2003, Healthy ageing: a new approach on older people's health and well-being. In: Liamputtong P & Gardner H (eds), *Health, Social Policy, and Communities*, pp 182–205, Oxford University Press: Melbourne.

Charlton F, Humphries S & Russell H 1996, Hostel or home? a study of Victorian ACAT Recommendations of hostel care plans, *Lincoln Papers in Gerontology*, No. 34, Lincoln Gerontology Centre, La Trobe University: Melbourne.

Commonwealth of Australia 2001, National Strategy for an Ageing Australia. An Older Australia, Challenges and Opportunities for all National Strategy for an Ageing Australia, The Hon Kevin Andrews MP, Minister for Ageing National Strategy for an Ageing Australia.

Commonwealth of Australia 2002, Intergenerational Report. Budget Papers, 2002–2003.

Davison B, Kendig H, Stephens F & Merrill V 1993, *It's My Place: Older People Talk about their Homes*, AGPS: Canberra.

Foreman P, Wells Y, Petralia W & Hamilton-Smith E 2002, *Promoting Positive Attitudes to Ageing by Health Professionals and Aged Care Service Providers*, Lincoln Gerontology Centre: Melbourne.

Gardner I, Brooke E & Kendig H 1998, *Improving Social Networks Report*, Department of Veterans' Affairs: Canberra.

Griffths J 1998, Meeting personal hygiene needs in the community; a district nursing perspective on the health and social care divide, *Health and Social Care in the Community*, 6(4), pp 234–40.

Harrison J 1997, Social policy and Aboriginal people. In: Borowski A, Encel S & Ozanne E (eds), *Ageing and Social Policy in Australia*, pp 119–36, Cambridge University Press: Cambridge.

Howe A 1992, *Housing for Older Australians: Affordability, Adjustments and Care*, The National Housing Strategy Background Paper 8, Commonwealth Office for the Aged, Commonwealth of Australia.

Hughes A & Alexander L 1995, *The HACC Program: Improving Access for Homeless People*, Prepared for the RDNS Homeless Persons Program, Royal District Nursing Service: Melbourne.

Kendig H 1995, Costs of community care for older people, *Proceedings of the Australian Nursing Federation Gerontology Special Interest Group*, 2nd National Conference, Perth, Western Australia, 23–26 July 1995.

Kendig H & Brooke E 1997, Australian research on ageing and social support, *Australian Journal of Ageing*, 16(3), pp 127–30.

Kendig H & Duckett S 2001, *Australian Directions in Aged Care: the Generation of Policies for Generations of Older People*, Australian Health Policy Institute, University of Sydney, Commissioned Paper Series 2001/5, p 113.

Kendig H & Russel H 1998, Aging, ethnicity, and health policy in Australia. In: Wister A & Guttman G (eds) *Health Systems and Aging in Selected Pacific Rim Countries: Diversity and Change*, pp. 19–42, Simon Fraser University Press: Vancouver.

Kendig H, McVicar G, Reynolds A & O'Brien A 1992, *The Victorian Linkages Evaluation: Executive Summary*, Department of Health, Housing and Community Services and Community Services, Victoria.

Kendig H, Parker J, Scotton R & Hay B 1992, *Evaluation of 24 hour Home Nursing Services*, for the Health Services for Older Persons Unit, Health Department, Victoria.

Kendig H, Davison B & Walker-Birckhead W 1993, Meanings of health in later life, *Proceedings of the International Congress of Gerontology, Budapest*, July 1993, pp 1553–8.

Kendig H, Helme R, Teshuva K, Osborne D, Flicker L & Browning C 1996, *Health Status of Older People Project: Preliminary Findings from a Survey of the Health and Lifestyles of Older Australians*. A joint publication of the Victorian Health Promotion Foundation, Lincoln Gerontology Centre, Faculty of Health Sciences, La Trobe University and the National Ageing Research Institute, The University of Melbourne.

Kendig H, Browning C & Teshuva K 1998, Health actions and social class among Older Australians, *Australian and New Zealand Journal of Public Health*, 22(7), pp 808–13.

Kendig H, Browning C & Young A 2000, Impacts of illness and disability on the wellbeing of older people, *Disability and Rehabilitation*, 22(1–2), pp 15–22.

Mathers C 1994, *Health Differentials among Older Australians*, Australian Institute of Health and Welfare, Health Monitoring Series No. 2, AGPS: Canberra.

McCallum J 2001, Health in the 'grey' millennium: romanticism versus complexity?, *International Journal of Law and Psychiatry*, 24, pp 135–48.

Minichiello V, Browne J & Kendig HL 2000, Perceptions and consequences of ageism: views from older persons, *Ageing and Society*, May, pp 253–78.

Pickard S & Glendinning C 2002, Comparing and contrasting the role of family carers and nurses in the domestic health care of frail older people, *Health and Social Care in the Community*, 10(3), pp 144–50.

Reynolds A & Kendig H 1997, *Community Care for Older People with Complex Needs*, Report for the Aged Care Special Initiatives Program, Department of Health and Community Services Victoria, Victorian Department of Human Services, Melbourne.

Russell C & Oxley H 1990, Health and aging in Australia: is there culture after sixty? *Journal of Cross-cultural Gerontology*, 3, pp 5–50.

Schofield H, Murphy B, Herrman H, Bloch S & Singh B 1994, *Family Carers; Adult Offspring, Partners and Parents*, Paper presented at the 29th Annual Conference of the Australian Psychological Society, Wollongong, September 1994.

St John W 1998, Just what do we mean by community? Conceptualisations from the field, *Health and Social Care in the Community*, 6(2), pp 63–70.

Walker-Birckhead W 1996, *Meaning and Old Age: Time, Survival and the End of Life*, Lincoln Papers in Gerontology, No. 35, Lincoln Gerontology Centre, La Trobe University: Melbourne.

Wells Y & Kendig H 1996, Changes in carers' capacity and motivation to provide care, *Journal of Family Studies*, 2(1), pp 15–28.

Wells Y & Kendig H 1997, Health and well-being of spouse caregivers and the widowed, *The Gerontologist*, 37(5), pp 666–74.

Wells Y, Kendig H & Swerissen H 1999, Client Outcomes in case-managed care: Who benefits most?, *Australasian Journal on Ageing*, 18(2), pp 79–85.

Wells Y, Petralia W & Foreman P 2002, *Older Italian-Australians' Use of and Satisfaction with Health and Community Services. A Pilot Collaborative Project*, Lincoln Gerontology Centre, La Trobe University in collaboration with Co.As.It, Final Report.

Wenger C, Grant G & Nolan M 1996, Older people as carers as well as recipients of care. In: Minichiello V, Chappell N, Kendig H & Walker A (eds), *Sociology of Aging: International Perspectives*, pp 189–207, International Sociological Association Research Committee on Aging: Melbourne.

World Health Organization 2002, *Active Ageing: A Policy Framework*. A contribution of the World Health Organization to the Second United Nations World Assembly on Ageing, Madrid, Spain, April 2002.

CHAPTER 8

Rural gerontic nursing in Australia

ELIZABETH LAVENDER AND HELEN KELEHER

INTRODUCTION

Since the mid-1980s, health issues for rural and remote Australians have achieved a high profile on the national political agenda (Siegloff & Buckley 1998). In particular, the health needs of older Australians are highlighted because of rising costs associated with care and management of chronic illnesses associated with ageing and the proportion of people over 65 years of age increasing by about 8% each year. It is paradoxical that general medical practice has been highly politicised, while rural nursing issues remain relatively invisible and small rural health services—primarily staffed by nurses—struggle for adequate funding to meet the needs of ageing populations.

This chapter examines issues for rural nursing, arguing that the predominant populations requiring health services in rural Australia are older people. Although rural nurses are primarily involved in issues of ageing, they are poorly prepared for this reality. This chapter argues that these issues have particular relevance for rural nurses, who need to be skilled in both public health and gerontic nursing in order to meet current needs. A further concern of this chapter is that the literature on the health issues of older rural Australians makes little distinction between them and their metropolitan counterparts, as if their needs are the same. We begin with an outline of demographic and health-status issues for rural and remote populations, before discussing the scope of practice for rural nurses and the implications for nurses' education.

RURAL AND REMOTE POPULATION HEALTH

The demographic profile of rural and remote Australia leans heavily towards an ageing population (AIHW 2002; Frager et al 1997). The impact is magnified because although many small country towns have a declining population, the proportion of aged people in those towns is increasing (Department of Human Services [DHS] 1996a). Typically, in small and medium-sized towns at least 30% of the population are over the age of 60 years and at least 10% are over the age of 75 years. Population projections are for about a 20% decrease in the 0–14 years age-group and a 51% increase of people over 65 years of age (DHS 1996a). These trends call for innovative approaches to the delivery of programs and services to meet the needs of older rural people (Department of Health and Family Services [DHFS] 1996).

According to Buckley (1997), the term 'rural health' is used variously, to refer to:

- the health-care needs and access of rural Australians;
- the health differences of rural Australians; or
- the roles of the various health-care providers.

For planning purposes, classifications of rurality are based on distance, population size and density (DHFS 1994). The ARIA (Accessibility/Remoteness Index of Australia) classification subdivides rural areas by stressing known transport links as a means of access to health services, and considers settlement at five levels. At Level 1, which is for populations of between 200 and 5000, there are 1500 settlements in rural Australia. Level 2 settlements have between 5000 and 17,999 people. Level 3 classifies settlements with populations over 18,000, going up to Level 5 for settlements of over 250,000. About two million Australians live in localities that are defined as having fewer than 200 people. Many older Australians choose to live in rural areas, in or near communities with which they are familiar, close to friends and relatives, and in a social infrastructure that has meaning and cohesion for them. Small towns experience retirement by migration from metropolitan and surrounding rural areas, with steady increases in the number of 1–2 person households linked to increasing demographic in the 60+ age groups. Small towns typically have below-average income levels, with most residents living on $25,000 or less per annum, and older people choosing to stay in small towns because of cheaper housing costs. However, small towns and sparsely distributed populations have a lack of health-service options, long geographic distances between health and community services, few social opportunities and low levels of employment, and a lack of transport options, which frequently results in isolation.

The focus of this chapter is mainly on rural nursing in relation to ARIA Levels 1 and 2. These are the townships which have a health service that is likely to be a mix of acute, chronic, palliative, high- and low-dependency nursing-home type beds, as well as Community Aged Care Packages (CACP), respite care beds, and an emergency department. Rural health services are dependent on medical general practice, although it becomes uneconomic without income subsidy for populations below about 1200 people. Thus, small townships are increasingly dependent on the services provided by a clinical nurse practitioner (Best 2000), who is sometimes called a 'bush nurse' or remote area nurse practitioner.

Compared with their counterparts living in metropolitan areas, many rural residents experience significant problems of inequity in the provision of, and access to, health-care services (DHFS 1994). The major issues continually identified are the shortage and maldistribution of health-care providers, above-average ratios of population to health-care providers, high turnover of workforce, and inaccessibility of needed services.

HEALTH PROFILE OF RURAL OLDER PEOPLE

There is increasing evidence of differences between the health problems of rural people and the health problems of metropolitan people. In terms of morbidity and mortality, rural older people have a significantly worse health status (AIHW 2002). VicHealth lists the most common preventable health issues in older people as being: diabetes, depression, poor mobility, inappropriate medication use, falls and injuries, poor cardiovascular health and poor nutrition (VicHealth 1996). Death rates from ischaemic heart disease, stroke and cancer are higher in rural areas, and the morbidity statistics are equally worrying—with hospital separations for stroke, diabetes and asthma all significantly higher than metropolitan levels (Carson 1997). Even though cancer and heart disease are the main causes of mortality in rural areas, emotional and mental health issues are a major cause of morbidity. Suicide rates and injury rates, especially among males (AIHW 2000), are noteworthy for their higher incidence in rural and remote areas, with consequences for the health of whole families and communities. Humphreys & Rolley (1991) contend that there are four groups who experience special problems associated with living in the country: the aged, the poor, women and Aborigines. This creates special problems for older people, who are often poor and more likely to be women, and therefore also creates special challenges for health professionals.

The health issues evident for the rural population as a whole are compounded and exaggerated for older people. Nevertheless, most rural older people perceive themselves as healthy (VicHealth 1996). Indeed, most live independent and satisfying lives in their own homes, no differently from older people in metropolitan areas. Older people can look beyond their physical-health status, and subjectively describe their health and well-being in positive terms.

Health and social issues associated with ageing are major issues for rural Australia. Providers talk of the overloading of systems and problems associated with meeting needs for issues of ageing and extended care. District nurses are 'run off their feet' trying to cope with elderly people with complex health conditions being managed at home and who are thought to need hospitalisation or are waiting for a bed to become available in residential care. Thus, rural older people are being managed at home with high acuity, occasionally receiving treatment in accident and emergency departments and then sent home to the care of district nurses, who express concerns about the numbers of older people living in fairly isolated conditions without access to transport. As people age and become less mobile or without private transport, they become isolated and reliant on health services for all contact, including social interaction. Providers commonly raise perceptions about the coping skills and low levels of self-care knowledge of older people in relation to self-management of chronic disease. The health of many older people is characterised by poor mental health related to chronic unhappiness and depression. Associated issues include those of physical and social isolation, such as lack of connection, low levels of income, lack of transport options and issues arising from caring responsibilities.

Rural older Indigenous people

Indigenous people comprise 2.1% of the total Australian population, but a greater percentage (42.3%) live in smaller urban centres than do non–Indigenous people (23%). Moreover there are considerable regional differences, with about 50% of Aboriginal people in Western Australia living in rural or remote communities. So although the population of Indigenous people is spread across urban, rural and remote areas, often the problems associated with Indigenous health seem to be more visible in remote communities. Significantly, only 2.6% of the Aboriginal population are aged 65 years or older (Standing Committee on Family and Community Affairs, 2000). The health profile of Aborigines reflects their overall inequality in Australian society. Diseases of the circulatory system are the main cause of premature death (AIHW 1997), and effective strategies are needed to improve the overall health status of Aborigines— particularly in terms of diabetes, nutrition, asthma, renal disease and obesity (Crowe 1996). Unemployment, injury and violence are public health issues that require targeted strategies for use in rural Aboriginal communities. Information about older Aborigines is limited by poor identification of Indigenous people in data collected by aged-care agencies. The poor health of Indigenous people makes it more likely that they will need access to culturally appropriate aged care at younger ages (AIHW 1997). This presents particular challenges for rural nurses who have little, if any, access to cultural education about Indigenous ageing issues. Furthermore, there is an acute shortage of Indigenous registered nurses.

RURAL HEALTH SERVICES

Pressure on services

As previously noted, access to services is a recurring theme for older people in rural Australia. A vicious circle exists whereby, as services such as banks and government departments are withdrawn from country areas, young people seek employment else-where, leaving a smaller population with a disproportionate number of older people— who then have to travel to larger towns for essential services. This drifting away of family members can affect the psychological well-being of older people (VicHealth 1996). The stereotype of rural Australians, especially men—as stoic, independent, tough, healthy farmers who can look after themselves—may be an impediment to their seeking health care (Humphreys et al 1996). Rural counselling services are not only difficult to access, but are also expensive when they are available. Rural older peo-ple need enhanced health and medical information which is targeted, accessible and available in plain English. They also require health professionals who will support and facilitate the introduction of health-promotion programs and support groups for specific illnesses or diseases, to facilitate self-management. There are some indications that older rural women suffer from violence, loneliness and fear at higher levels than metropolitan older women, and that they have lower levels of schooling (Women's Health Australia 1997). Rural women have poor access to choice in reproductive services and child care, and poor access to emergency housing if the need arises.

A new phenomenon is the increasing number of elderly tourists—'grey nomads'—travelling in rural and remote areas, particularly in winter. Despite the joys of retirement and the realisation of long-held dreams, many have existing health problems that may develop acute exacerbations, or they may experience accidents or medical emergencies such as stroke or myocardial infarction. This further strains local health services and leads to new demands for care. General practitioners, especially female GPs, are in short supply in rural Australia, as is bulk billing. Dentists and publicly funded dental services are similarly sparse.

Service planning

The demographic and health profile of rural Australia therefore provides many challenges to health-service planners. Many rural and remote communities are at risk of falling below a critical threshold for the maintenance of viable health services (Humphreys et al 1996). In line with the National Rural Health Strategy, Commonwealth and State arrangements have embraced flexible approaches to funding and management of aged-care and health services in rural communities.

It is desirable that services be aimed at the population in their own environment, embracing the whole network of health and community issues (NRHA 2002). In an acceleration of change in the late 1990s, governments have closed or reduced the size of small rural hospitals and affiliated services, and have replaced them with new health-care delivery models (Siegloff 1997). Particular attention has been paid to alternative models for the provision of specialist medical care—although inpatient services do require people to travel long distances to reach regional hospitals. It should be noted, however, that many specialist services were not provided in small rural hospitals even before funding changes were introduced, because those hospitals were unable to provide the necessary medical technology and support services.

New models of aged and health care have been designed to introduce flexible funding models that target each community's specific needs, and to provide for a greater range of more cost-effective and better coordinated services than is possible with the usual restrictions of funding models (DHS 1996a,b). For example, within a multipurpose service facility—which can be a purpose-built service or an adaptation of an existing building—a range of services can be provided to a local area. These models mean that rural areas can have the mix and range of services that they need. Thus a community with a small, underused hospital and little or no aged-care and community-care facilities can redesign its funding allocations to provide a range of services not previously available. For older people this may include a variety of home and community care packages, allied health, community health, senior-citizen centres, health education, hostel and nursing-home beds.

These new funding arrangements demand that health professionals, especially nurses, be multiskilled in clinical and public health, able to work in collaborative teams, develop partnerships, implement health promotion and engage in intersectoral planning (Siegloff 1997). These skills are fundamental to the provision of flexible, integrated services as services are refocused from acute-care (or residential-care) activities to primary-health activities, community-care activities and health-promotion activities (DHS 1996a). Siegloff (1997) argues that these models provide opportunities for nurses to advance their practice, but that educational preparation at both the undergraduate and postgraduate levels is necessary. Older people commonly live in the community rather than in institutional settings, so it is important to consider relationships between nurses and older people in a range of settings and models of care other than hospital and nursing homes.

Health promotion is the most contemporary model of care that has emerged from the new public health movement. In this approach, people are seen not as the objects of care but as active initiators of their own health care, empowered to take control of the determinants of their own health. The creation of supportive environments for the creation of good health requires health professionals to adopt participatory ways of working with individuals and communities, as well as a shift in relationships that recognises the expertise of the latter. Rural nurses need health promotion skills as part of their toolkit for rural nursing practice.

RURAL GERONTIC NURSING

Before discussing gerontic nursing in rural Australia, we will consider issues relating to rural and remote nurses in general. The Commonwealth Government recently signalled its concern for rural nursing and held two national inquiries into nursing and nursing education, both of which explored issues relating to rural and gerontic nursing.

Rural nursing workforce

In its submission to the National Review of Nursing Education, the Association for Australian Rural Nurses (AARN 2002) observed that there is increasing community concern about the shortage of nurses in rural and remote areas, making this issue no longer just the concern of professionals and politicians. Indeed, the National Rural Health Alliance suggests that there is an emerging crisis in rural and remote nursing (NRHA 2002). Nurses provide the highest proportion of health care in rural and remote Australia (NRHA 2002), with 30.4% of nurses working in rural and remote areas (AIHW 2002). Despite this, there is a shortage of nurses, and an ageing workforce with an average age of 45–50 years. Many of these nurses will retire in the next ten years but only a small percentage of graduates are going into rural areas. The shortages are in many areas and many specialities, but the most urgent are in the aged-care sector (AARN 2002).

Handley (1998) draws attention to the difficulty of attracting health professionals to work in rural areas, and points to the shortage of GPs and medical specialists in particular. So although the rural health workforce comprises a range of health-care professionals, attention has centred on the perceived rural doctor shortage, and in the past few years much effort has been expended in securing the services of doctors, especially GPs (Best 2000). However, in recent years more Commonwealth funding has been directed towards the needs of rural and remote nurses. Currently the government funds the Australian Remote and Rural Scholarship Program, which provides incentives for people to pursue a career in nursing or for nurses to build on a career in this area. The program consists of four different scholarship schemes, including re-entry and upskilling, postgraduate, conference and undergraduate (DHA 2003). It is administered through the Royal College of Nursing Australia.

There have also been State and Territory initiatives to develop the role of nurse practitioner in New South Wales, South Australia and Victoria, as well as isolated practice endorsement in Queensland (NRHA 2003). The federal government has also provided $104 million over four years for GPs to employ practice nurses (DHA 2003). This proposal is not without controversy and the AARN (2002) has voiced its concern that the deflection of resources to general practice could in fact make the shortage worse, especially in the public sector, and draw attention away from the needs of other types of nurses.

It is crucial to the health of rural people to have an effective nursing workforce. With the declining population base of rural areas, the traditional pool of women who continue to nurse at the local hospital is diminishing as the population shifts to regional centres. Another reason that rural areas may find it difficult to attract nurses is that better graduate programs are offered by metropolitan hospitals, with a perceived lack of opportunity to maintain knowledge and skills in rural areas

(AARN 2002). It is hoped that the provision of scholarships may go some way towards alleviating this problem.

Defining the rural nurse's role

There is no universally accepted definition of a rural nurse (Handley 1998). Most writers attempt to define the scope of rural nursing practice rather than the term 'rural nurse' itself. Central themes in most definitions are about the restricted access of nurses to other health professionals or a nurse's geographical location (Handley 1998, p 7). Kreger (1991) identifies the rural nurse as one who practises in an environment where the availability of medical practitioners (and other health personnel and support services) is not guaranteed. Thornton describes rural nursing practice as:

> the practice of nursing in a country community with population between 500 and 10,000 people who have access at most times to at least one medical practitioner living within the town.
>
> Thornton 1992, p 121

Another definition refers to:

> a nurse who works in a hospital where the support services are predominantly part-time or visiting services, and in the community or district-nursing role in a non-metropolitan area.
>
> Hegney, Pearson & McCarthy 1997, p 46

Rural nursing is practised in diverse working environments, and in degrees of isolation which may be both physical and professional because of the lack of immediate support available to the nurse.

Scope of practice

It is in this context of a lack of medical practitioners and allied health professionals that rural nurses have expanded their scope of practice. Some functions adopted by rural nurses that were identified by Kreger as early as 1991 include medical, pharmaceutical and allied health—in addition to the usual curative, maintenance, illness-prevention, health-promotion and community-development nursing responsibilities (Kreger 1991). Hegney (1997) also talks about the role of rural nurses in Australia, and how this is extended into medicine (including suturing, physical assessment and cannulation), pharmacy (dispensing and supplying) and all the other allied health disciplines (including radiography).

People living in rural and remote areas often depend on nurses for their health care—nurses are almost always the first point of contact for people in these areas seeking health care. These areas have a much lower provision of health-care workers and often extensive travel is required to reach support services at distant regional centres. Nurses frequently provide a range of primary health-care functions that would be provided by general practitioners and allied health professionals in metropolitan areas (NRNE 2002). The nurse's role is comprehensive, embracing: 'emergency care including dental, health promotion and illness prevention, managing chronic physical and mental illness, aged care, environmental and population health' (NRHA 2002).

The Review of Nursing Education (Steering Committee for the National Review of Nurse Education in the Higher Education Sector 1994) identified a need for specialist nurses across Australia, including rural and remote areas. There is, however, some difficulty with this. Hegney (1997) argues that rural nurses lose specialist skills due to lack of opportunity to practise and little opportunity for upgrading knowledge and skills (NRHA 2002). Handley & Blue (1998), however, point out that there is a reduced incentive for nurses to become specialists as complex cases are frequently transferred to other centres.

However, in recent years there has been a shift to multiskilling, as community-based and traditional health care is provided to people of all ages and across diverse social and cultural groups. Nurses are taking on leadership roles in the community through, for example, community development initiatives such as community building. These activities require some advanced skills but rural nurses have little opportunity for upgrading to such knowledge and skills (NRHA 2002). We are therefore building a picture of rural areas in which the traditional role of hospital-based nursing or community settings are primarily about aged care, with increasing emphasis on the expansion of community-based care. There is a need to move traditional hospital nurses into primary health care and population or community approaches, including health education, community and individual needs assessments and environmental scanning (NRHA 2002).

Francis et al (2001) have summarised the continuing challenges for rural nurses—these include issues of professional isolation, scarce resources for health promotion and public health, expectations of multiskilling rather than a focus on specialist skills, and a limited scope to specialise, legal implications of practising in an expanded role, and identifying professional boundaries of practice. As nurses working in rural and remote areas are currently working outside the scope of the law, the need for legitimacy of nurses' extended roles is vital (DHS 1996a).

As mentioned previously, the Commonwealth Government has recently made funds available to support GPs in employing practice nurses. While recognising concerns about the tendency to fund nurses through general practice, it does, however, provide an opportunity to provide elderly people with increased access to primary care. At present the role of the practice nurse is under-developed and there is little agreement as to what it involves. At present it seems to depend on how the particular GP views the role, and on the relationship between the GP and the nurse. The Royal College of Nursing Australia (RCNA) and the Royal Australian College of General Practitioners (RACGP) have recently united to conduct a joint project examining the roles of nurses working in general practice. It is funded by the Commonwealth Government and will include a national survey of nurses working in general practice, and joint nurse/GP workshops will be held around the country (RCNA 2003).

The paradigm of caring in contemporary nursing is a contested notion in relation to older people. Nursing care is more frequently given to the aged and to people with disabilities, but academic programs tend to emphasise technical nursing (Stevens & Couch 1998). Another disparity lies between the propensity of the nursing profession to adopt models of caring for the sick rather than models of public health or community nursing. This means that the care of older people is commonly cast in terms of geriatrics—influenced heavily by the biomedical model, which emphasises incapacity, decline and regression. Thus, caring and public health interventions—and their potential for positive outcomes in terms of quality of life, dignity, independence (however relative), and equitable access to health-promoting programs and services—may be excluded.

The present discussion rests on the premise that nursing education needs to be liberated from illness (and the technical aspects of care) to make way for a greater understanding of the significance of public health, as discussed above. This is especially the case for rural nurses.

The popular image of a rural nurse is dramatised by pictures depicting a nurse working alongside a flying doctor and saving a young person's life against the odds. Of course, the reality is quite different for the rural gerontic nurse who promotes the health of well elderly people or tends to the needs of the frail elderly. It seems that rural nurses in general do not identify themselves as gerontic nurses, nor do they acknowledge that they are primarily caring for old or very old people.

This lack of awareness has major implications for the care provided, because elderly people require specialised care by nurses—just as other age-groups, such as adolescents, require special skills and knowledge. There is also a problem in that the label of 'acute-care nurse' has a much higher status than that of 'gerontic nurse' (Nay 1992) and this problem possibly applies also to rural nurses. A browse through the Contents pages of standard gerontological nursing texts reveals that the needs of older rural people appear to have been entirely overlooked. There are some studies from the United States that deal with nursing care of older rural people. Lee (1993) identifies strategies for the delivery of nursing care to rural elderly individuals and Cudney (1991) reports on special approaches which she had developed to enhance the accessibility of continuing nursing education for rural nurses. Buckwalter et al (1993) report on the lack of services available to elderly people with psychiatric problems, and on the development of a nursing-outreach model. Johnson & Moore (1988) identify the drug-taking practices of a small group of rural elderly, and demonstrate that the problems were related to lack of access to the rural nurse.

Rural nurses' gerontic education

Undergraduate rural and gerontic nursing education

The National Review of Nurse Education (2002), in its consideration of rural nursing education, recommends that nursing programs be responsive to the competencies required for rural nursing practice, and to the problems of access to education and professional isolation (NRNE 2002, p 153). The Review found that there are a significant number of undergraduate nursing curricula which do not include coverage of Indigenous issues and rural and remote health issues. Yet, rural universities and campuses are in a good position to respond to local circumstances when designing the curriculum.

Nursing education has recently been identified as a national priority area and the Commonwealth is to increase its support to institutions offering nursing courses. It anticipates that the additional funding will go towards the cost of supporting clinical practice. Regional campuses will gain an extra 210 places by 2004, increasing to 574 by 2007. Nursing will remain in the lowest HECS band and universities will not be able to increase HECS for nursing courses. Furthermore, there will be additional financial support for regional universities based on their proximity to a capital city and the number of enrolled students (Commonwealth Department of Health and Ageing 2003)

Postgraduate rural and gerontic nursing education

Issues identified for postgraduate education include the following:

- It is inaccessible and expensive.
- New graduates are unable to cope with rural health service environments because they have inadequate specific undergraduate preparation.
- Access to professional development is limited (AARN 2002).

The rural-nursing literature (Hegney 1997; Hegney et al 1997; Duffy & Siegloff 1997) generally does not specifically acknowledge that older people comprise a significant proportion of a nurse's client-base in rural areas and that, as a consequence, nurses might require specialised knowledge and skills about older people in order to deliver effective interventions. Hegney et al (1997) refer to the education and training needs of rural nurses, but in the list of various nursing specialities the specialised care required for nursing older people is not mentioned. This study involved 129 rural health services with acute beds, with the majority (84) having 11–50 acute beds. The study did not include any stand-alone aged-care facilities, or any community-health services, district-nursing services or psychiatric-only services. Yet most patients admitted to these small acute facilities would have been over 65 years of age.

Thus, despite the growing strength of the rural-nursing movement, the reality of rural Australian health care in relation to older people has not yet been acknowledged. This may be due to the fact that rural nursing is a multiskilled role, thus blinding educators to the fact that aged care is a specialised area which warrants appropriate educational programs. When combined with nurses' propensity to see older people simply as diseased bodies, there is a lack of fit with the increasing focus on the provision of preventive, public and community-health services for rural Australia. Thus, the specific needs of rural older people in the provision of public-health services are not well understood among rural nurses.

We propose that rural nursing is actually an extended or advanced practice role that is congruent with a range of specialities—of which gerontic nursing, in a range of models of health provision, is integral. The nurse in this role is often the main health-care provider for a client, be it in the community or in the extended-care setting. In aged-care residential facilities or in the community, gerontic nurses are frequently involved in a range of activities, including:

- making certain medical diagnoses such as urinary tract infection (although anecdotal experience suggests that many nurses fiercely deny this diagnostic role);
- ordering the appropriate diagnostic tests; and
- initiating treatment.

Gerontic nurses often know their clients intimately because they have been caring for them over an extended period of time. Similarly, rural nurses know their patients well because they are often part of the same small community—which can present difficulties in the area of confidentiality. Rural nurses are, however, in an ideal position to provide comprehensive, holistic patient care. However, although rural and gerontic nurses have many skills in common, and although the rural nurse is of necessity a generalist, rural nurses still require adequate educational preparation for their specialist role in the care of elderly people.

In their pursuit of further education, rural nurses face barriers of distance, costs, lack of family support, family commitments and lack of confidence (Kreger 1991; Lampshire & Rolfe 1994). Rural nurses do not always see themselves as undergoing career development. Even when there are educational opportunities, rural nurses may be reluctant to pursue them—because of the stereotyped attitudes towards women's careers that are often prevalent in the country and because of the cost of postgraduate education. It may be acceptable for a woman to take on part-time nursing work to augment the farm and family income, but this does not always translate into support for her career development. Thus, rural nurses do not always translate their nursing work into a career—and perhaps this is not dissimilar to gerontic nurses in general.

Advanced practice for rural nurses

The knowledge and skills needed by rural nurses to respond adequately to the needs of older people comprise the elements of both an advanced practice nurse and/or a nurse practitioner. For the provision of credential education to meet the needs of nurses working in these roles, it is suggested that flexible, relevant learning be provided, and that:

> add-on specialist modules which meet the criteria for nurse practitioner accreditation be offered by service and education providers to provide the necessary context-based clinical knowledge, skills and attitudes relevant to particular areas of practice.
>
> New South Wales Department of Health 1995

Many rural nurses will work in small to medium-sized rural health services which require multiskilled staff. Although there has been considerable debate about the precise definition of a nurse practitioner, a rural nurse working with older rural people would encapsulate many of the dimensions of what is usually understood to be the role of the nurse practitioner. Nurses in rural and remote Australia are frequently required to be multiskilled in general nursing, midwifery and community health—which encompasses health-promotion programs, illness-prevention programs, community-support work, program planning, program implementation, program evaluation and (perhaps) research. Thus, a nurse in a sparsely populated area may have duties as the maternal and child-health nurse, but may also have duties involving health-program development and the care of older people.

For good health outcomes and quality of life, older people require the positive interventions that public health can deliver. We know that public health is practised by contemporary nurses in a wide variety of community-based settings because nurses are unique in their ability to combine clinical skills with community-based skills and knowledge. However, rural nurses are rarely defined as working in public health—although they are increasingly working in multipurpose models of service provision.

For the service models (now being established in rural areas) to work, they require staff who are flexible in working with different models of practice. The nurses who staff these new service models require education in public-health strategies such as:

- needs assessment, health needs priority setting and program planning;
- health education, health promotion (and program evaluation);
- illness-prevention programs;
- women's health, men's health; and
- leadership in chronic disease management.

As models of health care have broadened, recognition has been given to the importance of health maintenance, illness prevention, the restoration of health after illness, and health promotion for both young and old people. These are strategies of the public-health endeavour that comprise a public-health model of health-care delivery that is just as pertinent for older people as for other age groups.

> while some physical abilities deteriorate with age, the majority of health issues associated with ageing have the potential for successful preventative action.
>
> VicHealth 1996, p 3

There is increasing evidence that diet and exercise play an important role in the prevention of poor health in older people, and in the promotion of quality of life, just as they do for younger people. Indeed, there is evidence that much functional decline is due to lack of exercise (VicHealth 2003). Furthermore, VicHealth have identified social isolation and social connectedness as core determinants of physical and mental health conditions. This clearly illustrates that the advanced-practice nurse can accommodate public-health approaches, including client education and encouragement of healthy lifestyle practices. This is vital when older rural people are unable to access the usual range of preventive and curative services which are taken for granted by city dwellers.

CONCLUSION

Although the gerontic-nursing literature has largely ignored the special needs of the rural elderly, and although the rural-nursing literature has not addressed the ageing of the rural population (and its implications for nursing practice), this chapter has provided a framework for considering the work of rural nurses with older rural Australians. It has described an advanced-nursing practice role that integrates rural nursing practice and gerontic-nursing practice with public health. Nurses can provide innovative, flexible delivery of services in public health frameworks. In the face of some of the rural-health problems outlined in this chapter, the particular approaches to rural nursing described here can only enhance the health and well-being of older Australians.

References

Association for Australian Rural Nurses (AARN) 2002, Submission to the National Review of Nursing Education.

Australian Institute of Health and Welfare (AIHW) 1997, *The Health and Welfare of Australia's Aboriginal and Torres Strait Islander Peoples*, AGPS, AIHW Cat. No. 4704.0, AGPS: Canberra.

Australian Institute of Health and Welfare (AIHW) 2000, *Australia's Health 2000*, AIHW, AIHW Cat. No. AUS 19, AGPS: Canberra.

Australian Institute of Health and Welfare (AIHW) 2002, *Australia's Health 2002*, AIHW, AIHW Cat. No. AUS 25, AGPS: Canberra.

Best J 2000, *Rural Health Stocktake*, advisory paper to Commonwealth Department of Health and Aged Care: Canberra.

Buckley P 1997, A political profile. In: Siegloff L (ed), *Rural Nursing in the Australian Context*, Royal College of Nursing: Canberra.

Carson N 1997, Health status of rural Victorians: Strengthening health partnerships in your rural community. In: *Proceedings of the National Rural Public Health Forum 12–15 October 1997*, pp 62–8, National Rural Health Alliance, Commonwealth Departments of Primary Industries and Energy, and Health and Family Services.

Commonwealth Department of Health and Ageing (DHA) 2003, The Australian Remote and Rural Scholarship Program. Online: http://www.ruralhealth.gov.au/workers/nursing.htm, accessed 21 July 2003.

Crowe M 1996, Health promotion needs of older Aboriginal people, *Australian Journal of Ageing*, 15(1), pp 11–13.

Department of Health and Family Services (DHFS) 1994, *National Rural Health Strategy*, Australian Health Ministers' Conference, AGPS: Canberra.

Department of Health and Family Services (DHFS) 1996, *National Rural Health Strategy*, Australian Health Ministers' Conference, AGPS: Canberra.

Department of Human Services (DHS) 1996a, *The MPS Option: Health and Aged Care in Rural Communities*, DHS: Melbourne.

Department of Human Services (DHS) 1996b, *Summary of the Healthstreams Program and Co-operative Rural Health Planning*, DHS: Melbourne.

Duffy E & Siegloff L 1997, Models for health and nursing in rural communities. In: Siegloff L (ed), *Rural Nursing in the Australian Context*, Royal College of Nursing: Canberra.

Frager L, Gray ER, Franklin R & Petrauskas V 1997, *A Picture of Health? A Preliminary Report of the Health of Country Australia's Demographic Profile*, Vol 1, The Australian Agricultural Health Unit: Moree, NSW.

Francis K, Bowman S & Redgrave M 2001, *Rural Nurses: Knowledge and Skills Required to Meet the Challenges of a Changing Work Environment in the 21st Century: A Review of the Literature*, Department of Education, Science and Training: Canberra.

Handley A 1998, *Setting the Scene: Rural Nurses in Australia*, Royal College of Nursing: Canberra.

Handley A & Blue I 1998, *Education, Training and Support for Australian Rural Nurses*, Royal College of Nursing: Canberra.

Hegney D 1997, Rural nursing practice. In: Siegloff L (ed), *Rural Nursing in the Australian Context*, Royal College of Nursing: Canberra.

Hegney D, Pearson A & McCarthy A 1997, *The Role and Function of the Rural Nurse in Australia*, Royal College of Nursing: Canberra.

Humphreys J & Rolley E 1991, *Health and Health Care in Rural Australia: A Literature Review*, University of New England: Armidale, NSW.

Humphreys J, Mathews-Cowley S & Rolley E 1996, *Health Service Frameworks for Small Rural and Remote Communities: Issues and Options*, Department of Geography and Planning, University of New England: Armidale, NSW.

Kreger A and National Nursing Consultative Committee 1991, *Enhancing the Role of Rural and Remote Area Nurses*, Commonwealth Department of Health, Housing and Community Services: Canberra.

Lampshire H & Rolfe J 1994, *From the Lamp to the Laser: Educational Needs of Victorian Rural Nurses*, Department of Health and Community Services, AGPS: Canberra.

National Review of Nursing Education (NRNE) 2002, *Our Duty of Care: Final Report of National Review of Nursing Education*, Ausinfo: Canberra.

National Rural Health Alliance Inc (NRHA) 2002, *Nursing in Rural and Remote Areas* (Issues Paper), National Rural Health Alliance Inc: Canberra.

New South Wales Department of Health 1995, *Nurse Practitioner Project, Stage 3*, Final Report of the Steering Committee, NSW Department of Health: Sydney.

Royal College of Nursing Australia (RCNA) 2003, *Rural and Remote Nursing Bulletin*, 5(5), RCNA: Canberra.

Siegloff L (ed) 1997, *Rural Nursing in the Australian Context*, Royal College of Nursing: Canberra.

Siegloff L & Buckley P 1998, Nurse practitioners and workforce planning considerations. In: *Nurse Practitioners' Conference Proceedings*, Royal College of Nursing: Canberra.

Standing Committee on Family and Community Affairs 2000, *Health is Life: Report on the Inquiry into Indigenous Health*, Parliament of Australia: Canberra.

Steering Committee for the National Review of Nurse Education in the Higher Education Sector—1994 and Beyond, 1994, *Nursing Education in Australian Universities*, AGPS: Canberra.

Stevens J & Couch M 1998, Care—the guiding principle of nursing? In: Keleher H & McInerney E (eds), *Nursing Matters*, pp 157–66, Harcourt Brace: Sydney.

Thornton R 1992, Rural nursing practice. In: Gray G & Pratt R (eds), *Issues in Australian Nursing*, Churchill Livingstone: Melbourne.

Victorian Health Promotion Foundation (VicHealth) 1996, Older People, *VicHealth Letter*, (5), pp 3–13.

Victorian Health Promotion Foundation (VicHealth) 2003, Planning for Health, *VicHealth Letter*, (19), pp 1–24.

Women's Health Australia 1997, *Data Book for the Baseline Survey of the Australian Longitudinal Study on Women's Health*, University of Newcastle: Newcastle, NSW.

Woodward M 1996, Drug prescribing for older people: can we get it right?, *Australian Journal of Ageing*, 15(1), pp 11–13.

CHAPTER 9

Acute care of older people: a geriatrician's perspective

PHILIP STREET

INTRODUCTION

Younger people visiting an acute public hospital ward for the first time are often struck by the large proportion of older patients. In some areas, especially general medical wards, seeing a young or even middle-aged person is almost a noteworthy event. It is assumed by healthy younger people that older people are sicker than younger people, and for a diverse range of conditions which may lead to hospital admission, such as heart failure (Ho et al 1993), stroke (Wolf et al 1992), certain malignancies (Patterson & Calabresi 2000), pneumonia (Jokinen et al 1993) and hip fracture (Boyce & Vessey 1985), this assumption holds true. When combined with the effects of pre-existing disability and, to some extent, the ageing process itself, it is not surprising that sick older people are frequently admitted to hospitals and are over-represented in the hospital population.

The problems and needs of frail older patients pose a major challenge to the hospital system. There is increasing pressure on acute hospitals to treat more patients and to reduce length of stay, with an emphasis on discharging patients as soon as possible after medical or surgical conditions have been treated. Acute hospitals, which are geared towards treating acutely ill patients, are now caring for more older people, who may not conform to the usual picture of patients who are 'sick', but who still need to be in hospital for care related to their underlying disability. Physical and cognitive impairment may lead to stress on carers or other family members of older people, and the social situation may be tenuous. Patients awaiting permanent residential care in acute hospitals also cannot be discharged quickly to the community. All these factors militate against a short hospital stay and early discharge.

Generalisations cannot be made about all older people in hospital having a unique range of problems that unambiguously sets them apart from younger people. It is also important to recognise that older people do not form a single, monolithic patient population. Age alone is not the sole determinant of whether someone has problems typically associated with older people; and chronologically old but otherwise robust patients may have uncomplicated hospital admissions. However, increasing age is associated with a higher prevalence of cognitive impairment, physical disability and multiple medical conditions. It is vulnerable or 'frail' patients with these problems who are seen as requiring a specialised approach to care at an individual and health system level.

THE EFFECTS OF CHANGING DEMOGRAPHICS

Older people are admitted to hospital more commonly and have a longer length of stay than younger people. For the 2000/2001 financial year, in all Australian hospitals, people aged over 65, who comprise 12.1% of the population, accounted for 33% of hospital separations and 48% of hospital days. Their average length of stay (ALOS) was 5.3 days compared to 3.7 days for all patients (Australian Institute of Health and Welfare [AIHW] 2002). The hospital length of stay increases with age, and figures for public hospitals are shown in Table 9.1. The separation rate for older people is higher than for younger people and increases with advancing age, as shown in Table 9.2. On average, in the over-85 age group a male spends just over, and a female just under, seven days in a public hospital per year, compared to figures of about half a day for males and females in the 40–45 year age group.

Table 9.1: Public hospital admission rates and days data, Australia, 2000–01

	Age group					
	40–45 years		**65–69 years**		**85+ years**	
	Female	Male	Female	Male	Female	Male
ALOS (days)	2.8	3.2	3.9	4.0	10.9	9.2
Separation rate/1000	155	135	356	453	616	767
Hospital days/1000	438	434	1402	1794	6731	7082

Demographic changes in Australia within the coming decades will result in increasing numbers of older people, in both absolute and relative terms, being admitted to the hospital system. Various models, taking into account different fertility, mortality and migration rates, have been used to estimate population increases over the next century. Table 9.2 shows the estimated population increase of older Australians using a model which makes assumptions about population growth which lie between the highest and lowest scenarios (Australian Bureau of Statistics [ABS] 2000). Numbers in parentheses represent the percentage of the total population. The life expectancy of someone who reaches age 65 is expected to increase from 85 in the year 2000 to 95 in the year 2050 for females and from 81 to 94 for males over the same period.

Table 9.2: Projected increase in population of older Australians, 2000–51

	Projected increase (% total population)		
Year	**65+ years (%)**	**75+ years (%)**	**85+ years (%)**
1999	2.32 million (12.2)	1.03 million (5.4)	241,000 (1.2)
2020	4.22 million (18.4)	1.79 million (7.8)	479,000 (2.1)
2050	6.62 million (26.1)	3.70 million (14.6)	1,239,800 (5.1)

Disease prevention and health promotion strategies may have an impact on some conditions, but are unlikely to be able to compensate for the effect these demographic changes will have on hospital admission numbers. Encouraging trends have been reported in regard to the falling incidence of disabling diseases such as stroke (Jamrozik et al 1999; Thorvaldsen et al 1999) and, in some regions, myocardial infarction (Davidsen et al 2001), at least partly due to lifestyle changes. However, the projected increase in the number of older people admitted for stroke is greater than the declining incidence (Marini et al 2001), meaning that this disabling disease will be seen in increasing numbers in coming years. The situation for hip fracture is similar in that the effects of interventions to reduce osteoporosis or falls risk are likely to be more than overtaken by the increasing numbers of older people. Numbers of hip-fracture patients will therefore also increase substantially (Pocock et al 1999; Sanders et al 1999).

OLDER PEOPLE AND ACUTE ILLNESS

Patient characteristics: age or disability based

Chronological age is not the sole factor in determining whether a patient develops problems for which specialised aged care input may be required. Patients with an acute disabling illness, multiple medical co-morbidities, pre-existing physical disability or cognitive impairment are often targeted as being at risk of an adverse functional outcome during hospitalisation. Specialised aged-care services may be called to help manage these patients, most but not all of whom will be chronologically 'old'. Many older patients in an acute hospital, irrespective of age, will not have these problems and do not develop the complications for which aged-care input is sought.

The concept of 'frailty' may best define the group of patients who aged-care services see as their constituency. The term 'frailty' describes a state of vulnerability along a number of axes encompassing physical, cognitive, psychological and social parameters, without implying an underlying diagnosis. This places the person at risk of a number of adverse events including poor medical outcomes, further decline in functional and cognitive skills and increased likelihood of death or need for residential care. Frailty is the result of the cumulative effects of diminished physiological reserve and disease, interacting with other factors such as poor nutrition, physical inactivity and psychosocial problems. The frail older person is therefore more vulnerable to the insults of acute or progressive chronic disease, of external stress including trauma or the adverse effects of medications (Campbell & Buchner 1997). The frail older person is regarded as at best functioning close to a threshold level, with physical illness or psychosocial stress 'tipping the balance' and leading to adverse functional consequences. One component of frailty is muscular wasting and weakness. Someone described as being frail is usually thin and wasted, but non-physical components of frailty such as underlying cognitive impairment or tenuous social supports may also be important. Frailty better defines the patient population who will develop conditions typical of but not confined to older people, and who may benefit from aged-care assessment or intervention (Winograd et al 1991).

Acute care of older people: perception and reality

From a specialist aged-care perspective it is tempting to be over-critical and negative when considering the care of older patients in acute hospitals. This perception often arises from the less than ideal management of a relatively small number of older people, as a result of which aged-care staff in the hospital or community are 'left to pick up the pieces'. However, it should be acknowledged that these cases may give a biased impression, and that appropriately managed older or disabled patients do not come to the attention of aged-care staff. Acute hospitals are experienced in dealing with the needs of their older patients, including disability- and socially related issues, as well as with the acute medical illness. Staff working in the aged-care system tend to forget that only a minority of older people admitted to acute hospitals are referred for admission to a sub-acute aged-care ward.

Even in acute hospital units most attuned to the needs of older patients, there is still the potential for tension to arise between the needs of the individual patient and the needs of the hospital. Much of this centres around length of stay and the timing of discharge. Staff working in acute hospitals are under constant pressure for beds to be made available, and to discharge patients when it is deemed that they no longer need to be in hospital and can manage at home. A decision may be made to discharge an older person who seems medically stable, but who either has unrecognised medical problems, or would not manage because of impaired function or lack of adequate social support. If barriers to discharge are identified, especially after the discharge has been organised and the bed filled by a new patient, advocacy for the older patient within the acute hospital is not always an easy task.

PRESENTATION OF DISEASE IN OLDER PEOPLE

The way in which frail older people present with disease often differs from that of younger people. Elderly people may not present with specific localising symptoms when ill, and are more likely to have a non-specific disease presentation. Complaints may include falls, declining mobility, confusion or simply 'not coping' or being 'unwell'. Non-specific disease presentation is associated with the limited ability of frail older people to withstand external stress. Reduced mobility may be due to many underlying causes not directly related to neurological or musculoskeletal factors, such as a chest or urinary tract infection, cardiac failure or the effects of drugs. Age-related changes in mobility include reduced proximal strength due to Type II fibre atrophy, impaired balance related to slowing in the 'central processing' of visual, vestibular and proprioceptive inputs, and increased stiffness of the weight-bearing joints. These changes are accentuated by any pathology such as knee osteoarthritis, painful foot lesions or gait disorders related to cerebrovascular disease. The seemingly mild effects of a medical insult may therefore be sufficient to render an older person immobile, especially one who is functioning at close to the threshold of dependence. This in turn may be the main presenting problem rather than any local symptoms.

Another effect of this non-specific disease presentation is that functional and social factors may dominate the clinical picture, as one of the consequences may be increased dependency on others, and the possibility of underlying acute medical problems may not be considered. In the older patient presenting with immobility, for example, no obvious local weakness or other signs may be found to indicate any acute cause. If it has been difficult to take a history because of cognitive impairment, or there appear to be social factors contributing to the presentation, labels such as 'social admission', or the even more pejorative 'acopia' may be applied. A thorough and detailed assessment process should always be undertaken to exclude any organic problems before labeling a presentation as being due to a non-medical cause. Precarious social circumstances do not constitute a proper medical diagnosis, or justify the use of unhelpful and ageist terms.

RECOVERY FROM DISEASE IN THE FRAIL ELDERLY

Older people in general usually take longer to recover from illnesses or operations than younger people. A corollary of this slower recovery is that there is often a lag between clinical and functional recovery from the illness. Younger people with no pre-existing disability will have some functional effects from an acute illness—for example, leg weakness and reduced endurance after prolonged bed rest—but will usually regain sufficient function to enable them to mobilise as they recover from the illness itself. On the other hand, in frail older people the functional consequences of the acute illness persist for longer than the recovery from the illness itself. One important functional effect is impaired mobility, which results from a combination of bed rest, undernutrition and the catabolic effects of some illnesses on muscle strength. Improvements in cognition and continence may also be delayed after medical recovery. The functional lag is as important for conditions treated in acute medical wards, such as congestive cardiac failure and pneumonia, which may not seem to have as direct an effect on mobility as, for example, a hip fracture. Clinical improvement as assessed by physical examination findings or investigation results cannot therefore always be equated with concomitant recovery in physical or cognitive function.

In an acute hospital, a long recovery period is incompatible with a short length of stay. The delay between physical and functional recovery therefore has considerable relevance and highlights the importance of considering physical function in addition to medical parameters when planning for discharge. There will often be pressure to discharge an older person who seems to be 'medically stable' after an operation or illness, but in whom the functional consequences of the illness have not been considered. For example, after an episode of pneumonia, an older person may clinically not be tachypnoeic, have fewer chest signs, normal oxygen saturations, a normalising white blood cell count and improving chest X-ray appearance. The patient is 'medically stable' so plans may be made for discharge, not taking into account the patient's reduced mobility, urinary incontinence and ongoing delirium. This scenario is not uncommonly encountered in hospital practice and again demonstrates that the imperative of early hospital discharge can be at odds with the need of older people for a more prolonged recovery period.

The example below illustrates how illness may present, and how limited reserve in a number of body systems often interacts to magnify the effects of the underlying disease, with effects on physical and cognitive function.

Mrs S, an 85-year-old, is admitted to the hospital with a history of deteriorating function in the hostel where she resides. She is found to have pneumonia following an initial viral respiratory infection. She has been diagnosed as having an underlying early Alzheimer's dementia, and has a past history of osteoarthritis and hypertension. She normally ambulates the 20 metres between her room and the dining area using a four-wheeled frame and requires assistance in dressing and showering. Her arterial oxygen saturation is low and she is commenced on oxygen and intravenous antibiotics. Soon after her admission to the ward she becomes delirious and is treated with oral haloperidol. Her oral intake the next day is only 500 mL, leading to increasing renal impairment and electrolyte disturbance. As a result, Mrs S feels more unwell and is reluctant to ambulate. After five days of intravenous antibiotic treatment, her pneumonia improves and she begins to drink more. However, she remains very confused, and when seen by the physiotherapist she can only mobilise short distances with maximal assistance. She is also noted to have a small sacral pressure area and her family confirm continuing confusion. They are concerned that she will not manage at the hostel and may need to be cared for in a nursing home.

Mrs S is at greater risk of the development of both illness and declining physical function than a previously well younger person. Changes in lung structure and function leading to reduced clearance of lung secretions make her more susceptible to the development of pneumonia after a viral infection. Alterations in thirst mechanisms in older people, and age-associated changes in kidney structure (nephrosclerosis and tubular atrophy) and function (reduced glomerular filtration rate) make her more liable to develop acute renal impairment. This effect is magnified by any underlying pathology such as renovascular disease related to her hypertension. Mrs S is more likely to develop delirium as she has an underlying dementia, and changes in drug metabolism mean that she will be more sensitive to the effects of sedative drugs. Her limited ambulation prior to hospitalisation means that only a small reduction in muscle strength, on this occasion induced by bed rest, will be sufficient to render her immobile even though the pneumonia is improving. The bed rest has also led to the development of a pressure area. The combined effect has been to jeopardise her continued residence at the hostel.

This example demonstrates the cascade effect of an acute illness on a number of systems and on physical function. It also demonstrates the complexity of the relationship between acute illness, pre-existing conditions and age-related changes in various body systems. In a practical sense the concept that an older person is more susceptible to multiple otherwise 'subclinical' physiological disturbances, and that these interact with one another and have an effect on function, is essential to understanding disease presentation in older people. Recognising the clinical signs of these disturbances, anticipating their effects and attempting to prevent their future consequences lies at the heart of skilled nursing and medical care of sick older people.

GERIATRIC SYNDROMES AND ACUTE HOSPITALISATION

The increased incidence of medical co-morbidities, activity limitation and cognitive impairment in older people gives rise to a number of conditions which, although not occurring exclusively in the geriatric population, have been labelled 'geriatric syndromes' (Tinetti et al 1995). The problems that fall under this rubric include delirium, falls, impaired mobility, incontinence, pressure ulcers and polypharmacy. These conditions are not a normal part of ageing, but usually occur as a result of an interplay between the ageing process, illness, external factors (including drugs) and pre-morbid physical and cognitive function. They occur outside the hospital environment, but the medical problems leading to hospital admission, and the stress of the hospitalisation, mean that they often develop or are worsened by the hospital admission itself. It is important to have some understanding of the interrelationship between some of these 'geriatric syndromes' and the hospital admission, and to be aware of strategies for the prevention and management of some of these syndromes in hospital.

Delirium

Delirium is a transient disturbance in cognitive and attentional function, characterised by a fluctuating course and an alteration in the conscious state. It is much more common in older people and occurs in about 20% of all hospital admissions (Trzepacz 1996). The most important risk factor for the development of delirium is underlying cognitive impairment (usually dementia) with up to 40% of people with dementia who are admitted to hospital developing delirium, and 25% of patients with delirium having an unrecognised dementia (Fick et al 2002; Rahkonen et al 2000). Other risk factors are sensory impairments (hearing and visual) and advancing age. Any acute illness can precipitate delirium, as can the effects of certain drugs, pain and physical and psychological distress. Multiple causative factors are usually present (Rudberg et al 1997).

Diagnosing delirium is important as it may be the only clue to an otherwise unsuspected condition such as an infection. Nursing staff may be in a better position to suspect delirium than medical staff, who only see the patient for a short period each day and who have been shown to miss the diagnosis of delirium in up to a third of cases (Inouye 1994). Delirium should be considered in any older person hospitalised with acute illness, especially if there is a non-specific, otherwise unexplained deterioration in the patient's condition. A short, four-item instrument known as the Confusion Assessment Method (CAM), has been developed to help in diagnosis and has shown sensitivity and specificity of over 90% in clinical use (Inouye et al 1990).

Delirium has been associated with an increased hospital length of stay, an increased rate of institutionalisation on discharge, and possibly an increased mortality (George et al 1997), though the latter may be due to the severity of the underlying disease causing the delirium. Adverse effects can result from either the delirium itself or its treatment. Confused patients are at increased risk of sustaining injuries from falling, or by other means, especially if cot sides are used. In the acute hospital setting, powerful antipsychotic medications such as haloperidol may be used to settle the patient. This can cause excessive drowsiness, leading to poor oral intake and immobility with the risk of aspiration pneumonia, pressure sores and constipation. Antipsychotic agents may also cause extra-pyramidal or Parkinsonian side-effects, further reducing mobility and increasing the risk of muscle weakness (deconditioning) and falls.

The management of delirium is a good example of 'real-world' medicine often falling short of recommended best practice. Instead of non-pharmacological, environmentally or behaviourally directed measures implemented to prevent delirium, pharmacological agents such as benzodiazepines or haloperidol often form the mainstay of treatment of established delirium. Usually a junior doctor is called at night with a request to sedate an agitated patient. In this often emotionally charged situation, the ideal approach should be only to use sedatives if the patient cannot be calmed by reassurance and other means. Optimal use of sedatives (if they are to be used) in the elderly would be to first assess the patient for a possible reversible cause of the delirium, to use the minimum amount of medication to settle the patient, and to have patience in waiting for the sedative to work. However, the situation rarely proceeds as smoothly as this. Nursing staff will be familiar with the distressing scenario of an agitated patient not initially responding to escalating doses of neuroleptic agents administered by a harassed junior doctor. The drugs may then be given at progressively shorter dosage intervals, until the patient is finally rendered comatose. The full effects of the drug may only wear off after several days, with potentially dire consequences in terms of functional decline.

In contrast, strategies used to prevent and manage delirium have targeted the patients most at risk and concentrated on non-pharmacological interventions to both prevent and treat delirium. It has been shown that an intensive program of delirium prevention can reduce the incidence of delirium in a group of hospitalised patients from 15 to 10% (Inouye et al 1999). The major interventions, targeted at previously identified risk factors, were early mobilisation, prevention of dehydration, screening and providing assistive devices if necessary for hearing and visual impairment, avoidance of sleep deprivation and measures to minimise further cognitive impairment. Length of stay was not reduced. In those who did develop delirium, the severity was similar in treatment and control groups. The program was meticulously planned and evaluated, with substantial input from a large body of trained volunteers who were intensively supervised. A cost-benefit analysis showed that the program was not associated with increased costs to the hospital (Rizzo et al 2001). Although this program was successful, it is not clear whether it can be applied to all hospitals without the expertise, commitment and volunteer resources of the university hospital in which it was undertaken. At least one Australian hospital is now developing a similar multidisciplinary program. Studies targeting specific high-risk groups, such as hip-fracture patients who have rates of delirium of up to 25 and 65% (Inouye 2001) have also shown that the risk of delirium can be reduced by targeting risk factors and precipitating medical conditions (Marcantonio et al 2001). The risk of developing delirium can be reduced but not eliminated, and delirium will continue to be a major management challenge in acute hospitals. In a busy acute ward, environmental modifications such as providing a single room with muted lighting, having only a limited number of nursing staff consistently involved in the patient's care or minimising noise may be difficult to implement. There are other practical non-pharmacological measures which can be initiated by nursing staff. These include making a conscious effort to communicate clearly, ensuring that the patient has glasses or a hearing aid, and calling in the patient's relatives. Unfortunately, all too often these interventions are overlooked, and are usually implemented only in the setting of managing a behaviourally disturbed patient, rather than in trying to prevent delirium. Pharmacological agents will continue to have an important place in the management of delirium, but it is perhaps not too unrealistic to hope that, based on the findings of already published research, the focus will turn towards recognition of those at risk of delirium and the development of a practical program of behavioural and environmental interventions.

Falls

Falls remain a significant risk for older patients in acute hospital wards. Older people are more than twice as likely to fall when hospitalised than when living in the community (Mahoney 1998). Rates of between 4 and 12 falls per 1000 bed days, or up to 10 falls per month in a 25–30 bed ward have been reported (Mahoney 1998) and increasing age is associated with a greater risk of falling. Up to 10% of falls occurring in hospital may lead to serious physical injury, including fractures in approximately 5% of cases (Sutton et al 1994). Less immediately obvious but with potentially greater longer-term effects are the psychological consequences of falls, particularly the phenomenon of fear of further falling (Kressig et al 2001), which in turn may lead to less physical activity and social isolation. Patients who fall tend to have a longer length of stay (Bates et al 1995) and are at greater risk of institutionalisation. Adverse effects for the hospital include increased costs related to the greater length of stay, discharge to institutional settings, and the threat of legal action if a fall is perceived to be a result of the failure of care.

The identification of patients at high risk for falls in the acute hospital setting is important for the development of risk assessment tools and for targeted falls prevention measures. Falls are rarely due to one single, well-defined and identifiable medical cause and usually occur in older people with several risk factors. Those most consistently identified in the acute hospital setting include increasing age, cognitive impairment, medical diagnosis and co-morbidity, reduced mobility, medications, particularly tranquilisers and longer-acting sedatives, and a history of previous falls (Evans et al 2001). Environmental hazards such as slippery floors or obstacles play a part in approximately 10% of falls (Sutton et al 1994), and activity at the time of the fall is important, with up to a third of all falls occurring when a patient is trying to go to the toilet (Mahoney 1998). A number of brief falls risk assessment screening tools, usually completed by nursing staff, focusing on these and other risk factors, have been developed for use in hospital wards. Sensitivity and specificity of these scales is typically of the order of 80% (Oliver et al 1997; Perell et al 2001), although many scales overestimate the number of older patients at high risk of falling, potentially increasing the risk of complications related to bed rest and immobility.

A falls prevention plan should concentrate on risk factors identified for an individual patient, as well as more generally on the overall physical environment and culture of the ward. For example, a patient with delirium and urinary incontinence should if possible be moved close to the nurses' station, be nursed on a bed which can be lowered to the floor, and have a regular toileting regimen instituted. Possible medical causes for the delirium and incontinence should be investigated and treated. Measures to reduce the risk of injury if falls do occur, such as the use of hip protectors, which have been shown to reduce the risk of hip fracture in at-risk older people (Kannus et al 2000; Parker et al 2001), are also an important component of the plan. The environment of the ward is often less amenable to modification in the short term, but identification of potential environmental hazards such as poor toilet access or slippery floors (Healey 1994) may alert staff to the need for greater supervision when mobilising or the provision of appropriate aids. Other interventions include labels or wrist bands for high-risk patients, and use of bed and chair alarms to detect patient movement. If all other measures have failed, minimally restrictive forms of physical restraint, applied and closely monitored within the hospital's restraint policy, may be required. There is little evidence that restraints prevent falls, and restraints such as cot sides should not be used in a delirious patient as they may increase the risk of falls, injury and death (Bates et al 1995). A culture where there is a high awareness of falls prevention should help to promote active identification of those at risk of falling and the implementation of preventative measures as a normal part of ward practice. This is as applicable to medical as to nursing staff.

The evidence that hospital-based falls prevention programs work is not overwhelming (Gillespie et al 2001; Oliver et al 2000). Of the two randomised controlled trials, both of which used a single intervention (Mayo et al 1994; Tideiksaar et al 1993), neither showed a positive effect in reducing falls, and only trials comparing the intervention group with historical controls, most using a multicomponent approach to falls reduction, showed any effect, with a 25% reduction in the number of falls in the intervention group. No single intervention or class of interventions could be identified as being clearly essential for a successful program. However, there were limitations in subject numbers and duration, and limited ability to confine interventions to the study group. Thus it cannot be said that there is 'evidence of no effect', rather that there is 'no evidence of effect'. This should not therefore be grounds for a nihilistic approach to hospital falls prevention.

A fall can be an unpleasant and frightening experience for the older person, and may elicit negative responses from staff and families. One reaction is that falls should *never* happen, and to apportion blame if a fall does occur. After a fall, nursing staff often have to deal with the reaction of families, who may have understandable concerns that a fall has occurred in a hospital where patients should be monitored closely. Families may perceive that the fall has been the result of a deficiency in care. Although the implementation of falls prevention measures should be a priority in those identified at high risk of falls, a zero falls rate can probably only be achieved at the expense of an unacceptable use of physical restraints, and by a greater number of complications related to bed rest if patients are actively discouraged from mobilising. Falls should be regarded as an adverse event, and efforts made to minimise the number of older people falling in hospital. However, falls prevention measures must not be so restrictive as to infringe on the patient's rights and dignity and so hinder their functional recovery from acute illness. The philosophy that as part of this recovery, a patient should be allowed to take some risk, as long as this is clearly not unacceptably high, should not be used as a glib excuse to do nothing whenever a fall occurs, but implies that not all falls are a result of failings in patient care and that some patients will fall even when the highest quality care is being provided.

Acute hospitalisation and chronic disability

Acute hospitalisation may be 'good' for older patients' medical and surgical conditions, but paradoxically may be 'bad' for their chronic disability. There is an expectation that people admitted to an acute hospital for a condition will be treated for and possibly cured of that condition. Even if cure is not possible and treatment essentially palliates symptoms without having any lasting effect on the underlying chronic disorders, the decision to treat is made with the expectation that a positive effect on the medical or surgical conditions with which the patient presents justifies the intervention. Pre-existing chronic disability is seen in over 50% of older patients admitted to acute hospitals (Warshaw et al 1982) but is rarely the focus of management. The acute hospitalisation with prolonged bed rest and the attendant physical and psychological effects of the circumstances surrounding the admission can worsen the degree of disability, even when there are no direct effects of the acute illness itself and the more acute problems leading to admission have been appropriately treated. Hospitals cannot be 'blamed' for this, but worsening of physical function and loss of independence can be one unintended effect of hospitalisation (Creditor 1993).

The term 'deconditioning' refers to the deleterious effects of prolonged bed rest or inactivity on physical functioning, especially mobility (Siebens et al 2000), which is reversed by subsequent activity. Bed rest is a time-honoured measure commonly advised for a wide range of conditions, but evidence for its effectiveness is lacking and usually its adverse effects outweigh any benefit (Allen et al 1999). Younger people lose about 1% of muscle strength per day of bed rest. It is probable that losses for frail older people are similar and especially for those operating closer to the threshold of dependence in mobility, this will be of greater clinical significance. Although often limited to the effects of immobilisation on mobility, the term 'deconditioning' also encompasses adverse effects in other areas including bone loss, postural hypotension, hypoxaemia, balance and decreased cognitive function (Creditor 1993).

Studies have examined the risk factors and prevalence of functional decline associated with acute hospitalisation. Between one- and two-thirds of older people will have some loss of function, including mobility, during and after the hospital admission (Covinsky et al 2003; Hirsch et al 1990; McVey et al 1989; Sager, Franke et al 1996) and this may persist for months post discharge, especially in higher-level instrumental activities of daily living. The most important risk factor for functional decline is not the specific medical diagnosis, but a history of pre-existing functional disability (Wu et al 1995). Other risk factors include previous use of a gait aid, cognitive impairment, age 85 and older, and the need for hospital readmission (Covinsky et al 2003; Mahoney et al 1998; Sager, Franke et al 1996; Sager, Rudberg et al 1996). Risk stratification at admission using a simple three-item instrument based on these risk factors has been shown to predict in-hospital functional decline (Sager, Rudberg et al 1996).

As for hospital falls prevention, evidence for the effectiveness of early mobilisation and exercise programs specifically targeted to prevent deconditioning is not strong. A trend towards improved mobility was found in a trial examining the effectiveness of an acute care unit (Landefeld et al 1995). One trial providing twice-daily exercises supervised by physiotherapy assistants in hospital, and a self-directed home exercise program post discharge, reported some improvement in instrumental activities of daily living (ADL) function at one month after discharge, but with no effect on other outcomes such as measures of mobility (Siebens et al 2000). Length of stay was not reduced, a finding which, if replicated, will not favour development of similar programs.

In a practical sense, recognition of the potential effects of hospitalisation on pre-existing disability, and identification of those at high risk is important, even in the absence of clearly effective interventions. It is appropriate that early hospital management after an emergency admission should focus on the acute problem, but attempts should be made to begin mobilisation as early as medical or surgical factors will allow. The provision of care for sick patients is naturally regarded as the priority of an acute ward. This may mean that a frail elderly person who seems to be recovering from an episode of confusion and left ventricular failure, remains in bed for a few more days and becomes progressively more deconditioned. Given the seemingly more urgent competing demands of 'sicker' patients, it is not surprising that, in practice, mobilisation is often not begun early. Another factor often not considered is the attitude of patients and their families, who expect bed rest as part of the treatment of the illness and who may not respond positively to attempts to begin early mobilisation.

To tackle this problem, a number of hospitals are now establishing 'early mobility' or 'functional maintenance' programs usually as a physiotherapy or aged-care initiative, targeted to frail older or disabled inpatients. Using a model which incorporates aspects of the philosophy of a dedicated aged-care or rehabilitation ward, older patients are seen regularly for relatively simple and non-intensive interventions such as walking or group mobility activities. If an early mobility program is not operating as part of a controlled trial, it may be difficult to prove its effectiveness by showing improvements in outcome measures such as mobility or length of stay. Anecdotally, raising the awareness of medical and nursing staff about the adverse effects of prolonged inactivity does seem to be slowly changing attitudes at a ward level. The hope is that such interventions will eventually become as much a part of the activities and ethos of an acute ward as a rehabilitation ward, but even acknowledging that progress has been made, resource constraints and current work practices are a hindrance to the more widespread adoption of such programs.

Pressure ulcers

Pressure ulcers are the most stark illustration of the dangers of immobility and bed rest. Older people are particularly at risk, given the high prevalence of pre-morbid functional impairments, physical frailty, and age-related increased fragility and thinning of the skin. Iatrogenic factors may also play a part—for example, pressure ulcers may occur as a consequence of the use of sedation or physical restraint in the management of delirium. When a hospitalised older person is acutely unwell with a life-threatening illness, there is an understandable tendency to concentrate on the monitoring and interventions which may be necessary to save the patient's life. If resources are already stretched, pressure care may be difficult to implement. Monitoring for the development of pressure areas, especially over the sacrum, is practically difficult and time consuming in an immobile patient. For example, in an obese, delirious, non-weight-bearing patient recovering after a hip fracture operation, more than one person may be needed to help roll or stand the patient. Observing the sacrum and heels regularly is not an easy task, and may be impossible in some situations where absolute immobility is necessary, as after an operation for recurrent dislocation of a hip joint replacement.

Pressure ulcers are common in acutely hospitalised older patients. The incidence of new pressure ulcers developing during hospitalisation has been reported as being 10% (Cullum & Clark 1992) and overall up to 18% of hospital patients may have pressure ulcers (O'Dea 1993). In high-risk situations, such as after hip fracture, the incidence of pressure areas has been reported as being over 50% (Versluysen 1986). Pressure ulcers are regarded as one of the 'geriatric syndromes' with good reason, as over two-thirds of pressure ulcers occur in people aged over 70 (Barbenel et al 1977). Outside the hospital setting, the prevalence of pressure ulcers has been reported as being as high as 24% in nursing homes (Bates-Jensen 2001). The development of pressure ulcers is associated with poor outcomes, including an increased risk of death (LeVasseur & Helme 1991).

The risk of developing pressure ulcers is related to intrinsic and extrinsic factors. Intrinsic risk factors include increasing age, immobility, reduced conscious state, poor nutrition, incontinence and pain (Berlowitz et al 2001). Extrinsic risk factors are more difficult to study but the use of equipment such as hard mattresses or chairs and poor handling are likely to increase pressure ulcer risk. Risk assessment tools have been developed and some such as the Braden scale (Bergstrom et al 1987) have been validated in specific settings (Bergstrom & Braden 1992). The evidence that the use of a clinical risk scale is better than clinical assessment, or leads to improvement in outcomes, is not strong (Cullum et al 1995).

The cornerstone of pressure ulcer prevention continues to be 'pressure care' provided by nursing staff, with the use of pressure redistributing equipment as an adjunct. A randomised trial comparing no pressure care versus pressure care could never be supported ethically, so in a theoretical sense the practice of pressure care cannot be supported by the highest-grade evidence of a randomised controlled trial. However, the pathogenesis of ulcers is well understood, and this together with the practical experience and observations of staff provide ample, albeit not scientifically pure, evidence for the need for good pressure-care practices. High-risk patients are usually given two-hourly turning, but even shorter intervals of 1 to 1½ hours may be necessary (Knox et al 1994), an interval which would be very difficult to achieve on a busy acute ward. Pressure-reducing devices have been examined in a recent meta-analysis (Cullum et al 2000). This concluded that patients at high risk of pressure ulcer development should be nursed on high-specification foam providing constant low pressure, rather than standard hospital mattresses, and that pressure relief on the operating table also reduced pressure ulcer risk. It is not clear whether some of the more expensive alternating pressure mattresses are superior to constant low pressure devices, and there is also little evidence on the effectiveness of pressure-relieving cushions. Pressure-reducing devices are not a panacea. In one study, 25% of older patients admitted to hospital developed a pressure ulcer—over 90% of these had been nursed using a pressure-reducing device (Pase 1994).

Although pressure ulcer prevention has generally been regarded as a nursing activity, all staff involved in the acute care of older people should maintain a high level of awareness of the risk of pressure ulcer development and assume some responsibility for prevention. Medical staff should consider examination of areas of the skin at risk of pressure damage in the same light as listening to a patient's chest on a daily ward round or checking blood test results, and should attend to the management of associated factors such as undernutrition and incontinence. Therapy staff can encourage early mobilisation and provide advice on equipment to reduce pressure ulcer risk. In practice, however, despite optimal nursing and team practices and either 'low-tech' or 'high-tech' pressure-relieving devices, it is highly unlikely that pressure ulcers will ever completely disappear (Hagisawa & Barbenel 1999). Although it is recognised that not all pressure ulcers are preventable, and that pressure ulcers do not necessarily indicate poor quality care (Thomas 2001), the challenge is to minimise the development of pressure ulcers by recognising patients at risk, implementing appropriate preventative strategies and making pressure ulcer prevention the business of all members of staff providing care.

ALTERNATIVE CARE MODELS IN THE ACUTE HOSPITAL

Acute hospitals spend ever-increasing resources on the treatment of older people with acute illness. However, conventional medical and nursing models focusing on the episode of ill health often do not meet the many complex, although not strictly 'medical', needs of frail older people as exemplified by the risks of deconditioning and functional decline. Despite the best efforts of well-intentioned staff, it is usually not possible to offer a coordinated multidisciplinary assessment process and therapy program when operating within the requirements of the acute system. Staff who have worked in the aged-care or rehabilitation sector will recognise the deficiencies in assessment and care-planning processes for frail older people in acute hospitals, some of which are the result of length-of-stay pressures and the demands of a high patient throughput.

Dealing with the 'non-medical' needs of frail older people in acute hospitals demands a change in the philosophy of care. The multidisciplinary team approach practised in aged-care and rehabilitation units would theoretically seem to offer a more effective way of dealing with the functional, cognitive and social problems which often come to the fore as an older person recovers from an acute illness. In response to the recognition that frail older people do have special needs which are not met within the current acute hospital care model, acute aged-care units, sometimes known as Geriatric Evaluation and Management or GEM units, have been established in many hospitals. These units differ in the details of their operation but key components include a comprehensive assessment of disability and social factors, a nursing approach which aims to maximise patients' participation and independence, enhanced allied health involvement, specialised aged-care medical input and comprehensive care planning, including discharge planning, involving the patient and family or carers. Care is provided by a multidisciplinary team, usually within an identifiable area of the ward. Patients may be admitted either directly from the emergency department or soon after admission from hospital wards, and are often selected on the basis of their predicted needs for rehabilitation input and discharge planning. Such units are effectively running under an aged-care or rehabilitation model, but operating within the acute sector, and caring for older patients either when they are acutely ill, or in the early stages of recovery from acute illness.

As in other areas such as falls prevention where the intervention is complex and not applied uniformly across all patients, the evidence from controlled trials that acute aged-care units work is not dramatic or consistent. The outcomes which have been used to measure the effectiveness of the units are mortality, ADL function, need for institutionalisation, and hospital length of stay and costs. The initial report of a 50% reduction in one-year mortality in a GEM unit operating in a sub-acute setting (Rubenstein et al 1984) has not been replicated in further studies, although a recent study of an acute GEM unit showed similar mortality reductions at three months but not at one year (Saltvedt et al 2002). Improvements in ADL function and rates of residential care placement on discharge have been shown in some studies (Landefeld et al 1995; Rubenstein et al 1984) but not others (Asplund et al 2000; Counsell et al 2000; Harris et al 1991). In the study by Harris et al, patients were selected on the basis of age rather than disability. Depending on the model of care in the GEM unit, length of stay has been reported to be either increased (Rubenstein et al 1984; Saltvedt et al 2002), decreased (Asplund et al 2000) or unchanged (Counsell et al 2000; Landefeld et al 1995) in comparison to usual care.

Although the evidence is not compelling, the model of care adopted in acute GEM units seems to meet the disability and socially related needs of frail older people better than conventional care. However, one of the greatest barriers to the establishment of GEM units in acute hospitals is the need to operate within hospital length-of-stay constraints, imposed at least partially by casemix funding in States or countries where this operates. Age is taken into account when considering diagnosis-related group (DRG) weights, but it may still be difficult to meet length-of-stay targets for the DRG, especially if the GEM unit selects the most disabled and complex older patients. Anecdotally, some acute hospital GEM units have continued to operate successfully in what could be seen as this economically driven milieu.

Ideally, frail older people recovering from an acute illness who are assessed as requiring further care to maximise function and to plan for discharge should be transferred promptly to a non-casemix-funded, on-site GEM unit. In practice, delays often occur in acceptance and transfer to an off-site rehabilitation or aged-care facility. During this period, patients are not regarded as being a high priority for medical input or for therapy interventions. Therefore the problem of patients arriving in an aged-care or rehabilitation ward with unrecognised medical problems, and further deconditioned, is frequently encountered. Whether more GEM units will be established to help prevent this situation in the future will depend on research more clearly showing their effectiveness and on the willingness of hospital management to commit resources in already constrained financial environments.

DIAGNOSIS-BASED CARE: STROKE AND HIP-FRACTURE UNITS

Stroke and hip fracture are both examples of conditions whose prevalence increases exponentially with age, and which are associated with considerable disability. The majority of stroke and hip-fracture patients are older and the disabling effects of the acute event often occur on a background of pre-existing disability. Care models incorporating components of acute GEM and rehabilitation units would therefore seem ideally suited to the needs of patients who have just suffered a stroke or hip fracture. Hip-fracture or 'orthogeriatric' units are usually associated with hospital geriatric services in collaboration with orthopaedic surgeons, while stroke units are usually run by neurologists. Stroke and orthogeriatric units differ in their day-to-day operation, and in their patient mix, but there are similarities which go beyond the acute condition for which the patient is being treated. Both types of units employ a multidisciplinary approach, concentrate on disability as well as acute illness, and have a structured approach to the management of their patients. There is increased therapy provision and an emphasis on allied health and nursing involvement. Patients in stroke or hip-fracture units often have a number of disabilities and co-morbidities, but concentrating on one acute diagnosis promotes the development of expertise and enthusiasm in the management of these two groups of patients whose care in the past had generally not been perceived as being particularly 'interesting' or rewarding.

Evaluation of the effectiveness of hip-fracture units has been complicated by differences in the nature of the intervention and the model of care. Units vary in their location (either dedicated beds established off-site in a rehabilitation facility, rehabilitation beds in the acute hospital or beds in the acute orthopaedic ward), in their operation (either predominantly rehabilitation units or those managing acute medical aspects of perioperative care) and in the services they offer, particularly if they provide a domiciliary component to facilitate early discharge. After the publication of studies with positive outcomes in the 1980s (Gilchrist et al 1988; Kennie et al 1988), hip-fracture units were seen as an example of a successful aged-care initiative and many units were established in Australian hospitals. A meta-analysis of controlled trials, however, did not show clear evidence of their efficacy (Cameron et al 2001), at least partly due to the differences in the operation of the units. Another systematic review of hip-fracture rehabilitation has identified that programs involved in the acute care of hip-fracture patients and those providing support for early discharge lead to improvements in length of stay, return to previous residence and hospital costs. There was no evidence of reduced mortality in any of the models, and data on morbidity and function were inconclusive (Cameron et al 2000). From the acute hospital viewpoint, trends in reduced length of stay for hip-fracture patients, in association with a demand for increasing hospital throughput for all conditions, have occurred even in the absence of specialised hip-fracture units. As for other aged-care initiatives operating within acute hospitals, length of stay is a paramount consideration, and hip-fracture units will have to demonstrate that they reduce or maintain an acceptable length of stay, regardless of other positive outcomes they report.

Studies have confirmed that stroke units lead to improvements in outcome. Mortality is reduced by up to 20% in comparison with conventional general medical care (Stroke Unit Trialists' Collaboration 2000; Langhorne et al 1993). Stroke units also lead to reductions in the order of 25% in death or institutionalisation, and death or dependency, without increasing length of stay (Stroke Unit Trialists' Collaboration 2000). A multidisciplinary approach to care using many of the principles of comprehensive geriatric assessment and management has been identified as one of the most important factors associated with these improved outcomes (Langhorne & Pollock 2002). This is encouraging as it indicates that even relatively 'low-technology' interventions can be associated with positive outcomes, and it is likely that a greater number of stroke patients will derive more benefit from care in a designated stroke unit than from more aggressive interventions such as thrombolytic treatment (Donnan et al 2003; Szoeke et al 2003). In Australia, there are national initiatives to encourage the establishment of stroke units (Donnan et al 2003), and given the positive outcomes reported, it is probable that in the future, stroke units will become as accepted a part of hospital practice as coronary care units are today.

DISCHARGE AND POST-DISCHARGE INITIATIVES

Discharge planning has become one of the most discussed aspects of the hospital care of older people. Maxims such as 'Discharge planning begins as soon as someone is admitted to hospital' have now become part of the rhetoric of hospital-based staff involved in overseeing the discharge component of the admission. Discharge planning in the acute hospital may be fragmented and rushed, and there is rarely the opportunity to convene a case conference among all relevant nursing, therapy and medical staff to carefully coordinate a discharge and organise relevant post-discharge supports. In contrast to the aged-care or rehabilitation setting, discharge planning, if it is considered, may take place over the course of hours or days, rather than a period of weeks. The recognition of the often haphazard nature of discharge planning in acute hospitals has led to many hospitals appointing discharge coordinators or discharge planning teams to streamline the discharge process and to develop links with community agencies. This facilitates more intensive service provision for patients who have complex discharge planning needs. Part of the reason for the establishment of these teams has been to improve the care of the mostly frail older patients for whom discharge planning may have been inadequate in the past. The provision of funds for such initiatives is linked in part to the need to optimise hospital throughput.

The assumption that hospital-based discharge planning is effective has not been borne out by all controlled studies. Outcome measures used to assess the effectiveness of specialised discharge planning initiatives include hospital length of stay, readmission rate, discharge destination and health status. Some trials have reported slight reductions in length of stay of the order of one to two days (Naughton et al 1994), but this was not a consistent finding in other trials (Naylor et al 1994). One trial of comprehensive discharge planning for older medical inpatients showed a reduction in readmission rate (20% readmission rate at one week post discharge in control group versus 5% in the intervention group) at one week, but this difference was not maintained at two months (Kennedy et al 1987) and other controlled trials have not uniformly reported improvements in readmission rates. A study evaluating the effectiveness of a discharge coordinator for older medical inpatients reported increased patient satisfaction at one and three months post discharge (Moher et al 1992). A systematic review has concluded that hospital-based discharge planning may lead to some reduction in length of stay and readmission rates (Parkes & Shepperd 2000), but findings from controlled trials have not been consistent in showing clearly positive effects from more intensive hospital-based discharge planning programs.

The availability of increased post-discharge domiciliary support is one factor which may be important in enabling frail older people to be discharged home successfully. A number of programs which provide increased home-based care in the post-discharge period are now operating from acute hospitals, often as an integral part of an enhanced discharge planning service. The intervention may include medical treatment ('Hospital in the Home'), allied health visits, council services for personal care and monitoring of health needs by a community nurse. Some programs also have a case management component to liaise with the older person and family and to organise further assistance when necessary. A recent analysis of an

Australian program in which program coordinators purchased health and supportive services in the post-discharge period, showed reductions in total health-care costs and hospital bed-day use at six months, and increases in quality-of-life scores at one month in the intervention group (Lim et al 2003). While some studies have shown effects on reduction of readmission in the post-discharge period (Naylor et al 1999; Townsend et al 1988), this has not been shown consistently, even in studies specifically targeted to this outcome (Fitzgerald et al 1994). The outcome of functional status is similar in that some studies have shown improvements in mobility and ADL function after a home-based post-discharge program including physiotherapy (Nikolaus et al 1999), but this has not been a universal finding. A systematic review of post-discharge domiciliary interventions found that benefits were limited to cost savings and quality of care, and not other outcomes (Bours et al 1998).

Hospital in the Home programs focus primarily on medical treatment and have been established as an alternative to treatment in the hospital. They differ from programs providing increased post-discharge domiciliary support in that they replace a hospital admission, either completely or after a brief initial admission, with a period of time-limited medical treatment at home. However, there are programs which provide elements of both ongoing medical treatment and increased domiciliary support post admission, and the distinction is not an absolute one. Hospital in the Home programs operate in many Australian hospitals and may concentrate on patients with a specific diagnosis, such as chronic obstructive airways disease or stroke, or treat patients with a variety of conditions. Intravenous antibiotic treatment for some infections such as cellulitis, or heparin treatment for deep venous thrombosis, are examples of the treatments which can be given.

Most Hospital in the Home programs report at least some favourable outcomes. One of the main reasons for the introduction of such programs has been to reduce hospital utilisation, and this has been shown in reductions in length of hospital stay of the order of five to six days in some early discharge trials (Donald et al 1995; Wilson et al 1999) and in trials where all of the treatment has been given at home. An Australian trial reported fewer typical geriatric complications, increased patient and carer satisfaction and no increase in mortality for a program treating a range of conditions in which the majority of the patients were older (Caplan et al 1999). Costs of care have also been shown to be less in one trial (Jones et al 1999), but this has not been found in all studies. A systematic review of randomised trials concluded that Hospital in the Home programs treating patients who had a mix of medical conditions reduced hospital length of stay but were not otherwise associated with improved health outcomes, and nor were they cheaper than hospital care (Shepperd & Iliffe 2001).

Hospital in the Home and post-discharge support programs are likely to continue to operate within acute hospitals. The most important practical point is that older people should be assessed carefully for inclusion in the program. This is particularly true for Hospital in the Home programs, where informal and formal social supports must be adequate for the older person to remain at home while receiving treatment. At the ward level, there is little doubt that there is a perception that the availability of these programs has improved the level of support for older people in the post-discharge period, even if improved outcomes have been difficult to demonstrate.

VIGNETTE

Creating a hospital environment that promotes improved outcomes for the elderly

Margaret Winbolt

Frail older people are extremely vulnerable when admitted to hospital, particularly those with cognitive impairment or dementia. The physical risks include delirium, deconditioning, falls and loss of mobility and function. The psychosocial impact is less readily identifiable but fear, anxiety, isolation and grief are not uncommon. It is important that the role of the primary carer is recognised and valued, and that the carer is involved in care planning and decisions. A carer may have been providing care for many years and will have in-depth knowledge and understanding of the needs of the patient. Carers are often coping with high levels of stress, and an acute hospital admission increases stress dramatically.

For these reasons traditional ward structures and care environments can contribute to negative hospital experiences and reduced care outcomes for elderly people with dementia, and their carers. This is an account of how one hospital ward changed the underlying culture of care in order to create an environment more conducive to the needs of this client group. As with many hospital wards the culture was that of task-focused care, inflexible routines and a frantic, noisy environment. Care was delivered according to routines and was timed to meet the needs of the organisation rather than those of the client. Work allocation was by means of a patient allocation model, meaning that an individual nurse may be responsible for a different patient group each day. The focus was on getting the task done, with patients being identified as 'a shower', 'a feed' or simply a bed number. There was minimal understanding of the patient as a person, and nursing interactions with patients or carers was limited.

Rigid hierarchical management structures resulted in a disempowered staff group and inhibited change and the ability to develop practice.

The key aspect of the desired culture was the focus on respect for the patient as a person. A team-nursing model of care was implemented in order to facilitate closer relationships with patients and carers, as the importance of relationships and interaction when caring for frail elderly people cannot be over-emphasised. Patients, where able, and carers, were closely involved in all aspects of care, decision-making and discharge planning. The language used by nurses was altered to reflect the patient as a person. No longer were patients discussed in terms of being a task. Being 'a feed' became 'requires assistance with meals' and all nursing interventions were conducted in a way that promoted therapeutic interaction with the patient.

A total review of all nursing tasks was undertaken, asking: 'Why do we do this?', 'When do we do it?' and 'Do we need to do it at all?'. This highlighted the fact that many tasks are based on the way it has always been done, with little understanding of *why* it is done. Routines and rituals were reduced to a minimum, and the ensuing flexible work environment enabled nurses to deliver care in accordance with the needs of the individual, and allowed them to respond more readily to these needs. The flexibility led to a more relaxed work environment—there was no morning rush and the 24-hour nature of care delivery was emphasised, reducing the self-imposed pressure staff felt to 'get things done before the next shift arrives'.

The historical hierarchical management structure was replaced with a flatter, more open style of management with a focus on leadership, mentoring and coaching. This enabled nurses at all levels to work to their full potential and to actively participate in both clinical and administrative decision-making.

Underpinning the changed culture was the development of trust and respect across the nursing team—essential given the flexible nature of care delivery and work allocation.

While many difficulties remained, it was evident that this approach was able to create an environment that promoted improved outcomes for both patients and nurses.

CONCLUSION

The care of frail older people in acute hospitals presents challenges to health-care professionals looking after the individual older patient, and to the acute hospital system. Disease presentation often does not follow textbook descriptions and a lengthy, multifaceted assessment process may be required to reach a diagnosis and to identify the psychosocial and disability-related factors which have contributed to the hospitalisation. The acute medical illness may be appropriately managed, but admission to hospital for a frail disabled older person is often associated with complications such as delirium and with a worsening of underlying disability. Management of these problems is often not emphasised in the acute hospital. It requires skilled nursing and medical care and is often resource intensive. Older people with complex care needs often need to stay longer in hospital, and in an environment of financial constraint with intense pressure to discharge people quickly, this is not always feasible in the acute setting. Older people whose admission is prolonged because of social issues or disability can be seen as representing a threat to the capacity of a hospital or health-care system to deliver expected levels of emergency and elective treatment.

The increasing numbers of older people in the future will drive changes to their acute hospital care. Already, there is a greater presence of nursing, medical and allied health aged-care staff in the acute wards of many Australian hospitals than a decade ago. Despite a lack of unequivocal evidence of their efficacy, more specialised aged-care programs such as GEM and hip-fracture units, supported discharge schemes and interim care initiatives have been established in acute hospitals. Strategies to manage age-associated problems such as delirium and deconditioning will assume greater importance, and must be seen as the responsibility of more than specialised aged-care staff alone if acute hospitals are to continue to function efficiently. Unless there continues to be a commitment on the part of acute hospitals to adapt practice to identify and manage these problems, not only will more older patients receive less than optimal care, but hospitals will also find it increasingly difficult to satisfy the demands of society and government to treat sick patients of all age groups. How well older people are managed in acute hospitals will therefore have significant implications in the future for older people, their families and for all health-care consumers.

References

Allen C, Glasziou P & Del Mar C 1999, Bed rest: a potentially harmful treatment needing more careful evaluation, *Lancet*, 354(9186), pp 1229–33.

Asplund K, Gustafson Y, Jacobsson C, Bucht G, Wahlin A, Peterson J, Blom JO & Angquist KA 2000, Geriatric-based versus general wards for older acute medical patients: a randomized comparison of outcomes and use of resources, *Journal of the American Geriatrics Society*, 48(11), pp 1381–8.

Australian Bureau of Statistics (ABS) 2000, *Population Projections Australia 1999 to 2101.* Cat. No. 3222.0, AGPS: Canberra.

Australian Institute of Health and Welfare (AIHW) 2002, *Australian Hospital Statistics 2000-1*, AIHW Cat. No. HSE 20, Health Services Series No. 19, AIHW: Canberra.

Barbenel JC, Jordan MM, Nicol SM & Clark MO 1977, Incidence of pressure-sores in the Greater Glasgow Health Board Area, *Lancet*, 2(8037), pp 548–50.

Bates DW, Pruess K, Souney P & Platt R 1995, Serious falls in hospitalized patients: correlates and resource utilization, *American Journal of Medicine*, 99(2), pp 137–43.

Bates-Jensen BM 2001, Quality indicators for prevention and management of pressure ulcers in vulnerable elders, *Annals of Internal Medicine*, 135(8 Pt 2), pp 744–51.

Bergstrom N & Braden B 1992, A prospective study of pressure sore risk among institutionalized elderly, *Journal of the American Geriatrics Society*, 40(8), pp 747–58.

Bergstrom N, Braden BJ, Laguzza A & Holman V 1987, The Braden scale for predicting pressure sore risk, *Nursing Research*, 36(4), pp 205–10.

Berlowitz DR, Brandeis GH, Morris JN, Ash AS, Anderson JJ, Kader B & Moskowitz MA 2001, Deriving a risk-adjustment model for pressure ulcer development using the minimum data set, *Journal of the American Geriatrics Society*, 49(7), pp 866–71.

Bours GJ, Ketelaars CA, Frederiks CM, Abu-Saad HH & Wouters EF 1998, The effects of aftercare on chronic patients and frail elderly patients when discharged from hospital: a systematic review, *Journal of Advanced Nursing*, 27(5), pp 1076–86.

Boyce WJ & Vessey MP 1985, Rising incidence of fracture of the proximal femur, *Lancet*, 1(8421), pp 150–1.

Cameron I, Crotty M, Currie C, Finnegan T, Gillespie L, Gillespie W, Handoll H, Kurrle S, Madhok R, Murray G et al 2000, Geriatric rehabilitation following fractures in older people: a systematic review, *Health and Technology Assessment*, 4(2), pp i–111.

Cameron ID, Handoll HH, Finnegan TP, Madhok R & Langhorne P 2001, Co-ordinated multidisciplinary approaches for inpatient rehabilitation of older patients with proximal femoral fractures, *Cochrane Database of Systematic Reviews* (3).

Campbell AJ & Buchner DM 1997, Unstable disability and the fluctuations of frailty, *Age and Ageing*, 26(4), pp 315–18.

Caplan GA, Ward JA, Brennan NJ, Coconis J, Board N & Brown A 1999, Hospital in the Home: a randomised controlled trial, *Medical Journal of Australia*, 170(4), pp 156–60.

Counsell SR, Holder CM, Liebenauer LL, Palmer RM, Fortinsky RH, Kresevic DM, Quinn LM, Allen KR, Covinsky KE & Landefeld CS 2000, Effects of a multicomponent intervention on functional outcomes and process of care in hospitalized older patients: a randomized controlled trial of acute care for elders (ACE) in a community hospital, *Journal of the American Geriatrics Society*, 48(12), pp 1572–81.

Covinsky KE, Palmer RM, Fortinsky RH, Counsell SR, Stewart AL, Kresevic D, Burant CJ & Landefeld CS 2003, Loss of independence in activities of daily living in older adults hospitalized with medical illnesses: increased vulnerability with age, *Journal of the American Geriatrics Society*, 51(4), pp 451–8.

Creditor MC 1993, Hazards of hospitalization of the elderly, *Annals of Internal Medicine*, 118(3), pp 219–23.

Cullum N & Clark M 1992, Intrinsic factors associated with pressure sores in elderly people, *Journal of Advanced Nursing*, 17(4), pp 427–31.

Cullum N, Deeks JJ, Fletcher AW, Sheldon TA & Song F 1995, Preventing and treating pressure sores, *Quality in Health Care*, 4(4), pp 289–97.

Cullum N, Deeks J, Sheldon TA, Song F & Fletcher AW 2000, Beds, mattresses and cushions for pressure sore prevention and treatment, *Cochrane Database of Systematic Reviews* (2).

Davidsen M, Bronnum-Hansen H, Jorgensen T, Madsen M, Gerdes LU, Osler M & Schroll M 2001, Trends in incidence, case-fatality and recurrence of myocardial infarction in the Danish MONICA population 1982–1991, *European Journal of Epidemiology*, 17(12), pp 1139–45.

Donald IP, Baldwin RN & Bannerjee M 1995, Gloucester hospital-at-home: a randomized controlled trial, *Age and Ageing*, 24(5), pp 434–9.

Donnan GA, Davis SM & Levi CR 2003, Strategies to improve outcomes after acute stroke, *Medical Journal of Australia*, 178(7), pp 309–10.

Evans D, Hodgkinson B, Lambert L & Wood J 2001, Falls risk factors in the hospital setting: a systematic review, *International Journal of Nursing Practice*, 7(1), pp 38–45.

Fick DM, Agostini JV & Inouye SK 2002, Delirium superimposed on dementia: a systematic review, *Journal of the American Geriatrics Society*, 50(10), pp 1723–32.

Fitzgerald JF, Smith DM, Martin DK, Freedman JA & Katz BP 1994, A case manager intervention to reduce readmissions, *Archives of Internal Medicine*, 154(15), pp 1721–9.

George J, Bleasdale S & Singleton SJ 1997, Causes and prognosis of delirium in elderly patients admitted to a district general hospital, *Age and Ageing*, 26(6), pp 423–7.

Gilchrist WJ, Newman RJ, Hamblen DL & Williams BO 1988, Prospective randomised study of an orthopaedic geriatric inpatient service, *British Medical Journal*, 297(6656), pp 1116–18.

Gillespie LD, Gillespie WJ, Robertson MC, Lamb SE, Cumming RG & Rowe BH 2001, Interventions for preventing falls in elderly people, *Cochrane Database of Systematic Reviews* (3).

Hagisawa S & Barbenel J 1999, The limits of pressure sore prevention, *Journal of the Royal Society of Medicine*, 92(11), pp 576–8.

Harris RD, Henschke PJ, Popplewell PY, Radford AJ, Bond MJ, Turnbull RJ, Hobbin ER, Chalmers JP, Tonkin A, Stewart AM et al 1991, A randomised study of outcomes in a defined group of acutely ill elderly patients managed in a geriatric assessment unit or a general medical unit, *Australian and New Zealand Journal of Medicine*, 21(2), pp 230–4.

Healey F 1994, Does flooring type affect risk of injury in older in-patients?, *Nursing Times*, 90(27), pp 40–1.

Hirsch CH, Sommers L, Olsen A, Mullen L & Winograd CH 1990, The natural history of functional morbidity in hospitalized older patients, *Journal of the American Geriatrics Society*, 38(12), pp 1296–1303.

Ho KK, Pinsky JL, Kannel WB & Levy D 1993, The epidemiology of heart failure: the Framingham Study, *Journal of the American College of Cardiology*, 22(4 Suppl A), pp 6A–13A.

Inouye SK 1994, The dilemma of delirium: clinical and research controversies regarding diagnosis and evaluation of delirium in hospitalized elderly medical patients, *American Journal Of Medicine*, 97(3), pp 278–88.

Inouye SK 2001, Delirium after hip fracture: to be or not to be?, *Journal of the American Geriatrics Society*, 49(5), pp 678–9.

Inouye SK, Bogardus ST Jr, Charpentier PA, Leo-Summers L, Acampora D, Holford TR & Cooney LM Jr 1999, A multicomponent intervention to prevent delirium in hospitalized older patients, *New England Journal of Medicine*, 340(9), pp 669–76.

Inouye SK, van Dyck CH, Alessi CA, Balkin S, Siegal AP & Horwitz RI 1990, Clarifying confusion: the Confusion Assessment Method: a new method for detection of delirium, *Annals of Internal Medicine*, 113(12), pp 941–8.

Jamrozik K, Broadhurst RJ, Lai N, Hankey GJ, Burvill PW & Anderson CS 1999, Trends in the incidence, severity, and short-term outcome of stroke in Perth, Western Australia, *Stroke*, 30(10), pp 2105–11.

Jokinen C, Heiskanen L, Juvonen H, Kallinen S, Karkola K, Korppi M, Kurki S, Ronnberg PR, Seppa A, Soimakallio S et al 1993, Incidence of community-acquired pneumonia in the population of four municipalities in Eastern Finland, *American Journal of Epidemiology*, 137(9), pp 977–88.

Jones J, Wilson A, Parker H, Wynn A, Jagger C, Spiers N & Parker G 1999, Economic evaluation of hospital at home versus hospital care: cost minimisation analysis of data from randomised controlled trial, *British Medical Journal*, 319(7224), pp 1547–50.

Kannus P, Parkkari J, Niemi S, Pasanen M, Palvanen M, Jarvinen M & Vuori I 2000, Prevention of hip fracture in elderly people with use of a hip protector, *New England Journal of Medicine*, 343(21), pp 1506–13.

Kennedy L, Neidlinger S & Scroggins K 1987, Effective comprehensive discharge planning for hospitalized elderly, *The Gerontologist*, 27(5), pp 577–80.

Kennie DC, Reid J, Richardson IR, Kiamari AA & Kelt C 1988, Effectiveness of geriatric rehabilitative care after fractures of the proximal femur in elderly women: a randomised clinical trial, *British Medical Journal*, 297(6656), pp 1083–6.

Knox DM, Anderson TM & Anderson PS 1994, Effects of different turn intervals on skin of healthy older adults, *Advances in Wound Care*, 7(1), pp 48–56.

Kressig RW, Wolf SL, Sattin RW, O'Grady M, Greenspan A, Curns A & Kutner M 2001, Associations of demographic, functional, and behavioral characteristics with activity-related fear of falling among older adults transitioning to frailty, *Journal of the American Geriatrics Society*, 49(11), pp 1456–62.

Landefeld CS, Palmer RM, Kresevic DM, Fortinsky RH & Kowal J 1995, A randomized trial of care in a hospital medical unit especially designed to improve the functional outcomes of acutely ill older patients, *New England Journal of Medicine*, 332(20), pp 1338–44.

Langhorne P & Pollock A 2002, What are the components of effective stroke unit care?, *Age and Ageing*, 31(5), pp 365–71.

Langhorne P, Williams BO, Gilchrist W & Howie K 1993, Do stroke units save lives?, *Lancet*, 342(8868), pp 395–8.

LeVasseur SA & Helme RD 1991, A double-blind clinical trial to compare the efficacy of an active based cream F14001 against a placebo non-active based cream for the treatment of pressure ulcers in a population of elderly subjects, *Journal of Advanced Nursing*, 16(8), pp 952–6.

Lim WK, Lambert SF & Gray LC 2003, Effectiveness of case management and post-acute services in older people after hospital discharge, *Medical Journal of Australia*, 178(6), pp 262–6.

Mahoney JE 1998, Immobility and falls, *Clinics in Geriatric Medicine*, 14(4), pp 699–726.

Mahoney JE, Sager MA & Jalaluddin M 1998, New walking dependence associated with hospitalization for acute medical illness: incidence and significance, *Journals of Gerontology Series A—Biological Sciences and Medical Sciences*, 53A(4), pp M307–M312.

Marcantonio ER, Flacker JM, Wright RJ & Resnick NM 2001, Reducing delirium after hip fracture: a randomized trial, *Journal of the American Geriatrics Society*, 49(5), pp 516–22.

Marini C, Triggiani L, Cimini N, Ciancarelli I, De Santis F, Russo T, Baldassarre M, di Orio F & Carolei A 2001, Proportion of older people in the community as a predictor of increasing stroke incidence, *Neuroepidemiology*, 20(2), pp 91–5.

Mayo NE, Gloutney L & Levy AR 1994, A randomized trial of identification bracelets to prevent falls among patients in a rehabilitation hospital, *Archives of Physical Medicine and Rehabilitation*, 75(12), pp 1302–8.

McVey LJ, Becker PM, Saltz CC, Feussner JR & Cohen HJ 1989, Effect of a geriatric consultation team on functional status of elderly hospitalized patients: a randomized, controlled clinical trial, *Annals of Internal Medicine*, 110(1), pp 79–84.

Moher D, Weinberg A, Hanlon R & Runnalls K 1992, Effects of a medical team coordinator on length of hospital stay, *Canadian Medical Association Journal*, 146(4), pp 511–15.

Naughton BJ, Moran MB, Feinglass J, Falconer J & Williams ME 1994, Reducing hospital costs for the geriatric patient admitted from the emergency department: a randomized trial, *Journal of the American Geriatrics Society*, 42(10), pp 1045–9.

Naylor M, Brooten D, Jones R, Lavizzo-Mourey R, Mezey M & Pauly M 1994, Comprehensive discharge planning for the hospitalized elderly: a randomized clinical trial, *Annals of Internal Medicine*, 120(12), pp 999–1006.

Naylor MD, Brooten D, Campbell R, Jacobsen BS, Mezey MD, Pauly MV & Schwartz JS 1999, Comprehensive discharge planning and home follow-up of hospitalized elders: a randomized clinical trial, *Journal of the American Medical Association*, 281(7), pp 613–20.

Nikolaus T, Specht-Leible N, Bach M, Oster P & Schlierf G 1999, A randomized trial of comprehensive geriatric assessment and home intervention in the care of hospitalized patients, *Age and Ageing*, 28(6), pp 543–50.

O'Dea K 1993, Prevalence of pressure damage in hospital patients in the UK, *Journal of Wound Care*, 2(4), pp 221–5.

Oliver D, Britton M, Seed P, Martin FC & Hopper AH 1997, Development and Evaluation of evidence based risk assessment tool (STRATIFY) to predict which elderly inpatients will fall: case-control and cohort studies, *British Medical Journal*, 315(7115), pp 1049–53.

Oliver D, Hopper A & Seed P 2000, Do hospital fall prevention programs work? A systematic review, *Journal of the American Geriatrics Society*, 48(12), pp 1679–89.

Parker MJ, Gillespie LD & Gillespie WJ 2001, Hip protectors for preventing hip fractures in the elderly, *Cochrane Database of Systematic Reviews* (2).

Parkes J & Shepperd S 2000, Discharge planning from hospital to home, *Cochrane Database of Systematic Reviews* (4).

Pase MN 1994, Pressure relief devices, risk factors, and development of pressure ulcers in elderly patients with limited mobility, *Advances in Wound Care*, 7(2), pp 38–42.

Patterson VB & Calabresi P 2000, Cancer: an overview. In: Williams TF, Beattie BL, Michel J-P & Wilcock GK (eds), *Oxford Textbook of Geriatric Medicine*, pp 437–48, Oxford University Press: Oxford.

Perell KL, Nelson A, Goldman RL, Luther SL, Prieto-Lewis N & Rubenstein LZ 2001, Fall Risk Assessment Measures: An Analytic Review, *Journals of Gerontology Series A— Biological Sciences and Medical Sciences*, 56(12), pp M761–M766.

Pocock NA, Culton NL & Harris ND 1999, The potential effect on hip fracture incidence of mass screening for osteoporosis, *Medical Journal of Australia*, 170(10), pp 486–8.

Rahkonen T, Luukkainen-Markkula R, Paanila S, Sivenius J & Sulkava R 2000, Delirium episode as a sign of undetected dementia among community dwelling elderly subjects: a two year follow up study, *Journal of Neurology, Neurosurgery and Psychiatry*, 69(4), pp 519–21.

Rizzo JA, Bogardus ST Jr, Leo-Summers L, Williams CS, Acampora D & Inouye SK 2001, Multicomponent targeted intervention to prevent delirium in hospitalized older patients: what is the economic value?, *Medical Care*, 39(7), pp 740–52.

Rubenstein LZ, Josephson KR, Wieland GD, English PA, Sayre JA & Kane RL 1984, Effectiveness of a geriatric evaluation unit. A randomized clinical trial, *New England Journal of Medicine*, 311(26), pp 1664–70.

Rudberg MA, Pompei P, Foreman MD, Ross RE & Cassel CK 1997, The natural history of delirium in older hospitalized patients: a syndrome of heterogeneity, *Age and Ageing*, 26(3), pp 169–74.

Sager MA, Franke T, Inouye SK, Landefeld CS, Morgan TM, Rudberg MA, Sebens H & Winograd CH 1996, Functional outcomes of acute medical illness and hospitalization in older persons, *Archives of Internal Medicine*, 156(6), pp 645–52.

Sager MA, Rudberg MA, Jalaluddin M, Franke T, Inouye SK, Landefeld CS, Siebens H & Winograd CH 1996, Hospital Admission Risk Profile (HARP): identifying older patients at risk for functional decline following acute medical illness and hospitalization, *Journal of the American Geriatrics Society*, 44(3), pp 251–7.

Saltvedt I, Mo ES, Fayers P, Kaasa S & Sletvold O 2002, Reduced mortality in treating acutely sick, frail older patients in a geriatric evaluation and management unit. A prospective randomized trial, *Journal of the American Geriatrics Society*, 50(5), pp 792–8.

Sanders KM, Nicholson GC, Ugoni AM, Pasco JA, Seeman E & Kotowicz MA 1999, Health burden of hip and other fractures in Australia Beyond 2000. Projections based on the Geelong Osteoporosis Study, *Medical Journal of Australia*, 170(10), pp 467–70.

Shepperd S & Iliffe S 2001, Hospital at Home versus in-patient hospital care, *Cochrane Database of Systematic Reviews* (3).

Siebens H, Aronow H, Edwards D & Ghasemi Z 2000, A randomized controlled trial of exercise to improve outcomes of acute hospitalization in older adults, *Journal of the American Geriatrics Society*, 48(12), pp 1545–52.

Stroke Unit Trialists' Collaboration 2000, Organised inpatient (stroke unit) care for stroke, *Cochrane Database of Systematic Reviews* (2).

Sutton JC, Standen PJ & Wallace WA 1994, Patient accidents in hospital: incidence, documentation and significance, *British Journal of Clinical Practice*, 48(2), pp 63–6.

Szoeke CE, Parsons MW, Butcher KS, Baird TA, Mitchell PJ, Fox SE & Davis SM 2003, Acute stroke thrombolysis with intravenous tissue plasminogen activator in an Australian tertiary hospital, *Medical Journal of Australia*, 178(7), pp 324–8.

Thomas DR 2001, Prevention and Treatment of pressure ulcers: What works? What doesn't?, *Cleveland Clinics Journal of Medicine*, 68(8), pp 704–22.

Thorvaldsen P, Davidsen M, Bronnum-Hansen H & Schroll M 1999, Stable stroke occurrence despite incidence reduction in an aging population: stroke trends in the Danish Monitoring Trends and Determinants in Cardiovascular Disease (MONICA) population, *Stroke*, 30(12), pp 2529–34.

Tideiksaar R, Feiner CF & Maby J 1993, Falls prevention: the efficacy of a bed alarm system in an acute-care setting, *Mt Sinai Journal of Medicine*, 60(6), pp 522–7.

Tinetti ME, Inouye SK, Gill TM & Doucette JT 1995, Shared risk factors for falls, incontinence, and functional dependence. Unifying the approach to geriatric syndromes, *Journal of the American Medical Association*, 273(17), pp 1348–53.

Townsend J, Piper M, Frank AO, Dyer S, North WR & Meade TW 1988, Reduction in hospital readmission stay of elderly patients by a community based hospital discharge scheme: a randomised controlled trial, *British Medical Journal*, 297(6647), pp 544–7.

Trzepacz PT 1996, Delirium. Advances in diagnosis, pathophysiology, and treatment, *Psychiatric Clinics of North America*, 19(3), pp 429–48.

Versluysen M 1986, How elderly patients with femoral fracture develop pressure sores in hospital, *British Medical Journal (Clinical Research Edition)*, 292(6531), pp 1311–13.

Warshaw GA, Moore JT, Friedman SW, Currie CT, Kennie DC, Kane WJ & Mears PA 1982, Functional disability in the hospitalized elderly, *Journal of the American Medical Association*, 248(7), pp 847–50.

Wilson A, Parker H, Wynn A, Jagger C, Spiers N, Jones J & Parker G 1999, Randomised controlled trial of effectiveness of Leicester Hospital at Home Scheme compared with hospital care, *British Medical Journal*, 319(7224), pp 1542–6.

Winograd CH, Gerety MB, Chung M, Goldstein MK, Dominguez F Jr & Vallone R 1991, Screening for frailty: criteria and predictors of outcomes, *Journal of the American Geriatrics Society*, 39(8), pp 778–84.

Wolf PA, Cobb JL & D'Agostino RB 1992, Epidemiology of stroke. In: Barnett HJM, Mohr JP, Stein BM & Yatsu FM (eds), *Stroke: Pathophysiology, Diagnosis and Treatment*, pp 3–27, Churchill Livingstone: New York.

Wu AW, Damiano AM, Lynn J, Alzola C, Teno J, Landefeld CS, Desbiens N, Tsevat J, Mayer-Oakes A, Harrell FE Jr et al 1995, Predicting future functional status for seriously ill hospitalized adults. The SUPPORT Prognostic Model, *Annals of Internal Medicine*, 122(5), pp 342–50.

CHAPTER 10

Public participation and individual control

BARB FIVEASH AND ROBIN WATTS

INTRODUCTION

Many older people are healthy and contribute not only to their own well-being but also to the community at large. However, for too long the aged have been grouped with the disabled and sick of society—age has been viewed as an illness (Neumayer & Goddard 1998). Along with the association of old age with illness and disability goes the notion that, even if articulate, the older sick person is dependent, voiceless and compliant with health-care requests. Although it is true that some older people require intensive health services, and that others live with chronic health disorders, some have no health problems at all and live their lives without the need for health-service intervention. Many older people make few visits to a medical practitioner, and many live their whole lives without major surgery or health intervention. As each cohort of older people age, they experience improved health outcomes and live longer than their predecessors (Neumayer & Goddard 1998).

In other words, some older people are sick and disabled, and some younger or middle-aged people are sick and disabled, just as some in both groups are well. The older person needs to be viewed as having the same rights to autonomy and a sense of control as the younger person. Each individual brings to their situation varying attributes and limitations, regardless of their age.

This chapter discusses client control over health at both the individual and community levels. Inherent to this discussion is the view that, whatever their age, people have the right—and should have the opportunity—to have control over their health, and to contribute to participation by the community in health. Although the arguments are relevant to any age, they are especially significant to care of older people, which has a long history of infantilisation, removal of choice, abuse of dignity, depersonalisation and a general lack of control by the older person.

It is acknowledged that there are situations of crisis and/or situations in which people suffer severe cognitive impairment that prevent clients from managing their own care. However, this chapter focuses on those people who are still capable of making their own decisions.

SOCIAL MOVEMENT TOWARDS INDIVIDUAL CONTROL

During the postmodern period, institutions and traditions stand to be challenged (Agger 1990). Postmodernists question 'truth' and 'reality' and seek to identify whose interests are being served in any particular situation (Calhoun 1996). At the same time, there is a social movement towards individual freedom and responsibility, and a decreased reliance on the 'expert' (Jewell 1994). This social change is seen in many areas of life such as management/industry, education and the general consumer perspective. Individuals are starting to represent themselves in courts of law. In higher education, with the movement towards student-centred and problem-based learning, there is greater student self-reliance and responsibility (Boud 1995; Biley 1998). In this situation, students are expected to explore databases for relevant information and to interpret, analyse and criticise accepted knowledge. The student makes choices about what information to access, and how to access it, and relies less on the teacher, the emphasis being on process rather than content (Boud 1995).

Similarly, in the work situation, although some employees are still represented by unions, others are more frequently expected to negotiate their own enterprise agreement with their employers—including salary and employment conditions (Teece 1995). There is a move towards decentralisation, participatory management, and the devolution of decision-making (Huber 1996). In this employment situation there is less management supervision and more personal responsibility and accountability for services provided.

There is a growing emphasis on self-management in health care. This is reflected in the rise in the fitness industry, the use of complementary therapies, and an emphasis on the relationships among nutrition, exercise, health, wellness and disease prevention. Similarly, there is growing awareness of the role of the individual in contributing to their own recovery (Jewell 1994).

Health-care clients are more likely to reach their health goals—and to positively influence health outcomes—if they actively formulate their own health goals and manage their care, than if they are the passive recipients of health care (Fiveash 1998). Positive health-care experiences for clients are associated with having a sense of control, feeling well informed, taking responsibility for their health care, having an opportunity to make decisions, and having their autonomy promoted—in general, situations in which clients feel that they are being treated as capable people. Where clients are involved in goal-setting there is an increased satisfaction with results. Some clients demand test results, seek explanations, ask questions, offer opinions, and assume responsibility for their health. Such informed people are then in a better position to identify health goals, seek realistic treatment, and share their health goals (Fiveash 1998).

Client control over, and input into, health provides an opportunity for the individual to accept the responsibility for personal health-care decisions. This also provides the basis for a preparedness to accept health outcomes (Fiveash 1998). Health is a very personal matter, and in no other area of life could it be more important or relevant to take control and have responsibility. Health is central to life. The capacity to work and learn arises from a positive state of health. Health care provided according to the person's health goals results in the person living with decisions made by themselves and a sense of ownership and control over their health.

Fiveash (1998) suggests that these social changes are congruent with:

- the principles of primary health care and public participation (Watts 1994);
- the changing nature of chronic illness and emphasis on wellness;

- the emphasis on the client's illness experience;
- the change from passive recipient of health care to active partner and consumer;
- the changing relationship between nurses and clients;
- changing health-care services;
- increasing access to health information; and
- the notion of client-managed care.

PRIMARY HEALTH CARE AND PUBLIC PARTICIPATION

Primary health care has been declared by the World Health Organization (WHO) as a means of addressing health for all by 2000 (WHO 1979). At the Declaration of Alma Ata in 1978, the WHO emphasised the need for people to take greater responsibility for their own health (WHO 1978). Nurses have been identified as key workers to develop and expand concepts of primary health care. Health-care workers have been asked to provide the public with information so that they can be self-determining and self-reliant, with more control and greater responsibility in health matters.

The primary health care movement encourages the provision of more information to, and increased involvement of, individuals and communities regarding their health care. Health is seen to be determined by economic, cultural, social, political, environmental, behavioural and biological characteristics of the individual and the society (Australian Institute of Health & Welfare [AIHW] 2002). Inequalities in health are reflected by these same factors. Baum (2002) describes equity in health as equity in health expenditure, income, access and use, cost and outcomes in regard to health services. Health is seen as more than an individual's responsibility, or as being predetermined by biological heritage, but also as a reflection of the social environment in which the person lives. Consequently, the nurse's role expands from a focus on the individual/family to include populations and social issues.

Baum (2002) describes other issues relevant to equity in health such as housing, education and income, and the need for affirmative action to distribute resources equally. She considers that the lack of resources also represents a lack of power, and that this lack of power is a major contributing factor in the health status of the person. Wealth is positively associated (and poverty negatively associated) with good health, power, prestige, life chance, education, ownership and control. Health influences social class, and social class is related to health status. The healthy are more likely to be upwardly mobile and the sick and disabled downwardly mobile (Schofield 1999). Given the impact of context and individual/community participation on health outcomes, the relevance of primary health care can be readily understood.

Watts (1994) describes a model of community involvement and public participation in health which addresses a continuum from individual decision-making to public participation in policy formulation. The same principles that underpin public participation in health are congruent with individual involvement in health (client-managed care). At all levels of participation, these principles include:

- democracy in health-care systems;
- equality of power between health provider and recipient in respect of outcome decision-making; and

- a positive view of the individual (whatever their age) as being capable and aware.

Participation in health care is unlikely to occur when there is a lack of democratic principles. This lack can be identified by an imbalance of power between health-care systems and the populations they serve, a lack of concern for the community's right to have input into their health care, and a lack of community knowledge of health care or strategies to facilitate involvement in health care. This level of public participation in health care provides an umbrella for the growth of not only individual involvement in health, but also individual control over health. In this way the model of Public Participation (Watts 1994) forms a framework that protects and facilitates clients who wish to have greater input, or even control, over their health. Such a model also justifies a nurse's activity that supports clients who wish to have greater control in this area of their lives. At the societal end of the continuum, where ill health may be the consequence of social circumstances, collective action can move towards changing those social circumstances.

CHRONIC ILLNESS AND CLIENT CONTROL

For most of their lives, the majority of people manage their health care and decisions about their best health interests outside the traditional organised health-care system. Indeed, if every health matter required a health professional, the health-care system would be overwhelmed and simply not cope with the workload. Today, with the emergence of new patterns of health and illness (and treatments) there is a need for people to manage sometimes very complex health matters over substantial periods of time. Added to this, many illnesses are chronic and require lifestyle changes to bring about an improvement in health. These issues increase the individual's responsibility for managing their health care because it is the individual, rather than the health-care worker, who can make the necessary lifestyle changes required.

Death is most likely to occur in very old age in Western societies. More than 30% of causes of death were related to coronary heart or cerebrovascular disease, and another 30% of deaths were related to the range of cancers. The leading causes of death in Australia in 2002 were ischaemic heart disease, cerebrovascular disease, lung cancers, breast cancers, chronic obstructive pulmonary disease, prostate disease, colorectal cancer, suicide, dementia, diabetes, pneumonia and influenza, land transport accidents, and diseases of arteries, arterioles and capillaries (AIHW 2002).

A number of conditions have been identified by the National Health Priority Areas initiative (AIHW 2002), which covers major diseases and conditions as well as injuries where there is the potential for health gain. This potential may be in areas of prevention with the identification of determinants and risk factors or with treatment and management. The six identified priority conditions where there is a potential for health gain include:

- cardiovascular health;
- cancer control;
- injury prevention and control;
- mental health;

- diabetes mellitus; and
- asthma.

In many of these disorders, both genetic and environmental factors contribute to the condition. It is possible that strategies can be used to address specific environmental risk factors that minimise the harm caused by these conditions. For example, some principle risk factors responsive to prevention include smoking, alcohol consumption, physical inactivity, exposure to sunlight and high-fat diet (AIHW 2002). People who are less well educated, unemployed or in low-income households report poorer health. Patterns of health and illness are often lifestyle generated, and reflect differences in wealth, opportunity, occupation and personal resources (Wilkinson & Marmot 1998).

It has been shown that individuals can not only bring about an improvement in their health through lifestyle changes but that they are also good predictors of their own health status. Self-reported health status has been shown to be the best predictor of the need for health-care intervention and survival (Idler & Benyamini 1997).

Where individuals require the assistance of health-care providers, several authors (Australian Nursing Federation 2001; Draper 1997; Lorig et al 1999) regard client participation as a vital element in the management of chronic illness—essentially, the health-care professional helps the client to help themselves. With the shift from acute to chronic illness, medicine simply cannot offer a cure for many lifestyle illnesses. In Britain the government has taken this participation to new heights by providing cash to health-care clients to purchase their own health-care services (client-centred funding) (Cohen 1995). The health professional may advise on care packages but users/consumers make the final decision about which product best suits them. The health-care provider is employed by the client. With this system, the professional can act as a service broker and identify the available services and payment required, and may or may not directly provide the service (Powell 1996).

THE NATURE OF HEALTH-CARE SERVICES

Even in cases of acute illness, the emphasis is on periods of brief hospitalisation and early discharge and, where possible, the nursing of the client at home (Reichley 1999). Clients nursed in their own home may be advantaged or disadvantaged, depending on a variety of issues. Some clients may be disadvantaged either because they have no family support at home, or because they have a family who are dependent on them for their daily functioning. Other clients, however, may find that they are advantaged because they can enjoy the independence of home, and are residing in a place where they feel comfortable. In this situation, they may be less likely to lose their sense of power and control over their health situation—a loss that often accompanies an admission to bureaucratic, rather impersonal hospitals.

EMPHASIS ON CLIENTS' ILLNESS EXPERIENCE

Individuals experience more than just the objective medical-disease diagnosis—they have highly personalised knowledge of their illness experience (Morse & Johnson 1991). Their way of knowing about their illness is through experiencing or living with it. This knowledge is not reduced to a set of problems, but is understood by the person in the context of their life. The understanding that the person has of their illness experience is likely to be substantially different from the health providers' knowledge of the illness (Redding 1995). People are the experts on how they feel in respect of their illness experience and the treatment regimen, and how much pain, disability and distress they are prepared to tolerate. Certain illness experiences are more shattering than others, and the impact of illness varies from person to person. One client may seek aggressive therapy for an illness, whereas for the same illness another may not. People vary in their assessments of the balance between benefits and burdens against their own value systems. They have different attitudes towards the maintenance of dignity, reduction in costs, lifestyle changes and family distress. These and other reasons affect their decision to accept or reject specific treatment for their illness (Gleeson 1995). Because of their subjective experience of the illness trajectory and knowledge of their personal circumstances, it is the client who, if adequately informed, may best judge whether the health care being offered is appropriate, and it is the client who is in the best position to make judgements about their own health.

RIGHTS AND RESPONSIBILITIES

Over the past decade or two there has been a move away from the client occupying a passive sick role (Crossley 1998) towards being more active consumers of health services. The Consumers' Health Forum was established in Australia in 1987 (Commonwealth of Australia 2000). This Forum was developed as an independent organisation representing community and consumer groups at a national level in health-related matters. It aims to establish a network of community and consumer groups, to develop position statements on policy, and to increase consumer decision-making on policy, budgets, regulatory and legislative matters, and research priorities. This organisation has identified a list of rights for consumers, including:

- appropriate and quality health care;
- the making of decisions about one's own health care;
- information by which to make decisions;
- privacy, respect and dignity;
- deciding who will be present during treatments;
- the seeking of information from others;
- the seeking of treatment from other health workers;
- confidentiality;
- access to, and amendment of, one's health records;
- avenues for comments and complaints about health care;
- compensation for damages; and
- refusing admission to and leaving a health facility.

The Forum also provided some questions which clients could ask of general practitioners, specialists or psychiatrists:

- What is my health problem?
- What information led you to this decision?
- What treatment options and alternatives are available in relation to:
  - purpose;
  - expected benefits and risks;
  - emotional, mental, sexual and social consequences; and
  - possible side-effects and after-effects?
- What happens if I don't receive treatment?
- Regarding the people who will be responsible for the treatment:
  - What is their role, qualifications and competence?
  - Will they be available over the period of treatment and afterwards?
  - Will they hand some of the treatment to others to perform?
- Is the suggested treatment a usual treatment or is it unusual or even experimental?
- What are the costs involved?

In Britain, client rights are defined in client charters and professional codes of ethics. Service-evaluation mechanisms have been developed into benchmarks for quality control and standards of care (Jones 1993). Consumer rights include self-determination, access to relevant information, input into health services, the right to health protection, access to prompt high-quality services and equitable distribution of health resources—as well as the right to receive reasonable health care, to consent to treatment, and to access health records and have health information kept confidential (Jones 1993; Dimond 1993). Client responsibilities include being honest in their transactions with health providers, producing relevant information and accepting responsibility for their own health-care decisions, carrying out instructions on treatment and care responsibly, carefully keeping appointments, being considerate towards other clients and staff, and reporting complaints (Jones 1993; Dimond 1993).

Issues of informed consent, autonomy and client rights are central to client-managed care. The principle of autonomy described in the ethics literature is concerned with independence, self-determination, privacy, self-worth, dignity, accepting responsibility, and the freedom to act (Thompson et al 2000). In 1991, the United States introduced a Client Self-Determination Act (Weiler 1993). The intent and spirit of the legislation was to assist clients to exercise autonomy in health care. Health-care professionals are required to provide the client with written information about their disease, treatment and rights, including advance directives (living wills) or legal-substitute decision-maker (power of attorney). This legislation requires the health professional to deal with the issues of client rights and to document care options for their clients (Weiler 1993).

Autonomy is concerned with the right to make choices according to one's own values and beliefs, and the right of individuals to act according to their own free will, even when their decisions are not the ones that the health provider would consider to be in the client's best interest (Kerridge et al 1998). Respect for autonomy is central to the decision-making process for both the client and the nurse. Clients have a right to be informed, to act voluntarily, and to make decisions about health care—whether or not others view the decision as wise or foolish. For those people who are capable of making their own decisions (in the context of this discussion), there is no law that requires a person to maintain their health or seek health care when sick.

Central to the nature of autonomy is the client's sense of personal control (Dworkin 1988) and right to make decisions (Oddi 1994). The fundamental moral principle is autonomy—a person's freedom to take whatever action they wish, provided they do not violate others—by which the client chooses and the health provider supports and facilitates that choice (Johnstone 1989). Mills (1962) asserts that there is no way that power can reasonably be used over a member of a community against the person's own will unless it is to prevent harm to others. The health professional's perception of benefit to a client is not an adequate reason.

Client-managed care could be another emerging form of client autonomy by which health professionals advise clients, and by which the client seeks from the range of service providers available, obtains information from a variety of sources, and make choices about care options according to their own health goals. From this perspective, client rights, autonomy, control over health care, accountability and self-responsibility prevail.

ACCESS TO HEALTH INFORMATION

Clients respond differently to the health-care worker when they are adequately informed (McCahon & Larsen 2002). People are gradually becoming more informed and aware of their right to information. Over recent years, the general population's knowledge of health matters has improved through the distribution of information in the print and electronic media (Shepherd et al 1999). An educated, confident and articulate person can access information about their illness through their social network, magazines/newspapers and texts, television documentaries and the internet. An informed consumer has more chance of having their needs met than an uninformed consumer. It is anticipated that the more informed a person is, the less likely they are to view the health-care system with awe. Rather than placing their total trust in a system, they are more likely to question the success or otherwise of treatments on offer (Miller 2000). Such people are also more likely to exercise their freedom and to refuse treatments. Health-care workers' control over clients is reduced when the clients have information about their health condition and how to care for themselves, because the individual has more knowledge available to them, and can either make the choices themselves or know the appropriate questions to ask others.

Over the past decade there has been an emergence of consumer health information. Web-based health information in particular has flourished (Commonwealth of Australia 2000). There are a range of free sites on the web, including the Cochrane Collaboration, Medline, Psych INFO and CINAHL databases. Health information is also available through the Consumer's Health Forum of Australia. In this situation, information strengthens the person's capacity to care for self—and self-care does not necessarily replace traditional health services, but complements it.

Information contributes to reducing stress and increases a sense of control because it provides clients with an opportunity to adapt to changing circumstances and, in this way, promotes recovery (McCahon & Larsen 2002). According to Petersen:

> It has been found that clients who are given sufficient knowledge about their treatment (and condition) recover more quickly than those without the knowledge.
>
> Peterson 1994, p 91

Clients need information about their body and how it functions, how to prevent illness and cope with disease, how to use health-care systems, and the social, political and environmental influences on health.

NURSE AND CLIENT RELATIONSHIP

Apart from the changes with respect to primary health care, there have also been other changes in recent years, particularly with regard to how nurses are viewed and their relationships with clients. During Nightingale's era, nurses reflected the Victorian approach—reserved, conservative, rigid, with a rather puritanical approach to the client. This approach required obedience to the doctor, and this type of dominance prevailed until quite recent times—in some places it may still prevail. Over the past two or three decades, nurses have moved from viewing the client as a biomedical, mechanistic, passive recipient of care to a holistic, active consumer. There is increasing recognition of the client as a whole, humanistic individual. Similarly, the nurse is recognised as being human, with both positive and negative attributes, and as a person who experiences emotions the same as any other (Taylor 1994).

In nursing today, more attention is given to the nature of the experience of the client and the nurse (Taylor 1994). Stories of nurses and clients can encourage nurses to 'relinquish some of [their] professional control and strengthen the client's sense of power' (McCurdy 1990, p 111) and allow nurses to learn from each other and, more importantly, from clients. Clients' stories:

> serve to explain and support the choices [that] clients make. Respectful, empathic attention to stories can help caregivers understand and appreciate those choices and the person making them.
>
> McCurdy 1990, p 112

When nurses are informed of the client's experience of health and illness, they are more able to offer care which is congruent with the client's perspective. Similarly, if the nurse is informed of other nurses' experiences, they have the opportunity to learn from those experiences. The real issue here is the shared humanity between nurses and clients, as well as between nurses.

Nurses vary in how they relate to clients. Some nurses take over the client's care and expect the client to follow, whereas other nurses ask the client to explain their health goals, and ask them what services they require. It is true that, in the past, nurses have expected clients to follow orders. This remains a real problem in relation to care of older people, because of the ageist perceptions of old people as being in 'their second childhood', 'senile', 'daft', 'dependent' and so on. The categorisation of clients according to their 'obedience' is reflected in nurses' descriptions of 'good patients'.

A 'good patient' has been described by Remen (1980) as one who:

- is totally cooperative;
- implicitly trusts the professional carer and does not question the reason or purpose of management;
- is not curious;
- does not make demands on the professional's time;
- has no relatives who may become emotional or demand explanations;
- has their own emotions under control, and is stoical about pain;
- is a thorough and accurate observer of symptoms and an accurate historian of the past;
- heals quickly and does not develop complications;
- has a bodily disease which can be diagnosed and cured; and
- doesn't become chronically ill or die.

Although this is a satirical description of a 'good patient', it does reflect the expectations which a number of health-care providers have of the elderly. These expectations are not only unrealistic, but they also fail to reflect any concern for the client's experiences or wishes. There is no recognition of the client's capacity to contribute to their own health, or any concern for the client's health goals or human rights. Human rights extend beyond legal and professional barriers (Driscoll 1997). Issues such as client dignity, and protecting the client from harm, are considered central to these rights. Although the Consumer Health Forum of Australia has identified guidelines for health-consumers' rights, little has been done to ensure that these rights are protected on an individual level in everyday clinical practice (Driscoll 1997). When nurses relate to clients in a way that ignores their experience, rights and goals, the client quickly appreciates that this nurse does not want to know about their condition and they keep their thoughts and feelings—and sometimes the private nature of their health problem—to themselves.

CLIENT-MANAGED CARE

In Australia, there is much debate about who will manage the client's health—the doctor, the nurse, or one of the other health-care professionals. This chapter suggests that the most appropriate person to manage the client's health is the client. Client-managed care rests on the idea that all people who want to have control over their health should have that right and be supported in their choice. At the individual level, the person can even move past the level of being *involved* in their care towards *control* over and *self-management* of their care. At this level the individual is an active consumer of health services, and has authentic control over their health.

Client-managed care is not the same as self-care. Self-care implies that the person looks after their own interests and welfare and addresses their own needs themselves. It is possible for the client to provide their own self-care under direction from the health professional without actually managing or having control over their own care. The client may simply be performing certain tasks as directed by the health-care worker, and in this way self-care can be imposed on the client by the health-care worker.

Client-managed care may or may not include self-care, but does include client control, choice and decision-making about health care. In client-managed care, management and coordination of the person's health care rests with the person. Health care is not directed from the health professional to the client, but from the client to the health professional. When health-care workers are involved, they advise, consult and provide services where desired (rather like any other professionals) and the decision to take the advice or the service from the professional rests entirely with the client. With client-managed care, clients select and determine their care—according to their own goals—from the range of services offered, and decide whether or not to self-care. The health-care expert does not take control. It is the individual who requires relevant health information, formulates decisions and manages their health care over time. The emphasis is on the development of personal responsibility and control over health.

Everyone manages his or her own health care to some extent. People manage their health care in a variety of ways. When a person is sick and requires health care they may seek assessment and treatment from a range of health-care providers, including 'natural' therapists, family, friends and pharmacists as well as members of the organised health services. Most people initially consult a GP, who may offer treatment or referral to another health practitioner. Others may directly access a range of health professionals, such as physiotherapists, speech pathologists or nurses (either in hospital or at home in the community). Clients may directly access nurses involved in client education, and community nurses involved with mental health, child health, diabetic care or palliative care. In this way, people may manage their health care themselves by making decisions about what they want from the range of health-care services available.

Client-managed care is different from client collaboration, involvement or partnership in health care. Collaboration in health care is not client-managed care (Cahill 1998). Collaboration implies that two or more individuals cooperate in some kind of mutually responsive way. Client-managed care is not necessarily about close nurse–client interpersonal relationships, mutual nurse–client goals, shared understandings, negotiation, empowerment, or giving clients a voice. For many clients, their only goal is the fastest pathway to health, and some care little about engaging in a close relationship with the health-care provider.

Client-managed care is not about offering choices, or providing an adequate amount of information at the optimum time. It is about the client taking charge of their health care and exerting their right to act autonomously. Client-managed care is more than involving the person in their care at bedside handovers, through self-medication or via input into choice of menu—as useful as that involvement may be as an underused resource (Saunders 1995; Watkins 1995). Client-managed care is more than simply participation in decision-making—it is the client identifying their health goal according to their needs, and having genuine power and control over their health (Ashworth et al 1992).

In client-managed care, the client is in control and makes decisions about whether they want to engage with nurses in a close therapeutic relationship. In this situation, the nurse is neither enabling (Buchanan 1995) the client to health nor allowing them to be active in various ways, but is serving or providing services to the client. In client-managed care, the client directs the health service according to their needs, rather than the health-care workers deciding what they will 'allow' the client to do in respect of this or that matter. The underlying assumption is that the illness state belongs to the client, and that the nurse's role is to support the client's choice. The nurse's role is not to be a partner in care, but to deliver nursing services congruent with client-identified goals.

With client-managed care, the client advises the nurse of their broad health goals, and the nurse provides the nursing services that meet the client's needs. The nurse provides these services—assuming that they are not requests outside the law, or against the rights and personal safety of the nurse (Dimond 1993; Morgan 1996), or against the nurse's ethical practice—whether or not the nurse agrees with the client's decision. The nurse does not believe that he or she knows what is best for the client, because the nurse is not in the historical, social, cultural and personal life position of the client. Although the nurse can advise the client of the services available, and can give them information and support them in their goals, the nurse is not the client and does not know what is the right action for the client to take. However, the nurse does know a variety of ways of navigating a way through the health service, and can offer nursing care congruent with the client's wishes, and can also inform the client of ways of getting their health-care needs addressed. The nurse promotes client efficacy, control and autonomy at every opportunity. Nurses organise their work to support clients' control over their health, and question their own motives underpinning their practice—and do not seek a power relationship with clients. Rather, they stand back and support the client in forming and articulating the client's own view. Neither do nurses fear viewing their clients as people, or themselves as emotional human beings.

In this way, client-managed care is supported, and it is not possible for the client to be 'non-compliant', or for the nurse to 'allow' the client to perform some activity—because it is the client who decides on the health-care service. Nurses, rather than directing their energy to the needs of the doctor or the health-care system, concentrate on addressing the client's needs.

Barriers to client control over health

Within the health-care system there are many factors that reduce a person's sense of autonomy and control over health. These include:

- the impact of illness on the client (for example, pain or unconsciousness);
- the client's fear of entering a strange environment (such as a hospital);
- the client being psychologically located in the beneficence/paternalistic model and expecting that others will necessarily act in their best interests;
- the client's lack of knowledge about their illness, prognosis, treatment and rights;
- the bureaucracy of the health-care system;
- the nurses' and other health professionals' willingness or otherwise to respect the client's autonomy;
- the costs of health care;

- the health-care worker's philosophical and practical perspective;
- health-care workers' lack of knowledge in respect of legal and ethical aspects of practice;
- the gap between the knowledge of health-care workers and that of clients;
- tradition; and
- health-care workers' concern for professional influence and income.

Strategies to overcome these barriers need to be developed in order to find pathways for clients through the organised health-care services. For nurses, substantial work is needed to address the contextual barriers of hierarchy and paternalism that constrain them in their efforts to meet clients' health needs.

Benefits of client control over health

There are substantial benefits to the client when they have a sense of control, and manage their own care. Such a practice offers the client:

- an opportunity to identify and articulate their own goals based on their experience of the illness, treatment and sociocultural family circumstances;
- an opportunity to make decisions and take responsibility for their own health which offers the client an increased sense of control over their health;
- increased satisfaction because the person's own goals are used and so they are more likely to accept health outcomes;
- increased knowledge about their own health, which provides the person with a greater opportunity to adapt to changing health circumstances;
- access to their own health information, which puts them in a better position to make decisions and maintain confidentiality and continuity of care;
- the opportunity to exit the health service with less of a sense of indebtedness; and
- choices when there are limited funds and resources.

Health-care clients have the right to control over their health. Control over health has positive health outcomes for the individual because it locates the responsibility and accountability with the individual and serves the interest of the person with the health concern.

CONCLUSION

Changes in individual and social values, health-care needs and practices, and demography have been explored in this chapter to provide a context in which to present a new way of conceptualising managed care. The movement proposed is away from professional health management and towards client-managed care. At an individual level, the person strives to be informed, and to achieve and maintain control over their health. Where ill health is closely linked to social circumstances, collective participation can assist the population to bring about actions to address the social circumstances. Where ill health is linked to individual genetic circumstances, the person can work towards achieving and maintaining some control over the issues. Client-managed care is achievable and, it has been argued, is essential to nursing in the twenty-first century. This way of conceptualising practice is especially relevant in a health-care system with increasing numbers of older people who typically have suffered a reduction in choice, control, dignity and quality of life.

It was indicated at the start of this chapter that client-managed care was most appropriate for people who were still capable of making decisions. The vignette presented to conclude this chapter demonstrates how, even in cases where a client is demented, it is still possible for the wishes of the client to determine care strategies.

VIGNETTE

An informal network tailored to client needs

Barbara Potter

Miss Dee wore her 84 years proudly. She was a fit, healthy, active woman with a diagnosis of dementia—probably of the Alzheimer type. She was a retired secondary private-school teacher who had been used to being in charge as a capable decision-maker. She had not married, and was without siblings. Her mother had died when Miss Dee was 14 years old, and it troubled her greatly now that she had never known why. Miss Dee had travelled overseas frequently and her flat was full of mementos.

The difficulties with her current existence stemmed from complaints and concerns expressed by neighbours and home-care workers. These included:

- several times each week leaving generous amounts of rotting fruit and vegetables on neighbours' doorsteps;
- refusing to eat Meals on Wheels, and poking mouldy food into many nooks and crannies in her home;
- refusing admission to the home-help worker;
- sacking the council gardener;
- being away from home most days—where and with whom?
- muddles at the bank;
- muddles with medication—with a pillowslip half-full of prescription pills, potions and ointments (for herself and her late friend) ultimately being removed from her home;
- becoming increasingly unkempt—which was out of character;
- an urgent need for podiatry and dentistry;
- a lack of coordination in the formal and informal support network;
- a lack of understanding of the processes of dementia among the workers and neighbours; and
- refusing strategies which angered her.

However, Miss Dee also had identified strengths. She:

- was a charming, well-educated woman with a sense of humour;

- had some insight into her loss of memory and its impact;
- had general good health, and was a strong walker;
- had a loving god-daughter—the daughter of a school friend of 70 years ago—who had a family of her own, worked full-time and lived some distance away;
- had a strong family connection;
- had good friends, including ex-teachers and bowling friends;
- was a regular churchgoer at the same church for the past 38 years;
- owned her flat;
- had given her god-daughter enduring power of attorney;
- was able to allow trusted others to make tea in her house; and
- enjoyed food, but was unable to coordinate food preparation.

Miss Dee was referred to a Community Options Program. A care worker with interest in the arts—a person who was learning singing, loved poetry, and enjoyed reading and walking—was assigned to befriend Miss Dee. This care worker made visits, often walked with Miss Dee (allowing Miss Dee to lead and take the worker with her), received the Meals on Wheels, and prepared meals together. The method of providing the service/assistance was paramount to the success of the strategy.

Other aspects of the assessment revealed that the local Italian greengrocer and his wife made much of Miss Dee's visits with hugs, kisses and very warm welcomes—so much fruit was bought! But the hairdresser had given up because of lapsed appointments. The GP did not realise that Miss Dee was taking her late friend's medication. The bank teller was incredulous at having a bit of paper with numbers on it handed over in the expectation that he would return money. The minister was irritated by her flamboyant arrival in the middle of his sermon.

In summary, the informal network was extensive, and was rich and compassionate in dismay and concern for her.

It was decided, in consultation with the nearest and dearest, that a meeting of members of the network be organised for the purposes of:

- providing some information and awareness of the impact of memory loss;
- giving people an opportunity to express their concerns and annoyances;
- giving people a chance to know who else was in the network;
- giving people the 24-hour phone number of the care agency so that they did not feel that they were carrying the responsibility alone;
- congratulating the people on their support and concern over a long period of time; and
- thanking the people on behalf of Miss Dee—as she had lost the ability to do so herself.

Fourteen people came to the meeting in her local church rooms. Miss Dee was not present, but the intention of the meeting (that is, the promotion of her well-being) was described. There is no doubt that feelings of goodwill and support were there for their friend.

The format of the meeting was as follows:

- confirmation that all were concerned for the most suitable support for Miss Dee to remain at home for as long as she wished;
- 10–15 minutes' discussion about memory loss, its nature, impact and so on;
- each person invited to contribute to the meeting;

- some information given about Miss Dee's distorted perceptions; and
- problem solving, with people beginning to offer solutions to problems as various difficulties were raised, and offering various assistance, filling in the gaps in Miss Dee's own resources.

Examples of the services which were offered included:

- the fruiterers agreeing to remind Miss Dee that she had bought enough fruit and vegetables on the day before, but continuing to warmly welcome her and give the hugs and kisses that she so eagerly sought from them;
- two sisters down the road walking with her to church, and seeing that her dressing was dignified;
- two others taking her to their home for Sunday lunch, and walking with her to her own home afterwards;
- a local-hospital craft group agreeing to invite her as a helper and teacher, and for lunch, three times a week;
- the hairdresser phoning at a time suitable to the salon and saying, 'If you can come now I can do your hair' (thus giving as little time as possible for Miss Dee to forget); and
- her god-daughter organising the money and seeing to the payment of bills and some cash for Miss Dee to use.

There were many more arrangements slotted sensitively into the scheme that was to enable Miss Dee to stay at home long after it had been recommended that she go into residential care. Even the people who had struggled along did not feel—because they were friends—that residential care was appropriate for Miss Dee at that time.

The method of provision of the services by workers—with knowledge, insight and sensitivity—is imperative to the satisfactory tailoring of services to each individual, for each individual is unique in the way that dementia affects their lives.

In using the informal network, the participants in care should never be left without a 24-hour contact number of someone in the agency. The number is seldom used out of hours, but is imperative for participants to feel that they are backed up.

References

Agger B 1990, *The Decline of Discourse: Writing and Resistance in Postmodern Capitalism*, PA Falmer: Bristol.

Ashworth PD, Longmate MA & Morrison P 1992, Client participation: its meaning and significance in the context of caring, *Journal of Advanced Nursing*, 17, pp 1430–9.

Australian Institute of Health and Welfare (AIHW) 2002, *Australia's Health 2002*, AIHW: Canberra.

Australian Nursing Federation 2001, *Project to Support Nurses to Involve Consumers in their Health Care*, Australian Nursing Federation: Melbourne.

Baum F 2002, *The New Public Health*, Oxford University Press: Melbourne.

Biley EC 1998, The buck stops here: accepting responsibility for learning and actions after graduation from a problem-based learning nursing education curriculum, *Journal of Advanced Nursing*, 27(5), pp 1021–9.

Boud D 1995, *Enhancing Learning Through Self Assessment*, Kogan Page: Philadelphia.

Buchanan M 1995, Enabling clients to make informed decisions, *Nursing Times*, 91(18), pp 27–9.

Cahill J 1998, Patient participation—a review of the literature, *Journal of Clinical Nursing*, 7(2), pp 119–28.

Calhoun C 1996, Social theory and the public sphere. In: Turner BS (ed), *The Blackwell Companion to Social Theory*, pp 429–70, Blackwell: Oxford.

Cohen P 1995, Direct action, *Nursing Times*, 91(1), p 19.

Commonwealth of Australia 2000, *Improving Health Services through Consumer Participation, A Resource Guide for Organisations*, Brown & Wilton: Canberra.

Crossley M 1998, 'Sick role' 'empowerment': the ambiguities of life with an HIV positive diagnosis, *Sociology of Health and Illness*, 20(4), pp 507–31.

Dimond B 1993, *Clients' Rights, Responsibilities and the Nurse*, Quay Publishing BKT: Lancaster.

Draper M 1997, *Involving Consumer in Improving Hospital Care: Lessons from Australian Hospitals*, Commonwealth Department of Health and Family Services: Canberra.

Driscoll J 1997, In Defence of client/person human rights within National Health Care provision: implications for British nursing, *Nursing Ethics*, 4(1), pp 66–76.

Dworkin G 1998, *The Theory and Practice of Autonomy*, Cambridge University Press: New York.

Fiveash B 1998, Client managed care, *European Nurse*, 3(3), pp 186–93.

Gleeson G 1995, The 'Right' to Refuse Treatment: Autonomy vs Responsibility, *Bioethics Outlook*, 6(2), pp 1–2, 10–11.

Huber D 1996, *Leadership and Nursing Care Management*, Saunders: Philadelphia.

Idler EL & Benyamini Y 1997, Self-rated health and mortality: a review of twenty-seven community studies, *Journal of Health and Social Behaviour*, 38, pp 21–37.

Jewell SE 1994, Client participation: what does it mean to nurses?, *Journal of Advanced Nursing*, 19, pp 433–8.

Johnstone MJ 1989, *Bioethics: A Nursing Perspective*, Harcourt Brace: Sydney.

Jones GJ 1993, The client's charter in the accident and emergency departments, *Accidents and Emergency Nursing*, 1(4), pp 211–18.

Kerridge I, Lowe M & McPhee J 1998, *Ethics and Law for the Health Professions*, Social Science Press: Katoomba, NSW.

Lorig K, Sobel D, Stewart A, Brown B, Bandura A, Ritter P, Gonzalez V, Laurent D & Holman H 1999, Evidence suggesting that a chronic disease self-management program can improve health status while reducing hospitalisation—a randomised trial, *Medical Care*, 37(1), pp 5–14.

McCahon CP & Larsen PD 2002, Client and family education. In: Lubkin, IM & Larsen PD (eds), *Chronic Illness: Impact and Interventions*, Jones & Bartlett: Boston.

McCurdy DB 1990, Respecting autonomy by respecting persons: taking the client's story seriously, *Humane Medicine*, 6(2), pp 107–12.

Miller JF 2000, *Coping with Chronic Disease: Overcoming Powerlessness*, Davis: Philadelphia.

Mills JS 1962, Utilitarianism. On liberty—an essay. In: Warnock M (ed), *Bentham*, New American Library: New York.

Morgan D 1996, Respect for autonomy: is it always paramount?, *Nursing Ethics*, 3(2), pp 118–25.

Morse JM & Johnson JL 1991, Understanding the illness experience. In: Morse JM & Johnson JL (eds), *The Illness Experience—Dimensions of Suffering*, pp 1–12, Sage: Newbury Park.

Neumayer R & Goddard L 1998, Challenging the Myths of older adults with disabilities. In: Bevan C & Jeeawody B (eds), *Successful Ageing: Perspectives of Health and Social Construction*, pp 210–49, Mosby: Sydney.

Oddi LF 1994, Enhancing client's autonomy, *Dimensions of Critical Care Nursing*, 13(2), pp 60–9.

Petersen AR 1994, *In a Critical Condition—Health and Power Relations in Australia*, Allen & Unwin: Sydney.

Powell SK 1996, *Nursing Case Management—A Practical Guide to Success in Managed Care*, Lippincott: Philadelphia.

Redding P 1995, Science, medicine and illness: rediscovering the client as a person. In: Komesaroff PA (ed), *Troubled Bodies—Critical Perspectives on Postmodernism, Medical Ethics and the Body*, Duke University Press: USA.

Remen N 1980, *The Human Client*, Anchor Press/Doubleday: New York.

Reichley M 1999, Advances in home care: then, now and into the future, *Success in Home Care*, 3(6), pp 10–18.

Saunders P 1995, Encouraging clients to take part in their own care, *Nursing Times*, 91(9), pp 42–3.

Schofield D 1999, Ancillary and specialist health services: the relationship between income, user rates and equity of access, *Australian Journal of Social Issues*, 34(1), 79–89.

Shepherd S, Charnock D & Gann B 1999, Helping patients access high quality health information, *British Medical Journal*, 319, pp 764–6.

Taylor B 1994, *Being Human: Ordinariness in Nursing*, Churchill Livingstone: Melbourne.

Teece P 1995, *Bending Without Breaking: A Step-by-step Guide to the Successful Negotiation and Implementation of an Enterprise Flexibility Agreement under the Federal Industrial Relations Act*, Australian Library and Information Association: Canberra.

Thompson IE, Melia KM & Boyd KM 2000, *Nursing Ethics*, Churchill Livingstone: Edinburgh.

Watkins S 1995, Joint venture, *Nursing Times*, 91(16), pp 46–7.

Watts R 1994, Nursing theory and practice model of public participation. In: Greenwood J (ed), *Nursing Theory in Australia*, Harper Educational: NSW.

Weiler K 1993, Client self-determination: is anyone really listening? *Journal of Gerontological Nursing*, 19(10), p 42.

Wilkinson R & Marmot M 1998, *The Solid Facts: Social Determinants of Health*. World Health Organization: Geneva.

World Health Organization 1978, *Declaration of Alma Ata*, WHO: Geneva.

World Health Organization 1979, *Formulating Strategies for Health for All by Year 2000*, WHO: Geneva.

Part 2

Clinical issues and innovations

CHAPTER 11

Mental health issues

SALLY GARRATT

INTRODUCTION

The problem of defining 'mental health' and 'normality' as people age is complex and fraught with potential misinterpretation by health-care professionals. Establishing the signs and symptoms of mental *ill health* is relatively clearcut compared with understanding and unravelling what is meant by mental *health*. Most formal mental-health assessment protocols determine mental ill health by assessing such factors and abilities as cognition, intellectual ability, memory, life satisfaction, trait anxiety and depression against an established 'norm'. The difficulty with many of these assessments is that unless the person's cognition before they grew old is known, or unless there is evidence of gross abnormality in such parameters as memory loss, mistakes may be made that can affect care outcomes.

Many of the testing tools employed are culturally inappropriate, and do not interest the older person being tested. Translating testing tools into other languages is difficult, as the questions may be entirely rephrased during translation and lose meaning in the process. An example is the Folstein Mini Mental Health State Examination tool (Folstein et al 1975), which is routinely used in most aged-care facilities in Australia. Within Australia's culturally diverse population, some of the questions of this tool are inappropriate and may require amendments. For example, serial counting backwards by seven may not be in the repertoire of an elderly immigrant who did not attend school past grade three. Failing the test does not necessarily mean that the person has lost cognitive ability, but that they never mastered counting backwards. The assessor must be aware of these issues before using any normatively constructed tool.

In this chapter, an outline of possible factors involved in maintaining mental health is offered to assist nurses to determine whether they should be concerned about an older person's mental health status.

THE PROBLEM OF DEFINING MENTAL HEALTH

Defining something as intangible as mental health has occupied psychologists and sociologists for many years. A definition by Frieda Fromm-Reichman illustrates the complexity involved:

> these therapeutic goals (mental health) will be reached by the growth, maturation, and independence of the patient. Accomplishment will be further realised by his potential freedom from fear, anxiety, and the entanglements of greed, envy, and jealousy. This goal

will be actualised by the development of his capacity for self-realisation, his ability to form durable relationships of intimacy with others, and to give and accept mature love. I define 'mature love' in accordance with E Fromm and HS Sullivan, as the state of interpersonal relatedness in which one is concerned with the growth, maturation, welfare, and happiness of the beloved person as one is with one's own. This capacity for mature love presupposes the development of a healthy and stable self-respect.

Fromm-Reichman 1950, p xxvi

Another definition is offered by Freud:

the major determinants of mental health were the capacities to work and love, expressing the energies of aggression and eros.

Freud, cited in Ebersole & Hess 1981, p 471

To this, Ebersole & Hess (1981) added: 'the ability to enjoy leisure' as a third determinant of mental health.

Other authors have defined mental health from the perspective of gerontology social theorists.

Disengagement theory, developed by Cummings & Henry (1961), attempts to explain the withdrawal of older people from society as an inevitable and mutual disengagement. The older person and society interact less, resulting in perceived withdrawal by the older person from the mainstream activity which they once seemed to enjoy. Choosing to be alone is seen as a process of introspection and preparation for finalising those issues for which there was no time in earlier life. If this approach is used to understand mental health, a concerted effort must be made to distinguish between withdrawal as normal disengagement, and withdrawal as depression and loneliness.

The opposite theory to disengagement is the *activity theory*, proposed by Havighurst (1974). This approach suggests that old people need to remain active and enjoy social interaction to reach fulfilment in old age. Mental health, as defined using this approach, would suggest that if an old person remains active and socially engaged, they should be able to find contentment and enjoyment in life without seeking solitude.

Continuity theory (Atchley 1989) bases successful ageing—and, presumably, mental health—on adaptation to stress and development of coping mechanisms that remain throughout one's life. If the older person has had a successful pattern of coping throughout life, continuity theorists suggest that it is likely that this pattern will continue into old age. Life changes will be handled without excessive trauma, and adjustments will be made easily, due to established habits, customs, values and interests.

Most theoretical approaches have been challenged or supported by different authors. A final definition of 'mental health' is not possible, nor should it be attempted, because the interests of old people would not be served if one attempted to create a fixed, uniform definition of such a uniquely personal attribute. However, the view of mental health as a continuum—like health in general—may be useful for nurses (Ebersole & Hess 1981). One is never completely mentally healthy at all times, nor is one completely mentally unhealthy at all times, but one is always somewhere on the continuum—sometimes balanced, sometimes not. Mental health is as much a feeling as a state, a way of being rather than a definition.

APPROACHING AN UNDERSTANDING OF MENTAL HEALTH

Before making any attempt to ascertain the mental health status of another person, the health-care practitioner must know that person. Knowing the person means gaining an understanding of their life, the context in which they now find themselves, their relationships with others, their usual coping strategies, their ability to determine their own future, their own interpretation of what is happening to them as they age, and their sense of place in their world. The key to understanding these personal interpretations is observation of change in the way they live their life.

A change in attitude, behaviour, relationships, lifestyle and social interaction is often the clue for pursuing personal questioning further. For example, when an older person who has been living very well at home suddenly seems unable to make decisions, the family becomes concerned at the change. Does this change in lifestyle mean early dementia, depression, polypharmacy, dehydration or merely lack of interest in making decisions because other more pressing thoughts preoccupy them? Only by knowing the person can the assessor determine whether the change in mental health status is due to a conscious decision to cease concern with the small issues of day-to-day living—and to concentrate on bigger personal issues such as spirituality and inner peace—rather than evidence of mental pathology. Grappling with the philosophical realms of existence can make buying groceries and paying household accounts seem rather mundane. These personal ponderings are difficult for most people to explain to others, and an attempt at explanation may result in the person's being perceived as quite mentally unbalanced! Yet such mental activity is usual for older persons who have time to explore their thoughts about other realms of being.

ISSUES SURROUNDING MENTAL HEALTH STATUS

Facing the ageing process

The realisation that the physical body is ageing comes to people through the obvious signs of change that accompany physiological alterations. The hair turns grey, wrinkles appear, brown spots appear on the face and hands, the skin does not seem as supple, and so on. However, the self remains the same self that has developed over the years. How the person deals with this realisation of physical change shapes the way in which they will deal with end-of-life issues. When the self dictates to the body that it will not give in to ageing—that the 'I' is in control—body and self are at odds with one another. Gadow (1982) refers to this as 'disrupted immediacy', in which the body and self are acting upon one another, each determining mastery of existence.

> The self either controls the body through discipline, habituation and training, or it is controlled by the body through illness, awkwardness or disability.
>
> Gadow 1982, p 89

Eventually the body is seen as the source of impediment, restricting the self in the world and causing frustration, anger and denial. Older people who rail against their bodies as objects that will not physically do what they used to do, or because of pain will not permit the actions they desire, can either continue to be at odds with themselves or progress to what Gadow calls 'aesthetic immediacy'. As the ageing process encourages slowing, the opportunity for concentration on the body increases. Holding the body in aesthetic regard involves re-experiencing the body, neither despising it nor revering it, neither fearing it nor mastering it, but, rather, viewing it as an aesthetic object of value.

> The aesthetic relation can thus be characterised as a complex balance of form and freedom, in which both subject and object reciprocally affect and develop one another, the subject responding freely to the values expressed by the object.
>
> Gadow 1982, p 97

Aesthetic relation between self and body means listening to the body and working with it to bring an awareness of the body's own intrinsic value, not just being valued for its usefulness in allowing the self to take action.

Just as illness may render the body useless, ageing can be seen to do likewise. The dialectic of frailty and strength proposed by Gadow (1986) explains the dichotomy between a body seen as ugly, useless, dysfunctional and degraded, and a mind that still wants to experience life in all ways. The essential 'me' hasn't changed, but the shell around me deteriorates. Frailty that results in a disowning of the body is self-defeating, as the self or 'me' dissociates and regards the physical body as a loathsome object. Coming to terms with ageing may never happen, the self–body conflict may remain, and the results of this are apparent to those who care for old people who are at odds with themselves.

The perception of loneliness

Being alone does not mean that a person is lonely. To be alone is an act of physical or mental separation. Loneliness, however, is a feeling and a state of being. It can be experienced by any person, at any time, and in any situation. It is possible to be lonely in a crowd, just as it is possible to be alone, but not lonely, in a crowd. One chooses to be alone, but one does not generally choose to be lonely (Garratt 1984). The work of Sadler (1974), built on by Francis & Odell (1979), explores loneliness through four dimensions, all existential in origin.

The first dimension is cosmic in nature. This refers to an awareness of personal relation to the universe/deity/source of meaning. In this cosmic dimension, loneliness occurs when the person feels stripped of his or her identity with the natural environment or primal source. The American Indian and Australian Aboriginal cultures identify strongly with the earth, and trees, rivers and caves form an integral part of their existence. To take such people away from their land is to strip away identity and create soul-destroying loneliness.

The theme of loneliness runs through Judaeo-Christian scriptures. For example, the cry of Jesus Christ, 'My God, my God why hast thou forsaken me?' (Gospel according to Mark 15:34), reveals Christ's empathy with the intense cosmic loneliness which can afflict people.

Such cosmic dimensions of loneliness have a bearing on understanding the seeking of, and returning to, religious and spiritual practices/beliefs by old people. Such seeking can be interpreted as a healthy preparation for death, or alternatively as an unhealthy preoccupation with death, unless it is understood in the context of knowing the person.

The second dimension is one of cultural loneliness. The post-war patterns of immigration to Australia mean that many older people have been uprooted from their customs, beliefs and values, and forced to adapt to a new way of life. Second and third generations may or may not uphold the same cultural patterns of living that the older generation respects. Cluster groups in residential-care facilities based on ethnicity provide an anchor for some older people, but when illness or frailty compounds the ageing process, even such compatible social groupings cannot provide the sense of cultural belonging that the older person needs. Cultural estrangement affects the building of new relationships and the development of the trust that is necessary when dependence increases. Language and experiences are key determinants in understanding cultural loneliness. The ability to express cultural loneliness to family and friends may be difficult, as younger family members do not carry the same cultural memories and needs. In many situations, other carers cannot speak the language or know the culture well enough to determine what is happening. Feelings of devaluation may result from cultural alienation—even though the older person has lived in the new country for many years and managed very well.

By acknowledging cultural loneliness, the health professional indicates understanding and may help the older person to reach a stage of acceptance that will lessen the impact of the cultural loneliness. An acceptance that seeking a return to cultural values and ways of life is not abnormal will assist in the expression of need for meaning in ageing.

The third dimension of loneliness is social in nature. The establishment of a social personal identity that is known to others—and considered to be worth something—is necessary for establishing social relationships. Feelings of lowered self-worth can occur when the perceived value of what the older person offers others is diminished.

An example of such social loneliness is the story offered by a 90-year-old woman who was one of a group of quilters who met each afternoon in a nursing home to piece together handmade quilts. She was the last remaining member of the group able to continue the work—three others having died, and the fourth being too frail to contribute. The 90-year-old became withdrawn and distressed at the discontinuation of the quilting sessions. This was not because she was becoming frail herself, but because she could no longer give to the home. The quilts had been sold at the handicraft shop and, over some years, had raised considerable sums of money. This was her way of demonstrating economic worth and reciprocal care to those who provided care for her. This woman's social worth was constructed around the sewing work. She had an identity in the nursing home as the 'expert quilter'—an identity that was meaningful and gave her a sense of well-being. Her withdrawal was not depression, but rather a social loneliness generated from the loss of her group of cohorts, the loss of opportunity for reciprocity, and the loss of social identity. Understanding staff who grasped the significance of this woman's withdrawal would not intervene with antidepressants, but would assist the woman to work through her loneliness.

Sadler's fourth dimension of loneliness is interpersonal. This occurs when the person feels cut off from those they care about, and from those who genuinely care about them. This kind of loneliness relates to having another to love, another to need you—in an adult, mature love as described above by Fromm-Reichman (1950). This is not reciprocity in the sense of social loneliness, but rather the deep feelings of belonging and relating to another who returns the same feelings. Widowhood is prevalent in the older population and, as ageing progresses, deep feelings of yearning for the other may resurface and occupy the mind. Acknowledgement of the legitimacy of these feelings may not resolve the emotional pain, but may show an understanding of the need for a period of introspection over the loss. These feelings are not demonstrative of mental ill health unless they become overwhelming and render the person incapable of action.

All four dimensions of loneliness are useful in understanding the difference between depression and what may be considered 'normal' reactions to life events. When depression is accurately diagnosed, treatment is essential. However, non-recognition of the phases of the mental health continuum, and hasty recourse to antidepressive intervention, may be as detrimental as not treating depression.

Maintaining creativity

The creative abilities of human beings are endless, and ageing does not imply a loss of creative ability. In fact, many people begin the most creative phase of their lives after the age of 75 years. The US artist, Bill Fitzpatrick, rediscovered his creative talents later in life, finding that his talents had blossomed in age, and that anything was now possible. Fitzpatrick won many awards for his watercolours, and was still painting at 100 years of age (Goleman et al 1992).

Health-care professionals can forget that a person's need for creative expression does not stop as they age. In fact, it can become even more important. Because an older person wishes to attend painting classes and draw nude models does not mean that they are perverted, nor should it attract any other judgemental labelling. Conversely, the modern version of 'active ageing' that presents a distorted reality of bungee jumping and paragliding as normal activity, is not everyone's idea of expressing joy or creative living. Social expectations and stereotypical typecasting of the older generation often serve to suppress the creativity of older people. Physical restrictions may also hamper creative expression.

Struggling to find ways to continue to be creative can lead to despair, anger and frustration, and may mislead others into assuming that problems of mental ill health are present. Providing assistance in finding alternative outlets for creative expression in older people is a challenge for health-care professionals, who must broaden their thinking if they are to be successful.

How does mental health become mental ill health?

The difference between feeling 'low' or 'down' and the actual symptoms of depression is hard to define. Every human being at some point in their life has feelings of sadness, loss, grief, lack of interest and distress. These feelings may come as the result of some change in the life patterns such as moves away from home, loss of a person close to them, loss of job security, health changes that prevent physical action, and a host of other disruptive life events. Older people have endured many of these events over a lifespan of seventy years or more and have developed coping strategies that carry them over the low periods.

The Hammond Care Group was commissioned to undertake a project to examine depression in older people who were admitted to residential aged care. The report suggests that the use of the self-reporting Geriatric Depression Scale

(Yesavage 1988) identified 51% of people in high care and 30.2% of people in low care as having some level of depression.

When a person is faced with massive changes due to failing health that necessitates them moving to residential care, one could assume that a feeling of gloom and despair would be a usual, normal response. Sometimes, however, the feeling of relief that at last the difficult management of home and personal care matters has now been given over to others to deliver can bring initial positive responses.

Staff at the caring interface perceive the negative feelings exhibited by the older person as depression, and they are probably right. The initial response to loss and grief is a depressed mood and a feeling of the end of the world. Only when these feelings persist and become increasingly evident in a person's reaction to the environment and care can the diagnosis of depression be properly made.

In most cases the negative feelings are transient and can be deflected by activity and reconciliation, using the good things in life to counterbalance the bad. Older people have learned how to cope with this very well and can usually see the positives as well as the negatives, if given time.

The role of nurses in aged care is to recognise the potential for these feelings to become depression that requires more active intervention. Assessment of low mood, loss of interest in life, no enjoyment in any activity, loss of appetite and change in sleep patterns flag the changes that will lead to a diagnosis of the onset of a more serious problem. The astute practitioner will detect when the older person has moved from a position of possible reaction to events or feelings of gloom, to one of abnormal lack of interest in life. 'Many depressions seem understandable, and maybe that is one of the reasons why so often they are not identified as needing attention' (Challenge Depression Manual 2001, p 16). As Snowdon (1988) states, 'assessment is the vital first step in management of late-life depression' (p 57).

Some symptoms of depression are not as obvious as those mentioned above, and may consist of vague reports of anxiety, complaints about food, regular exacerbation of headaches and so on. These vague feelings of discontent may be masking the deeper symptoms that many older people do not feel they can disclose because it is not the 'proper thing' to discuss your personal feelings with others. Disclosure of inner feelings and thoughts about the end of life require a relationship with the carer built on trust. The integrity needed to establish trust in relationships takes time to develop. Often the ability to disclose what is really the main problem takes considerable effort on the part of the older person, who may also have physical disability that creates pain or other discomfort. It is impossible to run away for personal space if you are confined to a chair or wheelchair and totally reliant on others to meet your needs. The coping strategies that were used successfully in the past may, or may not, be able to be used now. Withdrawal may be the way to escape.

The role of the nurse is not to 'jolly' and cajole but to understand what may be happening and to recognise the need for making that understanding known—in other words, allowing for the reactive time and need for personal space to overcome the loss and grief if present, to give permission for the person to feel sad, to provide a good ear for listening without giving advice, and to observe carefully the reaction to this shared understanding. Over time the responses to others should be noted and if apparent changes are seen to be increasingly negative then further professional assessment needs to be sought.

Professional assessment should include the use of a screening tool that identifies the potential for depression in older people. A team approach to completing a thorough assessment requires all members of the care team to contribute, including the family if present. Reaction to medication for other conditions must be ruled out. Some frequently used medications can cause mood changes; alcohol or drug abuse can be identified after admission to a facility; and family interactions can be causal factors in creating depression.

The difficulty in determining depression when dementia is present is not insurmountable. Withdrawal and flattened affect may be present with either or both conditions but the key to ascertaining health status is observation and knowing the person. Most care staff can detect change in behaviour and relate to possible reasons for the change. The process of ruling out other reasons for behaviour begins by assessing for pain and other physical disorders. Commencing treatment for depression may be the only way to see whether the symptoms improve and the behaviour changes again.

Meaning in life

The mental health status of older people can be improved by creating opportunities to give meaning in the day. All people need to feel they have contributed and done something that gives pleasure both to themselves and to others. The reciprocity of giving and receiving makes for purpose in existence. Enabling activity that creates purpose is the challenge for carers. To have done some task or interacted in some way with another that has given pleasure is to enhance self-esteem and give value to the self. The opportunity to do this in residential care has to be sought. Care is given over twenty-four hours and most needs are met without necessarily allowing for the reciprocal act of giving back meaningful exchange. Yet, without being able to give, the value of one's presence is not felt—the person is a receiver only and that becomes burdensome. Where the person is valued, their world has meaning.

MENTAL HEALTH ISSUES WITH PARTICULAR GROUPS

The rural ageing population in Australia has the added burden of isolation from service provision available to metropolitan people. Gattuso (2003) found that older people who live in rural communities were being referred to psychiatric services because of their perceived lack of ability to deal with the challenges of ageing. They were presenting with depression and stress but not diagnosed psychiatric illness. A mental health promotion program was initiated in four rural centres, with a total of 103 older people taking part. While there were methodological issues with the study, the findings indicated a need for further work in assisting older people to modify their attitude toward ageing and to promote self-esteem. The outcomes of the project were to provide a successful intervention that gave the participants an opportunity to gain knowledge and insight into their feelings and improve their general health status.

Mental health in culturally and linguistically diverse groups also requires special understanding of the cultural differences and social expectations of ageing. For some cultural groups, mental health is not something that is discussed openly, even within the family environment. The expectations of the older family member may be to have continued devoted care at any price, as a right. Given the changing nature of work for women in particular, the use of age-specific services and residential care for family members is tantamount to failure. For other groups the use of care services is not seen as useful because of language difficulties and poor access capability. Mostly these issues are addressed by the voluntary sector that continues to provide specific care for their own cultural groups. Given the multicultural heritage of Australia, the needs of these groups must continue to be addressed by both community and government programs.

The mental health needs of family carers is often overlooked if the problem is not related to diagnosed dementia or psychiatric illness. There are support groups for most forms of mental illness, for carers to gain knowledge and understanding of their role in care. However, the carer of another older person may also be constricted in their own life because of the continual nature of providing 24-hour support. There is a caregiver burden for that family or other support persons who provide the avenue for the older person to remain at home. Shopping, cleaning and other activities of daily living require input from others, and access to services to assist in these activities may not always be available. The family member may find himself or herself in a relationship of dependence that can become very difficult to disengage from. Family life can revolve around whether the older member can participate, and who is staying home to provide care when others are away. Over time the dependence can become a burden that affects family functioning.

CONCLUSION

Mental health and mental ill health are serious concerns within an ageing population. This chapter has discussed some issues involved in mental health assessment and diagnosis in old age. Education of care staff who provide services for older people is essential to gain understanding and insight into the lives of others. Providing meaning and creating opportunities for purpose in life are the challenges for all those involved in care. Prevention of mental health deterioration is the key in ensuring that quality residential care is offered to a very vulnerable group within our society.

VIGNETTE

'Dorothy'

Maria McIntosh

Dorothy is an 84-year-old nurse who served in World War II and was admitted to a psychogeriatric unit because of her progressive dementia and inability to maintain her activities of daily living.

Her diagnosis of dementia seemed to be an addition to a pre-existing mental health problem but her personality was generally bright and happy. At times Dorothy became sad, distressed and very vocal in her demands. She created a noise level that was disturbing to others. The shouting and demanding could become abusive.

Dorothy had some insight into her mood changes and knew when she was unhappy and sad. The depressive mood changes could be predicted by her change in behaviour, and she seemed to know when this was occurring. She was also very active at night and would do her 'nursing rounds' to ensure others were asleep.

The staff were concerned about her distressed episodes and her nocturnal wandering. They determined to institute a plan to assist in keeping Dorothy on a more even plane. Medication did not seem to help her mood changes and the level of antipsychotic medication was kept at a minimum.

The staff found that Dorothy responded well to personal interaction and attention such as touch, voice contact and offering of food. It seemed that she found comfort in the one-on-one approach, and her behaviour could be ameliorated. This indicated a degree of loneliness and a need for human interaction when Dorothy became 'down'. Coca-Cola and Twisties snack food were very much in favour and seen as comfort food.

Every day at 4 pm the staff would give Dorothy special attention and offer food snacks, touch and conversation. This seemed to re-centre her day and she would then go about the other activities with a calmer disposition. Dorothy lacked the concentration or motor ability to do many coordinated activities but was physically strong and could walk all day.

The plan to offer her the attention needed to reassure her that her world was still intact worked very well, and her outbursts of noisy demanding behaviour decreased.

References

Atchley RC 1989, Continuity theory of normal ageing, *The Gerontologist*, 29(2), pp 183–90.

Challenge Depression Manual 2001, *The Hammond Care Group*, Commonwealth Department of Health and Ageing: Canberra.

Cummings E & Henry WE 1961, *Growing Old: The Process of Disengagement*, Basic Books: New York.

Ebersole E & Hess E 1981, *Toward Healthy Ageing*, Mosby: St Louis.

Folstein ME, Folstein SE & McHugh ER 1975, Mini-mental state: a practical method for grading the cognitive state of patients for the clinician, *Journal of Psychiatric Research*, 12, pp 189–98.

Francis G & Odell SH 1979, Long-term residence and loneliness: myth or reality? *Journal of Gerontological Nursing*, 5(1), pp 9–11.

Fromm-Reichman E 1950, Principles of intensive psychotherapy. In: Koenig HG (eds), *Ageing and God: Spiritual Pathways to Mental Health in Midlife and Later Years*, Haworth Press: New York.

Gadow S 1982, Body and self: a dialectic. In: Kestenbaum V (ed), *The Humanity of the Ill*, University of Tennessee Press: Knoxville.

Gadow S 1986, Frailty and strength: the dialectic of ageing. In: Cole TR & Gadow S (eds), *What Does It Mean To Grow Old? Reflections from the Humanities*, Duke University Press: Durham.

Garratt S 1984, *Old and Lonely: Not Always Synonymous*, unpublished paper, University of Colorado: USA.

Gattuso S 2003, Promoting mental health in rural elders: a pilot program, *Australasian Journal on Ageing*, 22(2), pp 76–9.

Goleman D, Kaufman E & Ray M 1992, *The Creative Spirit*, Penguin Books: New York.

Havighurst RR 1974, *Developmental Tasks and Education*, McKay: New York.

Sadler WAJ 1974, On the verge of a lonely life, *Humanitas*, X(3), pp 255–76.

Snowdon J 1998, Management of late-life depression, *Australasian Journal on Ageing*, 17(2), pp 57–62.

Yesavage JA, 1988, Geriatric Depression Scale, *Psychopharmacology Bulletin*, 23(3), pp 271–84.

CHAPTER 12

Dementia, mental health and issues of abuse in aged care

SARAH MOTT AND BETH KINGSLEY

INTRODUCTION

Australia is an ageing society. With a rapidly increasing population of people over the age of 65 years, a corresponding increase is to be expected in the number of older people with mental illness for whom health care must be provided. With more and more residential aged-care beds occupied by older people with dementia and other mental health problems, staff are faced with the difficulties of providing care to those residents whose behaviour presents special challenges.

This chapter describes the behaviours of people with dementia in relation to other mental health problems. It also discusses how residential-care agencies can aim for optimal outcomes of quality care by focusing on the selection, supervision, education and support of their staff.

DEMENTIA AND MENTAL HEALTH PROBLEMS

It is problematic as to whether or not dementia should be regarded and treated as a mental illness despite its being included in the fourth edition of the *Diagnostic and Statistical Manual of Mental Disorders* (American Psychiatric Association [APA] 1994). For the purposes of this chapter, dementia is addressed separately from other mental-health problems.

Dementia

Dementia occurs when changes in the brain result in confusion, loss of intellectual ability and memory impairment. Dementia can be a symptom of a number of conditions, including Alzheimer's disease, vascular dementia, Korsakoff's syndrome and Huntington's chorea (Eastley & Wilcock 2000). Although diagnosis of dementia has improved, the introduction of the term 'dementia of the Alzheimer's type' reflects the difficulty of precise diagnosis (Garratt & Hamilton-Smith 1995). The cause of this type of dementia, which affects more women than men, is unknown (Jorm & Henderson 1993).

As 'dementia of the Alzheimer's type' accounts for the largest proportion of people with dementia (O'Brien et al 1997; Mayeux 1993), much of the current literature concentrates on this condition. However, the changes characterised by global losses of intellectual and behavioural processes are common to most organic brain syndromes (Berrios 1995).

Demography of dementia

The life expectancy of both males and females has increased dramatically this century (Hugo 1986). The incidence of chronic disease and impairment rises with age, with the increase becoming more rapid after 75 years of age (Koch & Kralik 2001). In an ageing population, therefore, there will be increasingly greater numbers of people suffering from chronic disability, with an associated reduction in quality of life. Graycar sums up the situation as follows: 'in giving people more time to live, science and medicine have also given them more time to die' (Graycar 1986, p 8).

Demographic predictions indicate that there will be 174,300–194,200 people in Australia suffering from dementia by 2006 (Commonwealth Department of Community Services and Health 1990) and 459,000 in 2041 (Logiudice 2002). 'It is likely that an "epidemic" of dementia will be faced ... as the "baby-boomers" generation reaches retirement age' (Mayeux 1993). Currently, at least 60% of residents in nursing homes and aged-care units in psychiatric hospitals suffer from dementing conditions (Commonwealth Department of Health, Housing and Community Services 1991; Edwards et al 2003; Levesque et al 1993; National Centre for Health Statistics 1991; Spore et al 1991).

The prevalence of dementia is presented in Table 12.1. These figures show that the prevalence of dementia increases exponentially with age, with many more 'old-old' people being affected than 'young-old' people. Under the age of 50 years, dementia affects about one person in a thousand, and thereafter the chance of developing the condition rises steadily.

Table 12.1: Prevalence of dementia in Australia

Age group (years)	Prevalence (%)	Population (1000s)	Prevalence (per 1000)
60–64	0.72	731.2	5.26
65–69	1.42	653.4	9.28
70–74	2.82	476.3	9.28
75–79	5.60	370.2	20.73
80–84	11.11	211.1	23.46
85+	23.60	145.8	34.41

Source: Jorm & Henderson 1993, p 10.

Course of Alzheimer's-type dementia

Dementia of the Alzheimer's type has three stages, each with recognisable clinical characteristics (Reisberg et al 1999). The first stage is marked by mild memory loss and confusion, the next stage involves a further deterioration of the person's cognitive functioning and, in the final stage, the physical abilities of the individual fail, until total incapacity results. Each stage of the disease is examined below.

First stage

The early stage of Alzheimer's disease can progress quickly (over 2–4 years), or more slowly (over 15 years) (Storandt et al 2002). The first symptoms, an insidious development of absent-mindedness, emotional instability and lack of concentration, are often overlooked or dismissed as insignificant.

Signs in the later parts of stage one include increasing memory loss, spatial disorientation, lack of spontaneity, disturbances of perception, lack of care with hygiene/appearance and a tendency to blame others for an inability to perform everyday tasks efficiently. Depression is not uncommon at this point because the person knows that things are 'not quite right' (Katona 1994).

As the disease progresses into stage two, denial is a prominent defence mechanism, accompanied by emotional withdrawal. On occasions, however, anger, suspicion and transient crying episodes can occur (Eastley & Wilcock 1997). This stage may vary in length from 2 to 12 years. Progressive dementia, complete disorientation, dulling of comprehension and restlessness at night are typical occurrences during this period. Nocturnal awakenings can be particularly dangerous to the afflicted person and worrying to relatives. Forgetfulness of recent and more distant past events becomes more noticeable, and the individual may forget all personal details, intimate friends and close family (prosopagnosia). Further deterioration of the areas of the cerebral cortex that involve memory, language and motor functions results in loss of coordination and the abilities to write (agraphia) and speak (aphasia) (Tyler et al 1997). Perseveration, the continual repetition of a word or gesture, is common. The loss of coordination affects the ability to perform purposeful movements or tasks (apraxia) such as dressing or eating.

Second stage

People in stage two of Alzheimer's disease can no longer cope without assistance in the community (Griffith 2002). As levels of functioning deteriorate, they may have difficulty in carrying out simple tasks such as choosing clothing appropriate to the occasion or season without supervision, and may wear the same clothing day after day if not reminded to change.

The appearance of focal signs at this stage will vary depending on the brain areas most affected. Focal symptoms will include interference in direct sensory reception such as sight, hearing and pain. Other focal symptoms will result from deficiencies in association areas causing an inability to comprehend the sensations received. These symptoms may present themselves as visual disturbances such as homonymous hemianopia (the loss of half of the field of vision in both eyes) or decreased pain perception (Hayes 1995).

Loss of the ability to associate stimuli makes it difficult, if not impossible, for the person to recognise familiar objects by sight (alexia), or by touch (astereognosia), or to recognise familiar sounds or words (auditory agnosia) (Mayer & Darby 1995). The individual may also have problems in recognising his or her own face (mirror sign). There is increased muscle tension and a change in gait. A stiff, stooped posture and a wide-based stance, together with slow, shuffling steps, is typical. Individuals may cup their hands at their sides and limit arm-swinging. Problems with balance (ataxia) may occur, putting the person at risk of accidents or falls.

Constant movement and purposeless pacing are also characteristic of the second stage. Crump (1992) and Stokes (1987) consider that factors responsible for these movements may include:

- boredom—lacking exercise and interesting activities, the person may wander for something to do;
- searching—looking for a person, pet or place belonging to a world remembered from before the onset of the illness;
- forgetfulness—impaired short-term memory can lead to the person forgetting where they were going or for what reason;
- pain—sitting for long periods may cause discomfort, or exacerbate a minor problem; and
- enduring personality traits—lifelong patterns of exercising for enjoyment or stress-relief may not diminish in dementia.

Hyperorality—a need for oral stimulation, manifested by chewing or tasting whatever objects are available, however inedible—may be present at this time (Burns et al 1990). Neuronal damage blocks self-control, and the exhibitionism common among sufferers of Alzheimer's disease is often related to forgetfulness. Unable to locate the toilet, for example, a male may indicate the need to void by unzipping his trousers in the living room or the street. Similarly, a female may lift her skirt in the supermarket, indicating her desire to void. Urinary/faecal incontinence is likely to make its first appearance at this point in the disease (Boller et al 2002).

Third stage

The insidious progression of these symptoms continues as more and more neurons become affected, until the person reaches the third and terminal stage. This stage is usually the shortest one, lasting from six months to two years. People in the third stage of the disease lose the ability to speak and to walk. Before the complete loss of ambulation, the individual may be found on the floor, having 'forgotten' that they were walking and having sunk to the ground.

Denial appears to continue to protect the victim even in late dementia. The individual may continue to laugh, smile and appear to enjoy life as much as anyone else. They may be kindly and amenable, or recalcitrant and angry. Any emotional outbursts should be interpreted carefully, as they might be attempts to communicate needs, not merely an expression of anger (Lawlor 2002). Finally, the sufferer becomes completely unaware of the environment, and all motor abilities are lost. The end-stage of dementia is stupor and coma. Death commonly results from immobility causing such complications as pneumonia or thrombosis (Burns 1995).

With decreasing levels of cognitive and physical functioning, individuals lose their ability to live independently. Once they have entered stage two of the disease, it is highly likely that some type of care will be necessary. Depending on the availability of families and friends who can lend assistance, admission to residential care may be postponed until community care becomes inappropriate.

Mental illness

The most common mental illness of old age is depression, a disabling condition associated with increased mortality, through suicide or natural causes (Poole & Mott 2003). The prevalence of depression among people over the age of 65 has been estimated at 10–15% (Sadavoy et al 1995), rising to 30% for residents of nursing homes (Ames 1995). Depression may exacerbate cognitive disturbances, or may mimic states of pseudodementia. Untreated depression, wrongly diagnosed as dementia, may lead to inappropriate placement in aged-care facilities.

Other psychiatric disorders experienced by older people include those which have their onset in young-to-middle adulthood, such as bipolar-affective disorder (Broadhead & Jacoby 1995) and schizophrenia (Lacro & Harris 1995). Schizophrenia, although usually apparent before 45 years of age, may be of late onset (APA 1994).

BEHAVIOURS OF CONCERN IN RESIDENTIAL CARE

A major problem in the care of older people with mental health problems is that they are viewed as a homogeneous group. It is not uncommon for writers on aged care, or indeed those who develop aged-care policy, to lump all older people with mental illness and dementia into the same category (Gorman & Welch 1993; Ludwig 1993; McCullagh 1994; Ticehurst 2001). There is an indisputable need to advance a more precise classification of mental illness to make clear the differences among disorders such as dementia, depression, and affective and psychotic disorders. In Australia, the Victorian *Mental Health Act 1986* supports the requirement for care which both focuses on the individual needs of people and is delivered in the least restrictive environment.

Some mental illnesses and dementia need radically different approaches to care, and it is difficult to imagine how the needs of all individuals can be met if these groups are mixed together indiscriminately in the same environment (Lidz et al 1992; Mosher-Ashley et al 1991; Mott 1997). For example, the symptoms of schizophrenia—such as hallucinations, delusions and bizarre behaviour—may become less severe with age, leading to possible improvement in behaviour. Whereas people with dementia are on the inevitable road to cognitive decline, individuals with schizophrenia may seem to be improving (Krach 1993). Therefore, not only do the symptoms, behaviour patterns and care needs of these two groups differ, but they also change over time as the severity of the dementia increases, or that of mental illness increases or decreases. Of course it is not uncommon for a person with dementia to also have other mental illnesses such as depression, and it is important that changes in behaviour are thoroughly assessed and not just assumed to be a worsening of the dementia.

Dementia is responsible for up to 85% of behavioural concerns in residential aged-care facilities (Lawlor 2002), and much research considers the needs of nursing-home residents with dementia. However, there is scant research concerning the behavioural concerns of older residents who have a mental illness (German et al 1992; Vogel & Mercier 1991). The literature is also scarce on how the care needs of people with dementia differ from the care needs of people with a mental illness, and little has been written on the difficulties of caring for both groups in the one institution (Mott 1997).

The range of behaviours exhibited by mentally ill older people (who do not have dementia) is diverse—and these behaviours can be explosive and unprovoked, and can target more vulnerable people. Mentally ill residents with intact short-term memory are apt to bear grudges and seek revenge for real or imagined wrongs. The strategies needed to manage these behaviours differ markedly for each of the various mental illnesses. They also differ from strategies required for residents suffering from dementia.

Pacing, wandering and shouting are behaviours common to people with dementia, whereas irritability, abusive behaviour and paranoia are more likely to occur in someone with a diagnosis of mental illness (Santmyer et al 1992). Behaviours by residents that nursing staff see as disruptive include:

- trouble-making;
- irritability;
- explosiveness; and
- resistance.

All of these behaviours can alienate staff, and result in reduced staff–patient contact (Kikuta 1993; Stevens & Baldwin 1988; Winger et al 1987). When residents were asked in Mott's (1996) study to identify those behaviours of other residents which they felt disrupted their lives, they did not include trouble-making in their list of the ten most disruptive behaviours. Nevertheless, both staff and residents agree that disruptive behaviour—irrespective of the type or cause of the behaviour—is unpleasant, and reduces the safety of the living and working environment (Beck et al 1990; Carstensen & Fisher 1988; Kikuta 1993).

During the fieldwork in her study, Mott (1996) noted that people with dementia of the Alzheimer's type are not a homogeneous group, and that they also exhibit significant differences in behaviour (Gilley et al 1991; Teri et al 1990; Zubenko et al 1992). There is no clear reason for such differences existing. However, contributing factors may include:

- clusters of behaviours which change as the dementia progresses;
- the age of the individual at the onset of the disease; and/or
- the existence of other pathologies as yet unidentified.

The two distinct patterns of behaviour exhibited by residents with a primary diagnosis of dementia of the Alzheimer's type are those of sociable or solitary behaviour and are presented in Table 12.2.

Sociable behaviour

The sociable group of residents with Alzheimer's disease—male and female—move around in pairs or groups, or attach themselves to other residents or staff. They are rarely found on their own. However, when alone, the sociable residents approach anyone they see, and tend to follow this person if the other person does not stop to talk. The content of their speech can be:

- questioning—'Who are you, dear?'
- complimentary—'You look nice.'
- requesting—'Can I come with you?'.

Depending on the degree of dementia present, the words can be difficult to understand, but the inflection of the speech, as well as the non-verbal communication, lend clues to what type of remark is being made. These clues include the resident's touching of the other person's clothing or face, smiling, taking of the other's hand, or the giving of hugs.

Residents with sociable behaviour patterns interact frequently with the environment. These are the residents who rattle the door handle, tap on windows, pick flowers in the garden, and fiddle with their own (and other people's) possessions. They are not likely to be violent unless provoked. Such provocation usually comes when a member of staff attempts to pull them physically by the hand in a direction in which they do not wish to go—to the shower, for example. The aggression, if present, occurs in a reflexive and defensive manner that is aimed at allowing the resident to escape. Attacks from other residents, however, are poorly defended.

The sociable residents are easily distracted, and a resourceful nurse can achieve desired goals by employing diversionary tactics, whereas a direct approach invariably causes unnecessary confrontation. Residents with sociable behaviour have very revealing facial expressions and body language. Emotions such as happiness, confusion, distress and anger can be detected immediately. Whereas they do not seem to bear grudges towards other residents or staff—indeed the episodes seem immediately forgotten—altercations invariably produce facial expressions of distress. These seem to represent underlying thoughts that might be characterised as: 'I'm not sure what happened, but I feel unhappy'.

Table 12.2: Behaviour patterns of residents with dementia of the Alzheimer's type

Sociable	Solitary
Social—move in pairs or groups	Loners
Approach others	Do not approach others
Spontaneously touch or hug others	Do not spontaneously touch—avoid physical contact
Not violent unless provoked	Unpredictably violent
Easily distracted	Not easily distracted
Emotions clearly apparent through facial expression and body language	Lack of facial expression, body language 'tight'

Source: adapted from Mott 1996.

Solitary behaviour

The pattern of behaviour of both male and female residents in the solitary group with Alzheimer's disease differs recognisably from that of those with sociable behaviour. One of the most notable contrasts is the aloof nature of these residents; they tend to move through their environment on their own, not approaching anyone. They do not seem to avoid company, but rather pass it by as if it does not exist. The solitary residents do not spontaneously touch others; in fact, physical contact is avoided to the point of lashing out at a person who initiates such contact. Interaction with the environment is minimal, and tends to be destructive, such as pulling down curtains that are blocking the person's way. These residents lack mobile facial expressions, appearing blank and unemotional even during altercations. Their body language is invariably tense and, while walking, their fists are often clenched.

Aggressive behaviour is frequent in those with solitary patterns of behaviour. It is often unpredictable, but rarely personal. If a resident in this group, cruising around the corridors, has his or her movement restricted by a person or object, attempts are made to remove the obstruction, such as by pushing it out of the way. If other residents or staff approach a solitary resident using any form of physical contact, that person will be brushed or shrugged away. In the case of a sociable resident making an approach, a fall or a fight is a likely outcome. Solitary residents are more able than others to defend themselves in the event of an attack. Diversionary tactics are not successful, but pointing the resident in the right direction, and blocking off alternative routes, are more likely to get the person to the desired destination.

Staff attitudes

Staff tend to interact differently with different residents according to the residents' behaviour patterns. The differences in the activities offered by staff to individual residents have been documented by a number of research studies (Armitage & Champney-Smith 1990; Burgener & Barton 1991; Norbergh et al 2001, 2002). These studies found that nurses prefer to spend more time and seek more interactions with residents with higher cognitive and functional abilities than with those who have lower-level functioning. For example, when working with people with dementia, and those with other types of mental illness, staff choose to spend more time talking and socialising with the latter group, even though nurses find many of the behaviours of these residents to be unpleasant and disruptive (Mott 1996).

This evidence reinforces the need for staff training, in order that staff might consciously divide their time among residents on the basis of need, rather than on the basis of staff personal preference. The evidence also stresses the importance of staff members being educated, not only about the behavioural issues and care needs of residents with mental illness and dementia, but also about assessing and meeting the various needs of each resident, regardless of their level of functional, cognitive and social abilities.

The most important aspect of the care of nursing-home residents with mental illness is that staff recognise when to seek expert help from a psychiatrist or psychiatric/mental health nurse. Medical treatment of people with psychoses commonly involves the prescription of neuroleptic medication. As people with schizophrenia get older, their dosage requirements often tend to decrease (Tran-Johnson et al 1992). It is therefore vital that nursing staff be educated, informed and alert to the signs and symptoms of overdosage, so that dosage modifications can be made.

Research reported by Arthur et al (1992) indicates that nurses faced with uncooperative behaviours initially feel annoyed. When attempts fail to coerce the individual into submission, the resident is likely to be ignored. Behavioural-modification programs are more likely to include reinforcement of positive behaviours (Puckett 1993) than the ignoring of negative ones. However, the practice of ignoring undesirable behaviour must be based on a legitimate behavioural modification program, rather than being used casually as an excuse for abusive practices.

QUALITY OF CARE

All citizens have the right to live with dignity and independence, to be safe from threat or harm, and to receive high-quality health care. In 1982, these principles were enshrined in the United Nations *Principles for Older People* (Resolution 37/51), and they continue to apply to the care of seniors in both community and residential settings. All hostel and nursing-home residents have the right to be treated with respect and dignity, to live with optimal independence and choice, and to receive quality care that never harms—but always promotes—health and well-being. This topic is dealt with in more detail in Chapter 3.

Abusive practices

Quality care is provided by most residential-care staff most of the time. Nevertheless there will be instances where care is less than sympathetic. It is in the bedroom world of close, intimate care that mistreatment and punishing behaviours become an acceptable part of the daily routine (Lee-Treweek 1994, cited in Goodridge et al 1996, p 52).

The chilling fact is that, because of its hidden nature, the extent of resident abuse by staff is unknown. Nevertheless it is known that where people are frail, dependent or under the control of others, they are vulnerable to abuse (Eriksson & Saveman 2002). The abuse, by staff, of frail, dependent residents is a significant problem that is on the increase (Castledine 1994; Kapp 2002).

One very early study into staff–patient conflict defined 'abuse' as behaviour (by aides) which would result in negative sanctions if observed by a nurse (Stannard 1973, cited in Pillemer & Moore 1990). Other concepts of staff abuse of residents include the overt or covert misperformance of occupational duties as demonstrated by:

- physical, psychological, sexual or financial mistreatment/neglect; and
- inadequate, inappropriate, inhuman or abnormal expression of the caring role.

These types of abusive practices which harm, or are likely to cause harm, often result in the residents' needs for physical and emotional support being increased and/or ignored (Kingsley 2000; Meddaugh 1993; Payne & Cikovic 1995; Pillemer & Moore 1990). Abuse occurs when the older person is harmed because their needs, well-being and rights are deliberately or unintentionally ignored or dishonoured (Kingsley 2000).

Many factors affect the nature and quality of caring received by older residents. Some factors result in quality care, and should be developed and reinforced, whereas others contribute to poor care, and need to be identified and addressed. Kingsley (1997a) has suggested that three broad areas have a marked influence on the standard of service delivered to residents. These include:

- the functional status and behaviour of residents;
- the characteristics and attitudes of staff; and
- the philosophy and policies of the agency where care occurs.

Functional status and behaviour of residents

As discussed in some detail earlier in this chapter, resident characteristics and dependency levels will influence the nature and standard of care received by residents. Most staff have at some time been hit, had something thrown at them, or been sworn at by aggressive residents, especially those with cognitive disability (Goodridge et al 1996; Mercer et al 1993; Pillemer & Moore 1990). It is hard to provide quality care when residents with dementia or mental illness do not want to shower, go for a walk, have their clothing changed or take their medications. It is often residents who display challenging or erratic behaviour patterns who become unpopular with staff and are at risk of being neglected or even abused (Downing 1996).

Skilled staff are required to deal appropriately with behaviours of concern, yet the staff who give most of the complex personal care to physically and cognitively frail residents are unlicensed personal-care assistants. Assistants face a dilemma when confronted with 'difficult' behaviour, or when they have to choose between respecting resident autonomy and meeting individual resident needs on the one hand, or honouring the agency's requirements, time constraints and standards on the other (Goodridge et al 1996). The frailty of certain residents, and behaviours of concern of others, might explain why some receive less than ideal care, but resident frailty and the stresses of caring must never be used as reasons to blame the victim for any poor care which they might receive. Responsibility for the nature and quality of care will always lie with the agency and its staff (Penhale & Kingston 1997).

Staff characteristics and attitudes

The quality of life in any residential setting is largely dependent on the characteristics and behaviours of staff. Ideally, mature, advanced nurses who are skilled in aged care, and who enjoy working with older people, will centre their expert practice on the individual needs of each client (Sutton & Smith 1995). To achieve this, there is a need for nurses in aged-care settings to be educated in psychiatry as well as in gerontology (Gioella 1993; Hoeffer 1994; McBride & Burgener 1994; Mott 1996; Smith et al 1994). To enrich the care environment, it is suggested that the facility employ at least some nursing staff who have specialist education—preferably at postgraduate level—in gerontology, mental health and psychiatry. These nurses would be central to the organisation as role models, educators and clinicians.

However, this is not an ideal world, and some specific staff characteristics and attitudes have been associated with poor care, neglect and resident abuse (Pillemer & Moore 1990). Indiscriminate staff hiring, and the use of untrained staff, contribute to poor and abusive care (Uren 1996). Such untrained staff may be young, inexperienced and hold negative attitudes about old age and old people (Pillemer & Bachman-Prehn 1991; Pillemer & Moore 1990). Abusive staff often have poor stress-management skills, and are likely to respond inappropriately when confronted with stressful situations (Pillemer & Moore 1989). Some feel powerless and dissatisfied in their work, and others are at risk of burnout. Some dislike their work and think about resigning but stay for the convenient hours and location, or for job security (Meddaugh 1993; Pillemer & Moore 1989, 1990). Gender also seems to relate to poor-quality care. More male than female staff members perpetrate resident abuse;

although males are under-represented in staff numbers, they are over-represented in reported incidents of abuse (Payne & Cikovic 1995).

Such arguments do not conclusively prove a specific correlation between poor-quality/abusive care and the employment of any particular category of staff, such as assistants. However, Payne & Cikovic (1995) found that care assistants were accused of abuse more often than other employees, although this does not necessarily mean that they commit abuse more often. It may mean little more than that the bulk of research on this topic has concentrated on assistants, or that they have more close and personal contact with residents than other categories of staff.

Although it has been suggested that qualified nurses have more empathy towards residents than aides (Pillemer & Bachman-Prehn 1991), researchers have found that many qualified staff do have neutral attitudes (Treharne 1990) or, more commonly, negative stereotypical images of older adults. These attitudes are not conducive to empathetic caring, and they increase the possibility of staff members acting out their prejudices against older people rather than exploring possibilities of providing quality, individualised care (Armitage & Champney-Smith 1990; Bartlett 1993; Kujawinski et al 1993; Levin 1988; Ray et al 1987; Salmon 1993). Even so, this should not obscure the fact that a great deal of sympathetic caring is given by all categories of care staff (Foner 1994, cited in Goodridge et al 1996).

In an industry where profits are closely tied to labour costs, nursing homes rely heavily on the good attitudes of staff for the delivery of quality care (Tully 1986). To achieve a stable workforce that provides effective and efficient service, managers must provide a positive and nurturing environment that meets the needs of employees—and that also educates and supports in the provision of non-abusive quality care (La Rocco 1985).

Philosophy and policies of the agency

The living environment and quality of resident care are affected by:

- the quality of the institutional setting;
- the owners' philosophy of aged care;
- the owners' attitude towards clients and staff;
- the owners' budget and profit motive; and
- the agency's staffing, education and elder-protection policies.

A well-maintained home with proactive policies, and a supportive work environment which provides strong staff education and supervision, will promote and encourage high-quality resident care and staff satisfaction (Pillemer & Bachman-Prehn 1991). Conversely, La Rocco (1985), Mott (1996), and Paton et al (1994) concur that the risk of abuse and neglect is increased by:

- ill-kept premises with small bed-numbers and poor equipment;
- a mix of cognitively competent residents with those who have dementia or mental illness; and
- too few staff with too much to do.

Other factors related to resident abuse cited by Meddaugh (1993), and Pillemer & Moore (1990) include:

- high levels of conflict between residents, staff and management;
- a lack of staff development or supervision; and
- the use of untrained, unlicensed staff to give complex, intimate care.

Aged-care facilities are charged with providing a safe, homelike environment and quality care for residents. As with all nursing, the moral foundations of aged care demand interventions based on a framework that both honours the feelings and rights of residents, and meets ethical ideals and practice standards (Kingsley 1997b). This means that staff have a responsibility to provide a standard of care which ensures client well-being, and which honours their wishes and rights. Nevertheless, staff are not the only ones with responsibilities. Agency administrators also have an obligation to meet the needs of employees, to respect staff rights and to provide the necessary supervision and education to assist staff to give high-quality care (La Rocco 1985).

Supervision

Supervision in this context involves skills development to help staff build on their strengths, and to overcome any skills deficits. It involves mentoring new employees and teaching staff to be aware of client needs, and how best to meet them. It implies that senior staff will assess their own and others' work performance to ensure that all care is of a high quality that meets client needs and professional practice standards. Supervision also implies that staff are supported to learn how to manage difficult resident behaviours, to defuse staff–resident conflict, to develop positive attitudes towards residents, and to deal with personal stress and burnout. These factors are all related to resident abuse (Pillemer & Moore 1989, 1990), and must be addressed to ensure that duty of care is honoured and that residents receive optimal care.

Education

To ensure resident safety and to prevent abuse, supervision also means that agencies will educate and support staff to change negative attitudes/behaviours and make staff fully aware of the consequences of resident abuse or neglect. When first employed, staff should be given information about the agency's expectations for quality care. New staff must become familiar with agency standards and protocols. This involves knowing about abuse and what intervention protocols are in place. New staff should be informed of how suspected cases of abuse will be investigated, what level of staff will do this task, who will arbitrate on cases, and how disciplinary procedures will be carried out. This is not punitive—rather, it is a necessary preventive measure to encourage and support positive staff attitudes and practice.

Although it is not realistic to expect every registered nurse to have general, gerontological and psychiatric qualifications, it is feasible to suggest that all care staff should have access to a high-quality inservice education program. Education programs would include topics such as:

- normal and abnormal ageing;
- specific aged-care skills to meet residents' needs;
- evidence-based practice;
- environmental psychology; and
- models of care including innovative nursing practices and creative leisure and recreation activities to promote resident health and vitality.

In agencies where there is a mix of residents with physical and mental frailty, or with mental illness and dementia, specific staff education is required concerning the health problems of each group of residents, and the behavioural issues that arise from their cohabitation.

To ensure high-quality care, nursing practice must be firmly based in research, must honour 'duty of care', and must meet the needs and demands of aged residents. Nursing management must translate resident needs into staff education and mentoring programs (Uren 1996) which will support staff to give care that constitutes 'best practice', and thus reduce the level of poor care and abuse (Pillemer & Hudson 1993). In this way, a nurturing environment encourages all staff to achieve the highest possible standards of care (Batalden 1991; Eskildson & Yates 1991; O'Leary 1991).

CONCLUSION

With Australia's population growing older, aged-care facilities are becoming home for more people with dementia and mental illness. The care needs of these residents are disparate—indeed, within each group there are diverse care requirements. To provide an optimal environment it is essential that the resident mix and staffing mix are appropriate.

In this chapter, the behaviours exhibited by people with dementia or mental illness have been presented. That the conduct of these individuals places great strain on the staff of aged-care facilities is undisputed. However, the responses of professionally prepared nurses and personal-care assistants to such behaviour can make the difference between high-quality care and neglect or abuse.

It is timely for the residential-care industry to address a number of issues. These include the mix of residents, and the complex management and care implications that arise when residents with different physical and mental needs are housed together. Another consideration to improve quality care and to reduce the likelihood of resident abuse is for the industry to implement protocols to address both the prevention of abuse and the response to suspected cases. There is also a need for individual aged-care facilities to introduce safeguards and procedures to reduce the likelihood of poor work practices and to increase the level of safe, quality care.

Each health-care agency has a clear responsibility to recruit the most appropriate staff—that is, those people with a genuine liking for, and expertise in, aged care. Employees must be provided with supervision, support and education which enables them to provide high-quality care. In this way, people with dementia and other types of mental health problems will receive quality care that promotes health and well-being.

References

American Psychiatric Association (APA) 1994, *Diagnostic and Statistical Manual of Mental Disorders* (4th edn), APA: Washington DC.

Ames D 1995, Epidemiological studies of depression amongst the elderly in residential and nursing homes. In: Murphy E & Alexopoulos G (eds), *Geriatric Psychiatry: Key Research Topics for Clinicians*, pp 247–58, John Wiley & Sons: New York.

Armitage E & Champney-Smith J 1990, Primary nursing in long-term psychiatric care, *Senior Nurse*, 10(3), pp 4–6.

Arthur D, Dowling P & Sharkey R 1992, *Mental Health Nursing*, pp 3–8, WB Saunders: Sydney.

Bartlett H 1993, *Nursing Homes for Elderly People: Questions of Quality and Policy*, pp 155–68, Harwood: Switzerland.

Batalden E 1991, Organization-wide quality improvement in health care, *Topics in Health Record Management*, 11(3), pp 1–12.

Beck C, Baldwin B, Modlin T & Lewis S 1990, Caregivers' Perception of aggressive behaviour in cognitively impaired nursing-home residents, *Journal of Neuroscience for Nursing*, 22(3), pp 169–72.

Berrios G 1995, Alzheimer's disease: a conceptual history. In: Murphy E & Alexopoulos G (eds), *Geriatric Psychiatry: Key Research Topics for Clinicians*, pp 53–6, John Wiley & Sons: New York.

Boller F, Verny M, Hugonot-Diener L & Saxton J 2002, Clinical features and assessment of severe dementia. A review 1, *European Journal of Neurology*, 9(2), pp 125–36.

Broadhead J & Jacoby R 1995, Mania in old age: A first prospective study. In: Murphy E & Alexopoulos G (eds), *Geriatric Psychiatry: Key Research Topics for Clinicians*, pp 218–29, John Wiley & Sons: New York.

Burgener S & Barton D 1991, Nursing care of cognitively impaired institutionalized elderly, *Journal of Gerontological Nursing*, 19(4), pp 37–43.

Burns A 1995, Causes of death in dementia. In: Murphy E & Alexopoulos G (eds), *Geriatric Psychiatry: Key Research Topics for Clinicians*, pp 96–101, John Wiley & Sons: New York.

Burns A, Jacoby R & Levy R 1990, Psychiatric phenomena in Alzheimer's Disease: IV. Disorders of behaviour, *British Journal of Psychiatry*, 157, pp 86–94.

Carstensen L & Fisher J 1988, Perspectives from the inside: mental health problems of the elderly in nursing homes, *Behavioural Residential Treatment*, 3(3), pp 183–92.

Castledine G 1994, Elder abuse by nurses on the increase, *British Journal of Nursing*, 3(13), pp 331–7.

Commonwealth Department of Community Services and Health 1990, *Mid-Term Review of Aged-Care Reform Strategy 1990–1*, Commonwealth Policy and Programs for Dementia Care in Australia, Discussion Paper No. 2, CDSH: Canberra.

Commonwealth Department of Health, Housing and Community Services 1991, *Aged Care Reform Strategy: Progress and Directions*, AGPS: Canberra.

Crump A 1992, Restless spirits, *Nursing Times*, 88(21), pp 26, 28.

Downing J 1996, Patient abuse, Alberta Association of Registered Nurses Newsletter (AARN), November, pp 16–18.

Eastley R & Wilcock G 2000, Assessment and differential diagnosis of dementia. In: O'Brien J, Ames D & Burns A, *Dementia* (2nd edn), Arnold: London.

Edwards H, Courtney M & Spencer L 2003, Consumer expectations of residential aged care: reflections on the literature, *International Journal of Nursing Practice*, 9(2), pp 70–7.

Eriksson C & Saveman B 2002, Nurses' Experiences of Abusive/Non-abusive Caring for Demented Patients in Acute Care Settings, *Scandinavian Journal of Caring Sciences*, 16(1), pp 79–85.

Eskildson L & Yates G 1991, Lessons from industry: revising organisational structure to improve health-care quality assurance, *Quality Review Bulletin*, 17(2), pp 38–41.

Garratt S & Hamilton-Smith E 1995, *Rethinking Dementia: An Australian Approach*, p 5, Ausmed Publications: Ascot Vale, Victoria.

German P, Rovner B, Bertner L & Brant I 1992, The role of mental morbidity in the nursing-home experience, *Gerontologist*, 32, pp 152–8.

Gilley D, Wilson R, Bennett D, Bernard B & Fox J 1991, Predictors of behavioural disturbance in Alzheimer's disease, *Journal of Gerontology: Psychological Sciences*, 46(6), pp 362–71.

Gioella E 1993, Gerontological nurse education in the next millennium, *Gerontology and Geriatrics Education*, 13(3), pp 99–106.

Goodridge D, Johnston E & Thomson M 1996, Conflict and aggression as stressors in the work environment of nursing assistants: implications for institutional elder abuse, *Journal of Elder Abuse and Neglect*, 8(1), pp 49–67.

Gorman D & Welch A 1993, Effects of change of environment and nursing interventions on the behaviours of the chronically mentally ill, *Proceedings from Australia's First International Psychiatric Nursing Conference, Working With the Long-Term Mentally Ill*, Royal Melbourne Institute of Technology (RMIT): Bundoora, Victoria.

Graycar A 1986, Accommodation issues for elderly people, *Australian Journal on Ageing*, 15(4), p 8.

Griffith V 2002, Diagnose and treat mild to moderate Alzheimer's disease. *Nurse Practitioner*, 27(12), pp 13–25.

Hayes R 1995, Pain assessment in the elderly, *British Journal of Nursing*, 4(20), pp 1199–1204.

Hoeffer B 1994, Geropsychiatric nursing: essential curriculum content, *Journal of Psychosocial Nursing*, 32(4), pp 33–8.

Hugo G 1986, *Australia's Changing Population*, Oxford University Press: Melbourne.

Jorm A & Henderson A 1993, *The Problem of Dementia in Australia* (3rd edn), AGPS: Canberra, p 10.

Kapp M 2002, Criminal and civil liability of physicians for institutional elder abuse and neglect, *Journal of the American Medical Directors' Association*, 3(2), pp S77–S81.

Katona C 1994, *Depression in Old Age*, John Wiley & Sons: New York.

Kikuta S 1993, Modifying disruptive behaviour, *Canadian Nursing Home*, 4(1), pp 14–18.

Kingsley B 1997a, Resident abuse: an aged care tragedy, *Nursing Review*, October, p 21.

Kingsley B 1997b, The older client. In: Hawley G (ed), *Ethics Workbook For Nurses*, pp 181–92, Social Sciences Press: Wentworth Falls, NSW.

Kingsley B (ed) 2000, *Elder Abuse: Protocol and Policy Guidelines to Prevent the Abuse of Older People in Community and Residential Care*, Curtin University, Centre for Research into Aged Care Services: Perth.

Koch T & Kralik D 2001, Chronic illness: reflections on a community-based action research programme, *Journal of Advanced Nursing*, 36(1), pp 23–31.

Krach E 1993, Nursing implications: functional status of older persons with schizophrenia, *Journal of Gerontological Nursing*, 19(8), pp 21–7.

Kujawinski J, Bigelow E, Diedrich D, Kikkebusch P, Korpan E, Walczak J, Maxson E, Ropski S & Farran CJ 1993, Research considerations: geropsychiatry unit evaluation, *Journal of Gerontological Nursing*, 19(1), pp 5–10.

La Rocco S 1985, Patient abuse should be your concern, *The Journal of Nursing Administration*, 15(4), pp 27–31.

Lacro J & Harris M 1995, Late-life psychoses. In: Murphy E & Alexopoulos G (eds), *Geriatric Psychiatry: Key Research Topics for Clinicians*, pp 232–44, John Wiley & Sons: New York.

Lawlor B 2002, Managing behavioural and psychological symptoms in dementia, *British Journal of Psychiatry*, 181, pp 463–5.

Levesque L, Cossette S & Potvin L 1993, Why alert residents are more or less willing to cohabit with cognitively impaired peers: an exploratory model, *The Gerontologist*, 33(4), pp 514–22.

Levin W 1988, Age stereotyping: college student evaluations, *Research On Aging*, 10(1), pp 134–48.

Lidz C, Fischer L & Arnold R 1992, *The Erosion of Autonomy in Long-Term Care*, Oxford University Press: Oxford.

Logiudice D 2002, Dementia: an update to refresh your memory, *Internal Medicine Journal*, 32(11), pp 535–40.

Ludwig A 1993, Psychiatric health care for the elderly. In: Lieberman E & Collen M (eds), *Aging in Good Health: A Quality Lifestyle for the Later Years*, p 208, Plenum Press: New York.

McBride A & Burgener S 1994, Strategies to implement geropsychiatric nursing curricula content, *Journal of Psychosocial Nursing*, 32(4), pp 13–18.

McCullagh B 1994, A new age in aged care: a best-practice model for aged care, *Proceedings from Australia's Second International Psychiatric Nursing Conference, Mental Health Nursing in Transition: A Challenge to Practice*, Royal Melbourne Institute of Technology: Bundoora, Victoria.

Mayer R & Darby S 1995, Does a mirror deter wandering in demented older people? In: Murphy E & Alexopoulos G (eds), *Geriatric Psychiatry: Key Research Topics for Clinicians*, pp 169–74, John Wiley & Sons: New York.

Mayeux R 1993, Neurology of aging: the problem of dementia in the year 2000. In: Lieberman E & Collen M (eds), *Aging in Good Health: A Quality Lifestyle for the Later Years*, p 227, Plenum Press: New York.

Meddaugh D 1993, Covert elder abuse in the nursing home, *Journal of Elder Abuse and Neglect*, 5(3), pp 21–37.

Mercer SO, Heacock P & Beck C 1993, Nurse's aides in nursing homes: perceptions of training, work loads, racism and abuse issues, *Journal of Gerontological Social Work*, 21(1/2), pp 95–112.

Mental Health Act 1986, Victoria, ANSTAT, Government Printer for State of Victoria.

Mosher-Ashley P, Turner B & O'Neill D 1991, Attitudes of nursing and rest home administrators toward deinstitutionalized elders with psychiatric disorders, *Community Mental Health Journal*, 27(4), pp 241–53.

Mott S 1996, *Passing Time in Clifton Court: An Ethnographic Study of a Unit for Confused Older People*, unpublished doctoral thesis, Deakin University: Geelong.

Mott S 1997, Madness and mayhem: the place of people with dementia in a mental health setting, *Australian and New Zealand Journal of Mental Health Nursing*, 6(5), pp 102–12.

National Center for Health Statistics 1991, Mental illness in nursing homes, United States 1985, *Vital and Health Statistics*, Series 13, Data from the National Health Survey, No. 105, US Department of Human Services.

Norbergh K, Asplund K, Sandman P, Rasmussen B & Nordahl G 2001, How patients with dementia spend their time in a psycho-geriatric unit, *Scandinavian Journal of Caring Sciences*, 35, pp 215–21.

Norbergh K, Hellzen O, Sandman P & Asplund K 2002, The relationship between organizational climate and the content of daily life for people with dementia living in a group-dwelling, *Journal of Clinical Nursing*, 11(2), pp 237–46.

O'Brien J, Desmond P, Ames D, Schweitzer I & Tress B 1997, Temporal lobe magnetic resonance imaging can differentiate Alzheimer's disease from normal ageing, depression, vascular dementia and other causes of cognitive impairment, *Psychological Medicine*, 27, pp 1267–75.

O'Leary D 1991, Accreditation in the quality improvement model: A Vision for Tomorrow, *Quality Review Bulletin*, 17(3), pp 72–7.

Paton RN, Huber R & Netting EE 1994, The long-term care ombudsman program and complaints of abuse and neglect: what have we learned? *Journal of Elder Abuse and Neglect*, 6(1), pp 97–115.

Payne BK & Cikovic R 1995, An empirical examination of the characteristics, consequences, and causes of elder abuse in nursing homes, *Journal of Elder Abuse and Neglect*, 7(4), pp 61–74.

Penhale B & Kingston P 1997, Elder abuse, mental health and later life: steps towards an understanding, *Aging and Mental Health*, 1(4), pp 296–304.

Pillemer K & Bachman-Prehn R 1991, Helping and hurting: predictors of maltreatment of patients in nursing homes, *Research in Ageing*, 13, pp 74–95.

Pillemer K & Hudson B 1993, A model of an abuse-prevention program for nursing assistants, *The Gerontologist*, 33(1), pp 128–31.

Pillemer K & Moore D 1989, Abuse of residents in nursing homes: findings from a survey of staff, *The Gerontologist*, 29, pp 314–20.

Pillemer K & Moore D 1990, Highlights from a study of abuse of patients in nursing homes, *Journal of Elder Abuse and Neglect*, 2(1/2), pp 5–29.

Poole J & Mott S 2003, Agitated older patients: nurses' perceptions and reality, *International Journal of Nursing Practice*, 9(5), pp 306–12.

Puckett A 1993, *Community Mental Health*, WB Saunders: Sydney.

Ray D, McKinney K & Ford C 1987, Differences in psychologists' ratings of older and younger clients, *The Gerontologist*, 27(1), pp 82–6.

Reisberg B, Kenowsky S, Franssen EH, Auer SR & Souren LEM 1999, Towards a science of Alzheimer's disease management: a model based upon current knowledge of retrogenesis. *International Psychogeriatrics*, 11, pp 7–23.

Sadavoy J, Smith I, Conn D & Hall W 1995, Depression in geriatric patients with chronic medical illness. In: Murphy E & Alexopoulos G (eds), *Geriatric Psychiatry: Key Research Topics for Clinicians*, pp 191–200, John Wiley & Sons: New York.

Salmon P 1993, Interactions of nurses with elderly patients: relationship to nurses' attitudes and to formal activity periods, *Journal of Advanced Nursing*, 18, pp 14–19.

Santmyer K, Serafini G & Larson E 1992, Improving management of psychiatric and behaviour problems in long-term care, *Journal of Nursing Care Quality*, 6(3), pp 44–56.

Smith M, Buckwalter K, Garand L, Mitchell S & Albanese M 1994, Evaluation of a geriatric mental health training program for nursing personnel in rural long-term care facilities, *Issues in Mental Health Nursing*, 15, pp 149–68.

Spore D, Smyer M & Cohn M 1991, Assessing nursing assistants' knowledge of behavioural approaches to mental health problems, *The Gerontologist*, 31(3), pp 309–17.

Stevens G & Baldwin B 1988, Optimizing mental health in the nursing-home setting, *Journal of Psychosocial Nursing*, 26(10), pp 27–31.

Stokes G 1987, Managing the wanderer: first find out why, *Geriatric Medicine*, 17, pp 36–41.

Storandt M, Grant E, Miller P & Morris J 2002, Rates of progression in mild cognitive impairment and early Alzheimer's disease, *Neurology*, 59(7), pp 1034–41.

Sutton E & Smith C 1995, Advanced nursing practice: new ideas and new perspectives, *Journal of Advanced Nursing*, 21, pp 1037–43.

Teri L, Hughes J & Larson E 1990, Cognitive deterioration in Alzheimer's Disease: behavioural and health factors, *Journal of Gerontology: Psychological Sciences*, 45(2), pp 58–63.

Ticehurst S 2001, Is dementia a mental illness? *Australian and New Zealand Journal of Psychiatry*, 35(6), pp 716–23.

Tran Johnson T, Krull A & Jeste D 1992, Late-life schizophrenia and its treatment: the pharmacological issues in older schizophrenic patients. In: Alexopoulos A (ed) *Clinics in Geriatric Medicine*, pp 401–10, WB Saunders: Philadelphia.

Treharne G 1990, Attitudes in the care of elderly people: are they getting better? *Journal of Advanced Nursing*, 15, pp 777–81.

Tully C 1986, A proposal for a reinstatement rule in unfair labor practice cases involving patient abuse, *American Journal of Law and Medicine*, XI(3), pp 319–41.

Tyler L, Moss H, Patterson K & Hodges J 1997, The gradual deterioration of syntax and semantics in a patient with progressive aphasia, *Brain and Language*, 56(3), pp 426–76.

United Nations 1982, *Principles for Older People*, Resolution 37/51, United Nations: New York.

Uren J 1996, Unlicensed workers: we need hard data, *Australian Nursing Journal*, 4(1), p 3.

Vogel C & Mercier J 1991, The effect of institutionalization on nursing-home populations, *Journal of Gerontological Nursing*, 17(3), pp 30–4.

Winger J, Schirm V & Stewart D 1987, Aggressive behaviour in long-term care, *Journal of Psychosocial Nursing and Mental Health Services*, 25(4), pp 28–33.

Zubenko G, Rosen J, Sweet R, Mulsant B & Rifai H 1992, Impact of psychiatric hospitalization on behavioural complications of Alzheimer's disease, *American Journal of Psychiatry*, 149(11), pp 1484–91.

CHAPTER 13

The experience of chronic illness: a phenomenological approach

MARY FITZGERALD AND ELEANOR HORTON

INTRODUCTION

What is it like to be elderly and to have chronic illness? Attempting to answer this question helps us to understand other people's experiences. It means coming to know better the elderly people who require nursing assistance. Of course, people experience chronic illness in a variety of ways, but the phenomenon of chronic illness, as experienced by elderly people, is better understood as more experience is revealed. This chapter is based on a phenomenological study of eighteen people with chronic illness (FitzGerald 1995).

Chronic illness research over the past ten years has established a sound tradition of 'insider' research (Thorne & Paterson 2000)—that is, research that reveals chronic illness from the perspective of people who have experienced the broad range of chronic illnesses. Thorne & Paterson (2000, p 174) explain that the advantage of this perspective is that it shows the chronically ill as analysts of their experience, how they manage within their daily lives and how they can determine their own illness management and therapy. They also point out that this perspective demonstrates the degree to which professional health carers are limited in their ability to help with the illness experience.

A metastudy of 292 qualitative research papers relating to chronic physical illness has been conducted by a team of Canadian researchers (Paterson 2001, p 21). The metastudy does not focus on the elderly, although of course many of the participants in the various studies are older people. From this work, Paterson (2001, p 23) has developed a 'shifting perspectives model of chronic illness' that cleverly embraces the wide range of views and draws attention to chronic illness as 'containing elements of wellness and illness'. Thorne & Paterson (2000) and later Thorne et al (2002), drawing on the metastudy, remark on the extent to which the underlying assumptions of studies change. They note that 'the psychologists tended to focus on coping and adaptation, whereas sociologists oriented their studies around such phenomena as stigma and sick role—shaping the questions asked and answers obtained' (Thorne et al 2002, p 441). These authors also note a recent trend towards optimism and the substitution of concepts such as loss, burden and sorrow with those of transformation, courage and spirituality. This trend is also noticeable in the aged-care literature and, while the motives are laudable, reality checks with those who experience old age and chronic illness are necessary. Researchers are beholden to identify and critique the assumptions underlying their work and to assess the degree to which they relate to and affect the findings.

There is no doubt that chronic illness haunts elderly people. The incidence of chronic illness is highest among those over sixty years of age, and is complicated by multiple pathologies as age increases. Lingering ill health often heralds the onset of frailty, which may lead to dependence upon other people and government services. Anecdotally, people insist that they do not feel old as long as they remain healthy, but that they age quite quickly when they become ill. At least four of the younger participants in the study talked of chronic illness as something that had caused them to age. Chronic illnesses (that are severe enough to affect a person's ability to be independent) alter lives, and may be seen as 'the beginning of the end' by the person involved. Alternatively, some chronic illnesses are so common among elderly people that sufferers view them as an almost inevitable consequence of increasing age. One participant listed the friends he meets when he goes shopping:

> I was down buying fish the other morning and there were four arthritics ... buying fish with me, friends, and the one woman had had surgery to her leg and had had to have a series of operations. A man was having intensive ... thing for arthritis of his back ... there was me with my tablets and so on ...

It is sometimes also the case that chronic illness may not especially affect the older person's usual routine—as the above participant went on to say:

> people will say to me, 'You know you have got this arthritis, Bernard, what are you doing, you know, how do you keep yourself amused?' ... and they get surprised when I say I'm doing nothing ... *[pause]* ... because to me it's become very beguiling just to do nothing, just to sit and not have anything that I force myself to do.

The older people in this study were not in health-care institutions and, without exception, were rarely admitted to hospital. Indeed, they seldom accessed nurses at all—but they did use health services and they visited doctors regularly.

METHODOLOGY

Phenomenology was chosen as a research approach in this exercise, to illustrate the unique and shared meanings of the experience of chronic illness. This insight was achieved through meticulous attention to, and interpretation of, the everyday occurrences of the phenomenon. Kestenbaum (1982) dwells upon the connection between phenomenology and poetry by commenting on DH Lawrence's observation that poetry draws attention to things in a new way, and therefore helps people to see the familiar world in a new light:

> Like poetry, phenomenology makes a 'new effort of attention' by recovering and revealing the habitual structuring of our everyday experience, experiences of art and religion, and our professional experiences. Phenomenology enables us to see everyday and other realms of experience (science, fantasy, medicine, etc.) as constitutions of subject experience (not simply 'subjective' experience).
>
> Kestenbaum 1982, p 14

This way of researching lived experience is, as van Manen (1990) contends, a way for the researcher to become even more a part of the world. This type of engaged research is an act of caring. To care, in this instance, is to truly desire to understand others better. Originally this research was driven by a desire to benefit people who had chronic illness. For the purpose of this chapter, parts of the research that involved elderly people are now extrapolated from the whole set of data with the same intent—that is, to benefit elderly people who have chronic illness. Van Manen (1990) also states that knowing is not just a 'cognitive act' but involves a loving responsibility to find out what 'contributes to the good' of the people researched.

Phenomenology is now well established as an approach used by nurses in conducting research with elderly people (Nay 1993, 1996; Hudson & Richmond 1994; Pearson et al 1996). As part of the phenomenological approach, researchers write graphic interpretations that stir emotions and help people to come closer to the world of the elderly person.

To understand what something means is to reveal the nature of its existence. For example, to decide:

What is chronic illness in old age?

one asks:

What does it mean to be chronically ill in later life?

It means:

I have little chance of recovery.
I go towards the future filled with pain and contending with disability.
I have to ask other people to help me.

This is an ontological question (a question concerning existence), and one that can be answered only by turning to the reality of the experience of the sufferer of chronic illness: 'as lived, reality is the experiencing of the object' (Kestenbaum 1982, p 14).

It is impossible to speak, generically, of the chronically ill, elderly person. It is impossible to generate meaningful information that describes the experience of all those who have a long-term illness in later life. Indeed, Frank (1991, p 45) writes that 'care begins when differences are recognised'. However, chronically ill older people do share a world and culture. It is in this shared world and culture that the generally held attitudes, beliefs and practices constitute the situations in which people find themselves—and the ways that they learn to react to them. How people respond to these situations will always be complicated. Understanding these experiences is not concerned with simplifying and making abstract generalisations. Rather, seeing them in their concrete, complex situations is more likely to uncover the meaning these experiences have for people.

This existential view is not a popular one, for treating people as complicated beings is time consuming. As Frank (1991, p 45) points out, it is much easier to theorise and compartmentalise people into categories, each of which supposedly has its own slick solution. But solutions and treatment are not care. Such emotive knowledge is not generally regarded as appropriate in today's technological/bureaucratic health-care system. However, such knowledge is highly desirable, and the nurse who pays attention to the lived experience of people enhances the quality of what she or he does.

CHRONIC ILLNESS

Curtin & Lubkin (1990) offer the reader a range of definitions of chronic illness, dating from 1949 onwards. According to these authors, all the definitions have some problem or other, and the definitions reflect the changing prevailing attitudes towards chronic illness. For instance, a 1949 definition (not reproduced here) is dismissed by Curtin & Lubkin (1990, p 5) as being patriarchal, medically oriented and inflexible. Frustrated with the shortcomings of the available definitions of chronic illness, these two authors offer their own definition:

> Chronic illness is the irreversible presence, accumulation, or latency of disease states or impairments that involve the total human environment for supportive care and self-care, maintenance of function and prevention of further disability.
>
> Curtin & Lubkin 1990, p 6

The word 'chronic' derives from the Greek word χρονος *(chronos)*, which means 'time'. The *Shorter Oxford English Dictionary* defines chronic as 'lasting a long time, lingering, inveterate'. In turn, 'inveterate' is defined as 'long established; deep rooted, obstinate (now mostly of things evil)'.

In colloquial language, *chronic* is often used in a derogatory way to mean something which is not enjoyable and which has lasted too long—as in 'what a chronic day!'. Place (1992) found in her study that people who had a chronic illness resented the term 'chronic'—they felt that it was a derogatory word which should not be used to describe them. The participants in this study related more to their diagnostic group than to people with chronic illness generally. This propensity to dislike being grouped as chronically ill bears some similarity to elderly people's dislike of being grouped together as elderly.

The word 'illness' is also worthy of some analysis. It is a word that conveys the total experience of being unwell, rather than a state directly attributable to certain specific symptoms related to a disease. Helman makes this point briefly:

> Disease is something an organ has; illness is something a man [sic] has.
>
> Helman 1981, p 548

Kleinman remarks:

> By invoking the term illness, I mean to conjure up the innately human experience of symptoms and suffering. Illness refers to how the sick person and the members of the family or wider social network perceive, live with, and respond to symptoms and disability.
>
> Kleinman 1988, p 3

Indeed, there are some experiences of disease where illness is not a feature. Hypertension is an example of a disease that does not always correspond with an experience of illness. This difference between the experience of *illness* and that of *disease* is described by Kleinman (1988, p 4) as one of the 'principal difficulties' with which to contend. For example, rather than being bothered by asthma itself, the person experiences wheezing and embarrassment.

Brody (1987) undertakes a detailed investigation of the word 'sickness' in order to understand the experiential notion of not being well. He summarises the state of sickness in the following ways:

(a) To be sick is to have something wrong with oneself in a way regarded as abnormal when compared with a suitably chosen reference class.

(b) To be sick is to experience both an unpleasant sense of disruption of body and self and a threat to one's integrated personhood.

(c) To be sick is to have the sort of thing that medicine, as an evolving craft, has customarily treated.

(d) To be sick is to undergo an alteration of one's social roles and relationships in ways that will be influenced by cultural belief systems.

(e) To be sick is to participate in a disruption of an integrated hierarchy of natural systems, including one's biological subsystems, oneself as a discrete psychological entity, and the social and cultural systems of which one is a member.

Brody 1987, p 22

These statements are recognised by Brody as being short and rather general. However, he uses them as foundations from which to explore the complexity of the lived experience of sickness.

The cultural experience of illness constitutes the ways in which members of cultural groups organise their thoughts and construe their expectations of illness. However, these usual cultural patterns may be altered according to social circumstances and according to the particular life-history of the person involved (Kleinman 1988, p 5). These ideas are apparent in the present study. It is not possible to define the precise cultural values and beliefs which impinge on all the participants, but the differences which relate to the social circumstances of the participants, and to their particular histories, can be appreciated. Although illness trajectories are not—and probably never will be—predictable, it is possible to discover the source of many of the meanings which people make (and share) of their predicaments.

There is a tendency to view illness in terms of acute illness—thus relegating chronic illness to the margins of health-care interests (along with debates concerning the elderly and disabled). It is therefore necessary to consider the distinctive state of chronic illness. The question of who qualifies as chronically ill has expanded over the years. This is because of significant developments in the treatment of acute illnesses. Older people are the main 'benefactors' of these new treatments. However, the considerable successes of modern medicine have resulted in many more people joining the ranks of the chronically ill. Although modern medicine is often able to hold back death, it has not been similarly successful in finding complete cures for conditions such as heart failure, renal failure and liver failure. Frank explains the new dimension to chronic illness:

Disease used to be either critical, meaning life threatening but quick, or chronic, meaning long-term. Disease moved to a crisis from which the patient either recovered or died, or else the patient lived as an invalid, gradually wasting away. Medical technology keeps enlarging the numbers of those living 'normally' in remission; we have more and more of the 'chronically critical'.

Frank 1991, p 139

Although there are now many people who have survived acute illness, a proportion of them will reside in a state where the 'difficulties' referred to by Kleinman (1988, p 4) can be severe and last well into very old age. The need to have these 'difficulties' attended to is great, but in a health-care system which is geared to biomedicine, this is often given a low priority.

THE PAST

When the participants in this research first began to talk about their experience of chronic illness, they always went back to the time before the illness started. It appeared that their chronic illnesses, which were the focus of the narrative, could only be discussed, and made sense of, in terms of the context of their whole lives. Nurses who have experience of being with elderly people already know the importance of memories and histories to the current self-esteem and orientation of elderly people. The participants drew heavily on the past to establish their credibility and worth. Olson makes a similar deduction from her experiences as a person with renal failure:

> We search for the future through dialogue with what is past. We do not recall events that are over. Rather, our experience lives in us, making us what we are.

Olson 1993, p 69

A sufferer of chronic liver disease also contributes to this idea when she describes a persistent worry that 'your identity will be subsumed by your disease' (Register 1987, p 28).

In the present study, the participants relished the opportunity to tell their stories to an attentive listener. For example, Dr Craig, a retired man in his seventies, painted a satisfied portrait of his life. He had achieved a great deal in his life, fulfilling the promise of his natural abilities. Those achievements contributed to the construction of his self-concept. He valued his intellectual acumen and his achievements in his work. His illnesses did not cause him to retire early, or disturb his career or his sociability. Although the illness had brought about changes in his life, these did not involve the things he valued most. Other participants were far more unhappy about the changes brought about by chronic illness and wanted to paint a picture of themselves as they were.

When the participants described their lives before they became ill, they revealed the things they valued. Valuing things which are no longer attainable can make the burden of chronic illness greater, because people may construct and believe their own diminishment.

For example, Tom had had several strokes that left him with a severe dysphasia and marked weakness on one side. The first time that he was visited in the course of this study, his speech could not be readily understood, but there was no doubt about the achievements in his past that he valued—and that made his present so unpalatable. This excerpt from the fieldnotes shows how more was learnt about him and his loves through his past:

Mrs Palmer left us to it and went into the garden. I asked Thomas to tell me what having the strokes had meant to him. He launched straight into talk I could not understand and started to point to a photograph on the wall. The photograph was of a horse with a young man on its back. Remembering what his wife had said, I asked, 'You used to work with horses?'. He started to cry and got up. He clumsily walked into the hall. I followed him. He was standing and crying in front of more photographs of horses. I waited a while. He looked at me and I put an arm around his waist and said, 'Just tell me about them—I don't understand everything you say but it is nice to hear you talk of the horses'. He talked away, occasionally crying. We walked around all the photographs; I gathered that he had trained … ponies and coached a junior team which had been very successful.

On one occasion, when asked what he did now, Tom answered emphatically, 'I don't do anything'. Upon hearing this response, his wife, who was present, protested that he did a lot of things (Fldnte:2.4). She proved it the next week by making him write a list of the things he had done and the places he had been in the past week. As Tom dutifully handed over the piece of paper, he made a face indicating that he did not value these activities and that he stood by his original answer (Fldnte:2.5). He wanted to be driving a car and riding horses. He said that he still did drive a car and ride, which seemed incredible. It was explained that he visited his old horse on a property and that sometimes he drives on back roads.

A person's history is the key to his or her self-knowing. To gain any comprehension of the person's experience of chronic illness, some understanding and appreciation of a person's history and context is necessary. To draw upon people's memories is to know the person at a deep level.

> What makes time so valuable is that it is convertible into nourishing memory. Memory is where the proof of life is stored. It offers material for stock-taking and provides clues about where our lives are going.
>
> Cousins 1983, p 232

Learning from these elderly people allowed a contemplation upon how near or far was the observer from the perspective of each person. Dwelling with the data—and investigating them minutely—engendered a respect for the depth and influence of past experience. Learning about people's experience allows a better notion of the sources of their ideas, views and strength. Nurses who come into contact with elderly people with chronic illness need to listen to their histories, and to value the information contained in them—for this information leads to a better understanding of the person to be nursed.

The past is constitutive of the self-identity of the person, and reveals their values and the impact of chronic illness on their lives in terms of loss and missed opportunities. The specific illness history starts 'with the onset of the problems that mark the beginning of the illness trajectory. It is a path that entwines these people with the medical profession, and means their facing considerable change. In many instances, the illness heralds the beginning of old age—the time when they really begin to feel their age, begin to be inconvenienced by their bodies and fear losing independence. On the whole, this change is predominantly viewed in a negative light by the person, his or her relatives and the medical profession. It is certainly a path which they did not choose or deserve, although some elderly people are more philosophical about this change in health, especially if they have always had a positive view of their lives.

THE PRESENT

Following Gelven (1989), the key to the present was to ask the question, *What is being done?* The present actions and situations of the participants demonstrated accommodations for their illnesses, and the struggles they had to maintain their preferred lifestyles. In the report material, the present was written up in terms of the contributions made, by the people themselves, and by others, to the control and maintenance of their well-being.

The tasks or contributions that have been chosen for consideration in this chapter are self-care, maintaining independence, and socialising.

Struggle or fight in the present

The participants used the metaphor of *combating* the disease when talking about their day-to-day lives. Quite commonly they referred to 'refusing to be beaten', 'licking it' or 'keeping ahead of it'. They referred to their illnesses as if the illnesses were 'other' than themselves—malevolent things that needed to be controlled. Modern critiques of such metaphors (Sontag 1983; Ross 1993) suggest that metaphors of fighting perpetuate the common (although covert) conception of illness as an evil which is dealt out to people as punishment. Illness is thus seen as something alien that happens to the body—and which must be controlled, overcome, fought. Although these metaphors may contribute to generally unhelpful attitudes towards ill people and ill health, it does seem that some participants believe that this combative attitude has been an important means of surviving and living with chronic illness.

The elderly people in this study did not appear to choose one attitude towards their disease and the predicaments in which it put them. Nor did they describe phases of reactions to their illness—such as shock, denial, anger. Their moods and attitudes oscillated, altering the ways in which they behaved and coped with their illnesses. Several attitudes to illness emerged. There was the fighting spirit, the resigned/passive attitude, and an embracing attitude—the last being one in which the illness was accepted and a degree of peace attained.

Frank (1991, p 64) describes two types of emotional work that are involved in being sick:

- Trying to work out the meaning of the experience of illness—this is hard work which is best undertaken with other people who care, and who are prepared to hear about frustrations, fears, sadness and so on.
- Maintaining an emotional appearance that is socially acceptable—such as being cheerful, brave, uncomplaining and so on. For the chronically ill, this is not always just a facade or appearance—they can sometimes genuinely behave in these ways. However, the hard work of facing emotions and coming to understand the meaning of experiences is too often neglected.

Time and effort are expended by chronically ill people in maintaining their health and preventing their condition from deteriorating. In the present study, they did not differentiate between physical and mental efforts—when they were helping themselves, the right mental attitude was just as important as physical treatments. These efforts included complying with medical regimens, exercising, eating appropriate diets, engaging in some complementary therapies, and maintaining a positive attitude towards their lives in general.

There is a strong underlying social ethic that dictates that those who help themselves are worthy. Sarah (one of the participants) was blatant in denouncing other people with rheumatoid arthritis who could not (or would not) help themselves—and who therefore took up limited resources. When bemoaning the fifty per cent cut in home help which she had been forced to accept, Sarah made the following comments:

> there is such a demand for it [home help], I can't understand. You know, there are a lot of old people, really incapable people, who should be in a home. But, for instance, one lady who has chronic arthritis doesn't want to get out of bed, doesn't want to try, so the home care is there, twenty-four hours a day. And it is up to the doctor to say, 'No, you are going in a home'. But he doesn't, and the people who still want to get on with life, they're ... victimised.

Dr Craig, in contrast, explained how difficult it was to stick to healthy regimens—and how this type of 'work' can be really demoralising. He dreaded being a burden to his wife or his children. If keeping to a diabetic-control regimen would lessen this likelihood, he felt that he should comply. However, he resented the responsibility heaped on him, and he justified some non-compliance by being sceptical of the official word and faulty logic (as he perceived it) of the doctors:

> I find exercise is the biggest factor that can drop my blood sugar ... Now the trouble is—with the arthritis—often I am so sore that I can't exercise. ... there are various difficulties that occurred from this. First of all as far as the diets are concerned, I was previously on a gout diet, an arthritis diet, on a weight-loss diet and now on [a] diabetic diet—and that left me with about a lettuce leaf to eat.

Dr Craig demonstrated the important point that older people often suffer from a range of pathological conditions simultaneously—his arthritis and gout impeding efforts to exercise and control his blood sugars.

Sarah was a good example of vacillation in emotions and attitudes regarding her illnesses—and of the employment of self-helping activities. When Sarah read the first transcription of her interviews, she commented on how angry she sounded. She had not realised how palpable and recognisable had been the anger in her demeanour. Her anger was like a force which propelled her through life. She sometimes felt that she needed to fight for all her comforts—everything from her family's attention to support from social services. Although she voiced some surprise at the degree of her anger, she recognised it as an integral part of how she coped with life. She had had a life full of tragic loss, and she was used to railing against her lot. This reaction to life's incidents was one of her mechanisms for survival. Her antidote to the anger was a world of music, where she could distract herself from the frustrations, worries and pain that racks most of her time.

Sarah had studied pain management and had taught other people distraction-and-relaxation therapy. Intellectually she accepted and taught others that illness is a holistic concept. However, she found this way of living difficult and tiring:

> As you know, arthritis is a progressive disease which flares up at the most horrible, inopportune moments ... so what I have trouble with now, despite all my methods

[rueful chuckle] for control and management of chronic pain, is the progressive incapability of my body ...

That is not self-pity, it is just a matter—a fact—it is a matter of fact. And I think the mere fact that you are so tired, you think, 'What the hell, I am not doing it any more'. So you stay home—you are not going to the concert, you are not going to this, that and the other thing.

Self-help and a fighting spirit meant to Sarah that she needed to be resourceful and needed to expend vast amounts of her very limited energy—sometimes more than she thought she had. She also felt, to a certain extent, that to be resourceful and self-sufficient was to allow others off the hook. She was irritated by the inconvenience that her illness apparently caused to those who helped her, whether they were family, friends or members of the medical profession. The following excerpt from Sarah's transcript relates to the help she used to get from her home help. It reveals her anger and frustration with both the authorities and her daughter-in-law. She believed that the hours of her home help were reduced, in part, because she had tried to make herself look good each day. She dressed immaculately and always wore makeup.

I have a home care, daily ... who I have six hours a week who used to do my grocery shopping. That is now out *[clipped voice]*. They are not allowed to [do] my shopping anymore, so I am stuck with that. And now my daughter-in-law does it, under sufferance ... which makes me feel uncomfortable—not guilty, but uncomfortable. I cannot *[louder]* go and stand in queues. I cannot go and shop and reach for things because I drop things—and that's one [reason]. And I am on crutches—that's two [reasons].

Sarah's anger was directed at the people and organisations that she felt had let her down, rather than at the illness itself. This anger had energised her to face the authorities and people, and to demand what she needed. She had attended to her illness in the ways she had learnt (distraction, relaxation and the self-administration of narcotics), and had contributed to the welfare of fellow-sufferers through teaching and by being an official of the arthritis group. She helped to arrange and advertise an outing to the local museum and ensured that everyone who wanted to come would have appropriate transport. She did this in an efficient and kind way. Her anger was not overwhelming—rather, it was a part of her life which she managed to express.

On the other hand, Holly chose a different tack. The old maxim—laugh and the whole world laughs with you, cry and you cry alone—has a ring of truth. Holly, who remained remarkably cheerful on the surface despite years of pain from arthritis, explained that her cheerfulness was her normal facade. It made her popular, but this popularity did not make her life significantly easier to live. She put a great deal of effort into her cheerfulness and was sometimes disappointed by people's responses to her:

if people say to me, 'But you never complain', and I said, 'Well what's the point in complaining, people don't want to know about it', ... and sometimes, you know, somebody will come along and they will say 'Oh, how's your arthritis?'. [I reply] 'Oh, still there, you know, still with me, it's lovely.' *[Laugh]*

I'm not blowing my own trumpet, [but] somebody said [to me] once, 'Everybody loves you', and I said, 'Yeah, well, I love everybody'.

This was not always true and, when at home, Holly was apt to drop the facade of cheerfulness:

I am fairly placid. Well, I'm so placid I'm stupid, you know, and somebody once said, 'Do you ever get annoyed?'. I said, 'By Jove I get annoyed, sometimes I get really cranky'. *[laugh]* 'Oh, when?' [they asked]. 'Only with [my husband] Steve—he gets up my nose sometimes.' But ...

An examination (from the data) of the participants' ways of resisting the disabling effects of chronic illness reveals more examples of struggle than of fighting. There are extreme examples of struggle. Elizabeth put it this way:

Sometimes I think it is because you haven't got any choice but to cope. ...You either give in to it and you lose what goodness you have in your life, or you cope. You know you haven't got any choice.

The struggle was generally considered to be essential by those who engaged in it, but their stories revealed that it was hard work. Most of the participants' behaviour (in resisting or combating their diseases) involved energy and self-discipline. It was about the struggle involved in working to maintain a social life, a positive attitude, a healthy body, control in life, and so on. The people in the study found the struggle of everyday life very tiring:

The fatigue is incredible, and it is just as if you're going through a rice pudding, sometimes, pressing yourself to do things and to shift the system.

Sarah, a struggler *par excellence*, wrote this poem about the relief she felt when the responsibility of keeping going was taken from her for a while. This generally occurred when she was admitted intermittently to hospital.

Hospital

A sense of relaxed trust
In blurry faces poised over me;
A sense of powerlessness
Lying prone in the blue bed, and
Noises of caring floating around me.
A giving-in to the tiredness and pain,
Of holding myself erect
For the world and for myself.
Hospital—a last resource for me
To shed responsibilities—and rest.

Maintaining the everyday struggle was especially hard for those people in the study who were depressed. They had less inclination to struggle emotionally, physically and spiritually. Antidepressants could make them feel lethargic and unable to motivate themselves. Elizabeth referred to depression as 'this heaviness':

I can't explain this feeling inside of me, like it is in here, it's a heaviness and things that mattered to me before don't matter ... and the energy I had before, it's just not there, and I just can't get up and go.

The data revealed an anxiety that chronically ill people might be considered a social burden upon people. The Northcote Hydrotherapy and Massage Group (McDonald 1992) was a group of older women who had successfully maintained a hydrotherapy group after their physiotherapy was withdrawn. Their success was due to the commitment of the members, the fun they had together, and the contribution they all made to the group. Reading about the formation and conduct of the club revealed a sense of pride among the members. This was one of their most valuable assets, and ensured the continuance of the group.

Most people with chronic illness had to learn to accept help. The amount of help required was unique to each individual—and bore more relationship to the individual's makeup than to their specific illness or the type of disability. It was sometimes apparent to elderly people who were chronically ill that they had to do more taking than giving in their lives of illness. On the whole this imbalance was a strain for them. There are social pressures that expect social relationships to be based on the unwritten (but generally shared) rules of reciprocity. The people in this study who felt uncomfortable about the amount of help they had to receive were aware that they had broken the unwritten social rules—and they expected people to tire of their needs. In their experience, people generally could not, as Pauline (Pb:249) put it, 'last the long haul' with an ill person who needs help and attention.

Medical attention can be either a rewarding or a frustrating experience. There were plenty of anecdotes of both types. The relationship between the doctor and the chronically ill elderly person is a professional one. Therefore, the problems of an imbalance of giving and taking (which can occur with personal friendships) do not arise. The doctor is rewarded for attending to patients, and the provision of a service is therefore considered to be a duty. However, it is apparent that there are times when the patient's view of their 'due' is quite different from that of the doctor.

The relationships between medical practitioners and those involved in the study were very important. When the relationship was good, doctors were immensely helpful. They could make the person feel better even when medical treatments were not significantly affecting the disease process or symptoms of the disease. When the doctor–patient relationship broke down, the participants described feeling bereft, anxious and often angry.

When examples of good experiences and poor/bad experiences with doctors were examined, it became apparent that the length of the doctor–patient relationship was important. Chronically ill people have time to establish a rapport with doctors, often over a period of years. These chronically ill people should be well known to the GP and the surgery staff, because they are regular attendees over a long period of time. Continuity of care should ensure that doctors understand the person's story, and take into account their various diseases and the impact they have on the person as a whole.

The participants in the study referred to only a few long-established relationships with doctors, but these long-term relationships were examples of good work between patient and doctor.

Elizabeth had gone to the same practice for fifteen years. She always saw the same GP, and she really appreciated his care and attention. He would visit her at home if she was in pain. He was honest with her, treated her like a fellow human being and was welcoming. After she had seen a specialist—who had said that she complained too much—she had this to say about a visit to her usual doctor:

> When we went up to see my friend [the doctor] … and he talks to me and he is up-front and there is no mucking around with him and he said, 'Elizabeth, you are difficult to treat, you are a difficult patient'. He said, 'You are not a difficult person, you get all these unusual things wrong—and that is what makes it difficult' … I think he understands what is going on because he treats my everyday little aches and pains. I get phlebitis a lot, especially in my arm … it just comes. He treats that. He treats all these little unusual odd problems that I get—and he knows what happens in my day-to-day life. And I feel he is the one who should be getting the specialist fees because he is the clever one and he is the one who knows a little bit of everything—whereas if you go to a specialist who only knows one thing … [the specialist] can't connect one problem to another.

Her doctor maintained a relationship with Elizabeth no matter how difficult to treat she became—and she really appreciated this. She felt that he liked her and that he genuinely felt for her suffering. He liked her because he knew her. He listened to her and became her friend over the years. He knew what she had gone through. Other doctors appeared to regard her as a list of unsolvable problems, and they viewed her with frustration, which was sometimes manifested as irritation. Building this kind of professional relationship with a doctor can be one of the benefits of being chronically ill. Elizabeth enjoyed visiting this doctor, although she was careful with his time:

> You don't want to bother him too much; you don't want to be nagging at him all the time either.

> … but he really is a funny doctor. I went one day, and I walked in the room—he had called me in—and I went in, and I couldn't find him. I thought I must be in the wrong room and he went 'Boo!' from behind the door, *[laughter]* and he said, 'Oh, I knew Elizabeth was coming, so I hid'. *[More laughter]* See, you can handle that …

Medical diagnosis is very important to people. Receiving a diagnosis meant that they received medical attention and that their physical symptoms were not dismissed as 'simply old age'. The degree of responsibility that the individual had to take for the disease also depended upon the diagnosis. Dr Craig explained that he views arthritis as something that is not his fault:

> I know exactly why it happened to me. I chose the wrong parents … my mother's family, all of them, had arthritis … So I think there is a strong genetic … element in the thing.

However, he associated his diabetes with his weight, and he knew that control of it lay in his hands.

Accepting help from friends and others was viewed in a different light. If receiving help was seen as a necessity and something that signified the older person's dependence, it was viewed in a negative light. Even help from partners was difficult for some participants, although Tom (who had had a stroke) accepted help from his wife, and the impression was gained that he was always looked after at home. It was his wife who seemed to be stressed by the amount of care and attention he required and the effect this had upon her life.

THE FUTURE

How people view their future affects how they feel now. Sarah has fully equipped her bathroom so that she can be as independent as possible for as long as possible. She does not currently need to wheel the wheelchair into the bathroom, but it gives her great peace of mind now to know that she will be able to do so when this becomes necessary.

A marked difference between the younger and older people in the study was that the older people less frequently referred to future hopes and cures for themselves. There was, however, reference to more struggle, to death and loneliness, to worries about impending loss of independence, and to fears of losing loved ones.

Two aspects of the fear of future loneliness were expressed by older people in the study.

- They said their experience was theirs alone—other people, no matter how close or how sensitive they were, could not know exactly how they felt.

- Loneliness was described in terms of not being with people—either because they could not get to see people, or because people did not come to see them anymore.

When a person is lonely, others appear to be distant and the world of the ill person resounds to their own reflections and emotions. This feeling is hard to bear. Ill people often do not have the energy or the ability to keep up with well people, and get left behind. Molly Holden's poem (below) gives expression to this feeling of being left behind. This does not express a wish to curtail other people—it expresses the pain of being left behind.

Along the lane ...

Along the lane go two of almost
equal height, her arm
through his. She takes my place, so sweet
a surrogate, no harm
enters my mind. Yet I can hardly bear
to watch my daughter
on her father's arm. Salt in the wound.
Fate gives no quarter.

Molly Holden (1994)

It is good to have loneliness relieved by having people visit at home. Here, the ill person is more likely to be comfortable and able to enjoy company. Visits to participants in the study were appreciated, and a welcome and entertainment were always offered.

People were more often concerned about a future inability to look after themselves than they were concerned about death (although there were a few people who talked about death). A range of symptoms may ultimately affect the person's ability to move and help themselves. People who are chronically ill have plenty of time to study their diseases and to appreciate the difficulties they may face in the future. Dr Craig knew what his deteriorating eyesight meant—that the doctor might prescribe insulin and that, if so, he would not be able to give his own injections. He would have to rely on someone to help him, and this prospect was a source of anxiety now.

Apart from the notion that it is demeaning and embarrassing for any adult to require assistance with daily living activities, dependence is also feared because one may then become a burden upon others. Dr Craig would not have minded too much what was happening to him now, if only he could be sure that he would not become disabled in the future.

> So ... the thing that's threatening me ... in the [future] ... disabilities increasing ... that I am going increasingly to have, to have to give up control of my own life, really, and rely on other people ... that's a scary sort of ... situation.

He did not want his wife or his children to be inconvenienced by his disabilities. The prospect really worried him:

> It raises uncertainty. You just don't know what is ahead of you ... The future is uncertain, you just don't know the degree of disability again ... You don't know the amount of help you will need, or whether it is available or whether you can afford to get it if it is available ... I would not like to impose on my wife, who really doesn't like ... she had a ... stint of nursing during the war and really didn't like it—and she wouldn't like giving injections and she wouldn't like carrying bedpans and stuff like that ... I would also not like to look to my children to look after me. I think that's imposing on them too much, on them ... the future is uncertain, you just don't know.

These worries led him to try to comply with a medical regimen of medicines and diets which he hated, and which made him quite miserable at times. He felt guilty if he did not try—because of the repercussions for his family, rather than for himself.

These data have shown that, for most of the participants, the future contains more illness, struggle, loneliness and creeping dependence. However, when that future is faced with candour, it is possible to glimpse means of gathering support to lessen the struggle—ways of keeping company, and plans to maintain independence.

CONCLUSION

A conclusion to an interpretive phenomenological study is a strange concept, for interpretations are forever susceptible to further interpretation. In the case of the present study, the purpose of interpretation is to enrich our understanding of chronic illness as experienced by older people. However, it would be pretentious to suggest that definite conclusions have been drawn from this work. Rather, the meanings that the participants have revealed are contributions to the continuing search for a better understanding of the experience of chronic illness.

In what way is the understanding generated in this research useful to nurses who care for elderly people? To appreciate this type of research requires an understanding of underlying assumptions. For example, there is an assumption that an individual's own perspective of their experience is valuable, and that it contains insights and knowledge that are helpful to people at every level of the health-care service, from hands-on carers to policy makers. Writing specifically about women, Chin concludes that research that represents the experiencing person's perspective is:

> a significant shift from the usual and customary ways in which women are viewed and treated in the medical-care system and in medical research.
>
> Chin 1994, p v

This comment can be equally applied to phenomenological research on the elderly unwell person. It is equally important for elderly people to find a voice and be heard.

Parts of this study will confirm some of the things that nurses already value, including:

- respect for a person's history;
- regard for those aspects of personal life that are unique to the individual;
- regard for those aspects of life that are shared with others within the culture; and
- appreciation for the context and situation people are in, and how this affects their experience of health-related matters.

This chapter may also introduce some nurses to new perspectives, and help them to better understand each client. Nurses may be able to recognise those elderly people who need help before they present in desperate states. The participants in this study could have all been helped by nurses, but they did not have the knowledge or means of accessing nursing help.

In this context, it was disappointing to find that nursing did not feature strongly in any of the participants' stories. On the whole, participants were not offered a nursing service until they were in need of physical support due to disability or advanced age. As a result of visiting these people (and getting to know them), it was possible to describe the ways in which nursing care could have helped them to live with chronic illness (FitzGerald 1995, 1997). There were a significant number of participants in this study who were depressed and receiving no help.

Medical professionals may choose not to become involved with problems which are not directly associated with the diagnosis or treatment of the disease process. However, in this study, these problems often caused people the most distress. There was a dearth of care given to these people by health professionals. As noted previously, professional care does not have to be reciprocated in the same way that is considered the norm in relationships with friends and family. Professional care provides an opportunity for the person to receive care without feeling beholden or guilty. This would appear to be most welcome, given the participants' expressed concern about becoming a burden or a nuisance to other people.

The point is that treatment without care is poor treatment—and, in some instances, it is ineffective treatment. This was particularly evident when participants suffering from depression were treated only with antidepressants. The meaning of care in this context is professional concern for the person—a professional concern that incorporates a desire to help the person by understanding what matters in his or her life. Care is for the entire person (rather than relating merely to specific signs or symptoms of illness), and involves knowing and understanding all the problems which make the person's life difficult. Such problems as depression, poor self-esteem or difficult relationships make people just as uncomfortable as the symptoms of illness. Treating only physical problems is not an efficient way to help people who are chronically ill. Often there is not the opportunity to discuss these problems in the doctor's surgery. In contrast, seeing people's problems in the home context is very revealing.

The meanings extrapolated from the data collected from the participants in this study have been structured and represented as the past, the present and the future. This rich information is the material upon which nurses could base a caring service for individuals in the community. Two developments which have the potential to offer elderly people with chronic illness a nursing service that will have a positive effect on their overall well-being are the prospect of nurse practitioners, and a focus of care in the community.

VIGNETTE

One elderly man—and one nurse's experience of his haemodialysis

Craig Lockwood

Reg had been a front-bar man all his working life. He was wizened and tanned like leather, wore a black beanie and jeans in all weather, and had lively, blue, communicative eyes.

On meeting each nurse who was looking after him, Reg quickly and happily established that he would rather be at the pub. He seemed to feel more comfortable when talking, particularly about his past. This was encouraged because it helped us to understand where he was coming from and how he coped with renal failure and dialysis. It quickly became obvious that the restriction on fluid intake weighed heavily on him. If it wasn't a beer he craved, it was a cold can of coke with crushed ice. Reg freely admitted that he would find it impossible to stick to the diet and fluid allowance recommended for haemodialysis patients, and said that he felt a bit guilty but that he was going to enjoy himself anyway.

Older patients commencing dialysis often adapt poorly to the need for dietary changes, and Reg was a perfect example of this. Occasional cheating was important to him, and was good for his sense of well-being, if not for his health. Chronic renal failure presented a real threat to his sense of normality. It became apparent that the restrictive lifestyle seemed to highlight his problems, decreasing his self-esteem, sense of well-being and normality.

Elderly patients on dialysis have a number of common problems—they have grown up on a high-salt diet, have lost much of their functional capacity, are constantly fatigued by chronic anaemia and may take a day and a half to recover their energy from each dialysis session.

Fluid and dietary restrictions were not Reg's only problems. He was an honest stoic, openly admitting that he hated having needles put in, but bearing with it anyway. Talking was his way of coping. If he had a good rapport with the nurse he would joke that we enjoyed putting needles into him. When he was in a good mood, we would joke that he was a favoured pin-cushion, and he would pretend to run from the unit.

Secretly, he really would have loved to run away from all his troubles. On bad days he would be silent, as if his failure to share his difficulty made that difficulty less important. What made for a good day or a bad day was a mystery because we saw him only when he presented at the unit with the mood already established. Intuitively, I believed that his moods related to how he felt about himself rather than to his clinical status.

In my experience, the reaction of patients to needles varies—younger patients complain longer and louder at times, but older patients seem to actually grow older and shrink into themselves.

In Reg's case, he alternated between withdrawal and objection. He used to justify his pain by saying that we'd hurt too if someone stuck 'bloody great big needles' in us! If nurses reinforce the acceptability of responding to pain, this helps to validate the person's feelings and improves the nurse–patient relationship.

The nursing care for Reg was typical of many older patients on haemodialysis. These patients had to accept help to stand on the weigh scales, read the results, get off the scales, walk to their chair and sit down. Around them were younger, healthier patients performing these tasks with ease as the older patients had to accept extensive, time-consuming nursing care in a busy unit. Each visit accentuated their frailty or lack of health. The care during dialysis became more complicated as co-morbidities increase the effect of cardiovascular changes, and the body's coping mechanisms became less efficient. Thus, for example, the frail, elderly person may have needed to lose 1.5 kg, but was able to tolerate a loss of only 1.0 kg before significant hypotension occurred. This was a compounding problem in the elderly dialysis patient, and sometimes took several dialysis trips to correct.

To a certain extent, knowing how the person feels makes work in the dialysis unit more difficult, as different clients compete for attention and the nurse becomes more stressed trying to prioritise competing demands. However, knowing how these people feel helps us to judge the competing demands and helps to ensure that there is enough time to treat people as individuals. They require time to express themselves as human beings who have lives outside the dialysis unit.

References

Brody H 1987, *Stories of Sickness*, Michigan Book Crafters: Michigan.

Chin E 1994 (ed), *Developing Nursing Perspectives in Women's Health*, Aspen Publications: Maryland.

Cousins N 1983, *The Healing Heart: Antidotes to Panic and Helplessness*, WW Norton: New York.

Curtin M & Lubkin LCI 1990, *Chronic Illness: Impact and Interventions*, Jones & Bartlett: Boston.

FitzGerald M 1995, *The Experience of Chronic Illness in Rural Australia*, Health Care Studies, 289, unpublished PhD thesis, University of New England: Armidale, NSW.

FitzGerald M 1997, Nursing and researching, *International Journal of Nursing Practice*, 3, pp 53–6.

Frank A 1991, *At the Will of the Body: Reflections on Illness*, Houghton Mifflin: Boston.

Gelven M 1989, *A Commentary on Heidegger's Being and Time*, Northern Illinois University Press: Illinois.

Helman C 1981, Disease versus illness in general practice, *Journal of Royal College General Practice*, 31, pp 544–52.

Holden M 1994, Along the lane. In: Keith L (ed), *Mustn't Grumble*, p 60, The Women's Press: London.

Hudson R & Richmond RHJ 1994, *Unique and Ordinary: Reflections on Living and Dying in a Nursing Home*, Ausmed Publications: Melbourne.

Kestenbaum V 1982, *The Humanity of the Ill*, University of Tennessee Press: Knoxville.

Kleinman A 1988, *Illness Narratives: Suffering, Healing and the Human Condition*, Basic Books: New York.

McDonald M 1992, *Put Your Whole Self In*, Penguin Books Australia: Ringwood, Vic.

Nay R 1993, *Benevolent Oppression—Lived Experiences of Nursing Home Life*, pp 158–87, unpublished PhD thesis, School of Sociology, University of New South Wales: Sydney.

Nay R 1996, Nursing home entry: meaning making by relatives, *Australian Journal on Ageing*, 15(3), pp 123–6.

Olson C 1993, *The Life of Illness*, State University of New York Press: Albany.

Paterson B 2001, The shifting perspectives model of chronic illness, *Journal of Nursing Scholarship*, 33(1), pp 21–6.

Pearson A, Nay R, Taylor B, Tucker C, Angus J, Griffiths V & Ruler A 1996, *Relatives' Experience of Nursing Home Entry: Meanings, Practice and Discourse–Interim Report*, University of Adelaide: Adelaide.

Place B 1992, Living with chronic illness. In: *Extending Independence*, pp 145–51, University of New England Press: Armidale.

Register C 1987, *Living with Chronic Illness*, The Free Press: New York.

Ross J W 1993, In: Styles MA & Moccia P (eds), *On Nursing: A Literary Celebration*, pp 310–16, National League for Nursing Publications: New York.

Sontag S 1983, *Illness as Metaphor*, Harmondsworth: Middlesex.

Thorne S 1998, Shifting images of chronic illness, *Journal of Nursing Scholarship*, 30(2), pp 173–8.

Thorne S & Paterson B 2000, Two decades of insider research: what we know and don't know about chronic illness experience, *Annual Review of Nursing Research*, 18, pp 3–25.

Thorne S, Paterson B, Acorn S, Canam C, Joachim G & Jillings C 2002, Chronic illness experience: insights from a metastudy, *Qualitative Health Research*, 12(4), pp 437–52.

van Manen M 1990, *Researching Lived Experience: Human Science for an Action Sensitive Pedagogy*, State University of New York Press: New York.

CHAPTER 14

Medication issues

HELEN BAKER AND ADRIANA TIZIANI

INTRODUCTION

In general, older people consume a high proportion of all prescribed medications, as well as over-the-counter preparations, often in large quantities because of chronic illness and/or co-morbidities, putting them at risk of adverse drug reactions. Added to this, the drug-manufacturing business is highly profitable, and its products are marketed aggressively. Many medications are designed to treat the ailments of older people, and large businesses are based on their sales. This contributes to the pressure on prescribers and consumers to try new, and supposedly better, products in an attempt to reduce disease-related or medication-related symptoms. Television and other media news items about breakthroughs in drug therapies result in many people, not only the aged, approaching medical practitioners and pharmacists because they are convinced that the medication will reduce their problem symptoms.

The use of medication by old people should therefore be governed by great caution, as they are put at risk of adverse effects by a number of factors, including:

- age-related changes to pharmacokinetics and pharmacodynamics leading to altered responses to medication;
- age-related physiological changes;
- declining mental capabilities or altered cognition;
- social factors; and
- polypharmacy.

This chapter explores these issues.

PHYSIOLOGICAL CHANGES IN AGEING

As humans age and their bodies change, the way in which they respond to medications also changes. Although ageing is an individual physiological process, the following is a discussion of the common age-related changes that may affect the way an older body responds to medication.

Pharmacokinetics

Pharmacokinetics is the absorption, distribution, metabolism and excretion of a drug from the body. All these processes may be altered in the older person.

Absorption

Effects on absorption can include:

- increased gastric pH;
- altered gastric emptying and intestinal blood flow; and
- decrease in first-pass metabolism in the liver.

The net effects of these changes include unpredictable changes to dissolution and absorption of the drug, increased risk of stomach irritation (and potential ulceration), reduced effectiveness of short-lived drugs, and the possibility that enteric compounds will start their action earlier (that is, in the stomach, which the coating of the tablet is meant to bypass), causing gastric irritation and nausea.

Distribution

Altered body composition (decrease in lean body mass, increase in fat stores) may lead to increased storage of fat-soluble drugs (such as diazepam, lorazepam, haloperidol), leading to accumulation and higher than normal blood levels.

The decrease in total body water alters the distribution of water-soluble drugs (such as cimetidine).

A decrease in plasma albumin results in fewer drugs being bound, and subsequently a greater proportion existing as unbound (or free) drug, leading to an increased risk of adverse effects and toxicity. Many drugs used in the older person are highly bound to albumin—these include aspirin, warfarin, phenytoin, indomethacin, ibuprofen, naproxen, chlorpromazine, haloperidol, thioridazine, nifedipine, verapamil, frusemide and diazepam.

Decreased blood flow and cardiac output slow the drug, increasing the time taken to reach the target organs.

Metabolism

Decreased oxidative metabolism and decreased hepatic blood flow increase the half-life of a drug significantly in some cases (for example, the half-life of diazepam increases from 20 to 90 hours in an older person in their eighties).

Excretion

A decrease in the glomerular filtration rate slows excretion of the drug, resulting in some drugs being toxic within normal therapeutic range. Furthermore, there is an increased risk of kidney damage from those drugs considered to be nephrotoxic.

Pharmacodynamics

Receptor sensitivity and homeostasis are both altered by age-related changes, increasing the risk of adverse drug reactions and interactions in older people. For example:

- changes in receptor sensitivity in the cardiovascular system may reduce the effectiveness of adrenaline; and
- changes in receptor sensitivity in the central nervous system may increase the older person's sensitivity to psychoactive medications such as sedatives, hypnotics and tricyclic antidepressants (Newby 1999).

COGNITION

Sight and hearing

Sight and hearing both affect the ways in which older people manage their medications. The older person with a visual impairment may still be able to adhere to their medication regimen and maintain their independence, when some simple strategies are followed, including:

- using good lighting;
- using colour and contrast;
- using clear marking and labelling; and
- encouraging the person to use all their senses (Mowerson 2002).

Understanding and remembering

Elderly people who can see and hear well might still have problems understanding instructions, and remembering not only the instructions but also whether they have taken a medication. The cognitive effects of some medications can exacerbate these problems of understanding and remembering medications (e.g. anticholinergics, antidepressants, antipsychotics, antihistamines, anti-Parkinsonian agents, cimetidine, digitalis, hypnotics and sedatives). This can make it difficult for the prescriber to differentiate between cause and effect if problems arise—whether a deficiency in memory is the cause of problems in administration, or whether the medication itself has brought about changes which result in difficulty with self-administration. The National Health Strategy (1992) states that confusion is a recognised effect of inappropriate medication use in older people, and can be attributed to many groups of medications. It is also important to recognise that *non-comprehension* is a different problem from *non-compliance* and must be managed differently.

Manual dexterity

Reduced manual dexterity can cause problems for a person in dealing with the packaging of medications. Childproof packaging can be as impossible to open for an older person as it is for the child it is meant to protect! Removing a tablet from a sealed card might present a challenge to an older person, as might breaking a tablet in half; and peeling the backing from a medication patch can prove impossible. If packaging is a problem, there is a temptation to ask a relative or friend to help. Community nurses report finding medications mixed together on windowsills or benchtops. Medications packed in foil to exclude light are sometimes found in a saucer alongside those that should not be exposed to air until administration. Under these conditions, many of the medications in the mixture will have altered potency. This mixture of unpacked (and therefore unlabelled) drugs can prove hazardous to some consumers, as they rely on memory and visual recognition to select those required at a particular time. Identification of medications by others, such as nurses, can be almost impossible. Customised packaging by pharmacists is available to some, but is not necessarily the answer to this problem.

SOCIAL FACTORS

There is a common perception in Western societies that age should be equated with illness, or that old age is an illness in itself. As the 'baby boomers' (those born soon after World War II) approach young old age, they are slowly changing this perception, but among today's older aged, there is still an assumption for many people that age equates with illness and thus must be treated medically.

Advances in medical science have created expectations within the community that all illnesses can be cured. This expectation is reinforced by the plethora of medical programs—both real and fictional—presented in the media. This expectation includes cures or the relief of symptoms of chronic conditions that in the past were perceived as part of the normal ageing process. Many of these conditions are the result of long-established lifestyle patterns. Some members of Australian society, whether aged or not, believe that all unwanted symptoms are amenable to treatment, usually by means of medications, and that medical practitioners have not performed adequately if they fail to prescribe medications.

Self-medication

Australians often treat themselves with non-prescription drugs, including herbal preparations, vitamins and minerals. Healthy, active-looking, grey-haired celebrities advertising pharmaceutical products in the electronic and printed media promote this practice to older people. Stoehr et al (1997) link the wide use of over-the-counter (OTC) medications in the aged with a number of factors including the extent of ageing (that is, young aged or old aged), anxiety, income, gender and the number of symptoms experienced. The extent of the use of these OTC medications has been emphasised when faults are found in the manufacturing processes and consumers are alarmed at the abrupt withdrawal of their medications from the marketplace.

Over-the-counter preparations are readily available to all—from pharmacies, supermarkets and convenience stores, most of which offer no advice with the products. The two most common ailments treated with OTC products are indigestion and constipation, which also happen to be common ailments in the older person. Antacids in particular may alter the absorption of other drugs from the gastrointestinal tract and should not be taken within two hours of ingesting medications generally. Constipation is common in the elderly and may be the result of medication and/or lifestyle issues such as reduced mobility, reduced fluid intake and low-fibre diet. Rather than using laxatives, the older person should be encouraged to take a daily walk and increase their fluid intake. The diet can also be modified to include such things as stewed prunes, fresh citrus fruits, and wholegrain breads or cereals (Bryant et al 2003).

'Keeping it for a rainy day'

Many people are tempted to use prescription medications for purposes other than those for which they were prescribed, or to treat other people with medications prescribed for themselves, if they think they recognise symptoms similar to their own. As older people tend to take more prescribed medications, they have more opportunities to engage in this practice. In addition, because of financial constraints and a perception that frugality is a virtue, older people can develop the strategy of saving medications left over from one illness, to treat another.

Doctor and pharmacy shopping

Mobility is a feature of Australian society and this mobility among older people contributes to another medication-related problem. If their unwanted symptoms are not relieved after consultation with one medical practitioner, they can, and do, seek help from another. The problem may be further confused if they describe the symptoms caused by a new drug in addition to the original symptoms. Furthermore, it is common for Australians to deal with more than one pharmacist, and thus a client's medication record, as held by one pharmacist, differs from that held by another. Many efforts have been made to allow pharmacists to share such information, but the regulations with regard to privacy are still a barrier to such a provision, which might well protect consumers from adverse drug-related events.

POLYPHARMACY

'Polypharmacy' may be defined as 'the use of a number of different drugs by a patient who may have one or several health problems' (*Mosby's Medical, Nursing and Allied Health Dictionary,* 6th edn). Although polypharmacy tends to be associated with older people, it can (and should) be equated with anyone who takes more than two medications, prescribed or non-prescribed. The tendency to associate polypharmacy with older people comes from them having more co-morbidities and chronic illness treated by medication. The interaction between medications can be either *synergistic* (that is, working together or augmenting the activity of one of the medications) or *antagonistic* (working in opposition to each other) (Mosby's Dictionary). An example of this is warfarin, which interacts with some 250 different drugs (Myers 2002), including herbal preparations, that either increase or decrease its anticoagulant effect, potentially leading to an increased risk of haemorrhage or thromboembolic events.

The polypharmacy roundabout

The process leading to polypharmacy may be regarded as a 'roundabout', with many opportunities to enter, but few exit points. Some of these entry points include:

- the multiple health problems experienced by older people;
- resistance to therapy and the need to try other medications;
- prescribing by multiple physicians;
- the expectation of a 'pill for every ill' and receiving a 'treatment' during a consultation;
- physician and patient both being reluctant to stop old therapy;
- drug promotion (mentioned briefly in the introduction);
- treating side-effects of other medication;
- treating the symptoms rather than the cause of an illness;
- concurrent use of OTC and alternative medications; and
- a general failure to review therapy regularly (Newby 1999, p 68).

A study by Sloane et al (2002) found that the absence of weekly physician visits to review patients (and their medications) was one of the contributing factors to older patients in residential care/assisted living facilities being prescribed inappropriate medications.

Polypharmacy and adverse effects

Polypharmacy is associated with adverse drug reactions. In a study by Ali (1992), the potential for adverse drug reaction was found to be 6% when two drugs are taken, rising to 50% when clients are taking five drugs, and 100% when eight or more medications are taken together.

Admission to an acute-care setting for a serious adverse drug reaction is a common exit point from the polypharmacy roundabout. Martin et al (2002) carried out a prospective study of drug-related problems as a cause of hospital admissions and found that 11.9% of admissions during the period of the study were drug related, and that most of these were preventable. Guerra et al (2001) stated that greater use of prescription medicines was a predisposing factor in admission of older people to hospital, especially when associated with living alone, and financial constraints. Of course it could be argued that older people take so many medications because they suffer more co-morbidities, but it appears that highly educated women from higher socioeconomic groups are more likely to engage in polypharmacy than the rest of the population (Guerra et al 2001). Furthermore, there appears to be an increasing proportion of consumers taking both Chinese herbal medicine and traditionally prescribed medication. One estimate (Myers 2002) suggested that nearly 20% of the Australian population (3.7 million Australians) used prescription medication at the same time as complementary medicines.

Polypharmacy in other settings

Polypharmacy is not confined to the mobile, self-administering aged population. Older people under the supervision of community nurses, and those in hostels and nursing homes, are in as much danger of polypharmacy as those outside. The employment of unqualified and unregulated workers to administer medications increases the hazards of polypharmacy. Even if such workers conscientiously and correctly administer the prescribed medications, doing this without knowledge and an ability to evaluate the effects of those medications or changes in physical or mental status can lead to progressive under- or over-dosing, and has led to illness. For example, community nurses have reported incidents of older people who have a prescription for Lasix and another for frusemide and are taking both because they are unaware that this is the same medication—with the expected results. It is dangerous for clients to rely on the appearance of a medication to identify it, because the appearance can change at any time, depending on the source.

Exiting the polypharmacy roundabout

If the polypharmacy roundabout is interrupted by an admission to an acute-care setting, a rationalisation of medications usually occurs. However, this may be of short duration, as it has been known for patients to return to their GPs after discharge from hospital, requesting the accustomed medications that the hospital 'forgot' to reorder. An example of this is benzodiazepines that may have been ordered for patients who requested sedation, but who are also suffering from chronic respiratory conditions. Specialist respiratory physicians will almost certainly discontinue these, but the clients, believing that their short hours of sleep are insufficient (but perhaps normal for their age), or anxious about their health or social factors, may demand them from their GP soon after discharge.

This raises the question of whether a program of self-administration of medications for patients who are still in hospital would improve clients' knowledge of medications, and their ability to self-administer safely after discharge. Bird (1990) suggests that it does. Certainly, structured opportunities to learn about medications while still in hospital lead to better understanding of the medication regimen, and facilitate more successful self-administration after discharge (Fielo & Warren 1993).

COMPLIANCE, OR 'DOCTOR KNOWS BEST'

The term 'non-compliance' may be perceived as negative, and being 'non-compliant' as the responsibility only of the person who has not taken the medication. Shakespeare said, 'What's in a name? That which we call a rose by any other name would smell as sweet'(Romeo and Juliet, Act 2 scene 2) and one might question whether indeed there is any difference between the terms 'compliance' and 'concordance' (Rossi 2003). Rossi considers *compliance* to be a paternalistic term, while *concordance* refers to 'an agreement or partnership between patient and prescriber about obtaining the best use of treatment, compatible with what the patient desires and is capable of achieving. Non-concordance then relates to the patient–prescriber consultation, and not the patient' (Rossi 2003, p 105). Perhaps concordance is a better term as it suggests that the responsibility is a shared one.

A Western Australian study indicates that 17% of all readmissions to hospital are a result of non-compliance (Fremantle Hospital 1991). The incidence of non-compliance varies widely, but the range is commonly estimated at between one-third and one-half of all consumers, and this varies by only very small increments over many years (Pfister-Minogue 1993; Caserta 1987; Merkatz & Couig 1992). Conversely, there is a suggestion that older Australian people may be more compliant than overseas studies would suggest (Hopkins 2000).

Why then are consumers 'choosing' not to take their medication as directed? Hopkins (2000) perhaps controversially, suggests that 'in light of evidence about over-prescribing and polypharmacy, "non-compliance" may even represent a rational and responsible decision by the consumer' (p 103). A number of reasons have been postulated. Hopkins (2000) found that:

- consumers often wanted to ask questions about their medications but didn't feel able to;
- they wanted written information to read later;
- a communication barrier existed either because the doctor used medical terminology not understood by the patient, or came from a different ethnic background, or did not give an adequate explanation about what to expect;

- there were communication problems on discharge from hospital with changes to medication regimens;
- there were social barriers such as cost and access;
- no alternatives were suggested;
- the risks, when explained, deterred some people; and
- prescribers were not aware of the number of prescription and non-prescription medications taken by their patient.

Ebersole & Hess (1998) add a number of other reasons to this list, including:

- the medication being ineffective or perceived as no longer needed;
- uncomfortable side-effects;
- the drug regimen being too complicated for the person to maintain;
- duration of therapy;
- not having the prescription filled or refilled;
- physical limitations;
- misunderstandings about expected outcomes;
- inadequate directions ('take as directed');
- interference with lifestyle (e.g. 'Take three times a day with meals' when the person may only eat two meals); and
- when, where and how instructions were given.

This last point has particular relevance to nurses, who often 'educate' the patient about their medication on or before discharge.

The nurse's role and compliance

The nursing literature on the subject includes the notion that it is the duty of nurses to ensure that consumers adhere to their prescribed therapy—that is, that they be compliant. There is an assumption that compliance is good, and therefore desirable (Donovan & Blake 1992), and that deliberate non-compliance is irrational or deviant behaviour. Nurses who are familiar with particular client groups will recognise this as a false assertion. These nurses will agree with Holm (1993), who states that, although the medical practitioners are the experts on the diseases suffered by clients, the experts on the patients' lives and the ways in which they are affected by disease are the patients themselves. Many clients vary their own medication regimens for very good reason. Donovan & Blake (1992) apply the term 'reasoned decision-making' to the resolve of consumers to vary their medication regimen. This must be differentiated from those variations from prescribed regimens that are the result of failure to understand the instructions, forgetfulness, confusion over drug names, economic reasons for not purchasing medications—and a host of other reasons.

One of the methods recommended to nurses for ensuring compliance is to give consumers information about their medications. In acute-care and community settings, many nursing-care plans include sessions for education about medications. Pharmacists also claim that informing consumers about medications, whether in hospital or in the community, is within their professional domain. It is suggested that this information alone will ensure compliance, but this also appears to be untrue in many cases. Persons suffering from chronic disease, who know the most about their medications and their own disease, are the most likely to experiment, often seeking a narrow comfort zone between the symptoms of their disease and the side-effects of the therapeutic agents prescribed to control them (Donovan & Blake 1992).

INSTITUTIONALISATION

When older people are admitted to institutions for either acute or extended care, the issues related to medications are changed, but are still of concern. If they are admitted to an acute-care setting, the physiological factors of ageing may be complicated by acute illness. Admission to an extended-care institution presents its own set of problems.

In acute-care settings

Many older people are admitted from the community to hospital for acute illnesses or trauma, although they may also be admitted for exacerbations of chronic illness for which they have administered their own medications for many years. Over long periods, members of this group have established routines which suit them in terms of convenience, or as cues to self-administer, or (perhaps) to achieve reduction of side-effects to personally acceptable levels. When they arrive in hospital, the organisational norms generally take over. This means that, as far as possible, medications are administered as ordered, as interpreted in the hospital system.

Take, for instance, the case of an older person who has been taking medications ordered to be taken before meals and therefore on an empty stomach. For reasons of convenience, he has been taking these medications with his meals for some years. The GP has monitored his response to the drug, and has adjusted the dosage to obtain the required outcome. On admission to hospital, the medications are administered 20 minutes before meals, and the observed response is markedly different. This is reported to the medical officer, who adjusts the medication dosage. All is well, until the patient is discharged when, in spite of advice to the contrary, he returns to his old routine, probably arguing to himself that this routine has served him well for many years and should do so in the future. This change might require a readjustment of dosage by the GP but, in the worst cases, it may result in readmission to hospital, to the dismay of both the patient and the staff.

There are other problems arising from the admission of aged persons to acute-care facilities. New, unfamiliar medications may be ordered to treat a new or altered condition. The drugs the person has been taking may also be ordered, but by a different name. On discharge, confusion can arise over new or old medications, with difficult and sometimes serious consequences. Nursing authors suggest a program of education culminating in self-administration of medications by capable consumers while they are still inpatients (Bird 1990; Pearson & Baker 1992). This would provide at least a partial remedy for some of these occurrences, and would certainly allow for identification of potential problems in individuals. Nevertheless, the cultural environment discourages this as health-care disciplines defend their professional territory. Because they have difficulty in handing over responsibility for medications to the people who take them, they continue traditional procedures to avoid blame for errors. Self-administration programs are currently successful in rehabilitation settings, but they are yet to be accepted in acute-care settings (Merkenhoff H, personal communication, 1998).

With the change in environment and acute illness, the older person may experience acute confusion while in hospital. Add to this intravenous therapy to correct fluid and/or electrolyte imbalance or to administer medications and the nurse may be confronted with a confused and agitated patient who is trying to pull the intravenous lines out and/or trying to get out of bed. In times gone by, the answer was to 'restrain' the patient for his or her own good, so that they wouldn't hurt themselves and so that the lines remained in situ for the duration of the therapy. The challenge for nurses today when confronted with this situation is to explore options for treatment, resulting in the best outcome for both patient and nurse.

In extended-care settings

The problems associated with medication usage in extended-care settings are different from those in acute-care settings, but just as difficult to resolve.

One of the most basic problems is that of identification of residents. To create a homelike, non-medical environment, name bracelets and bed cards are not used. There may be photographs of residents supplied to those administering medications, but these can quickly lose their currency. Residents of extended-care settings are encouraged to be as mobile as their condition will allow, so there may be no clues to identify them in their immediate surroundings, and people with cognitive changes may ascribe incorrect identity to themselves or to others.

The changing physiology of older people requires constant sensitive evaluation of changed responses to medications. With staffing trends moving towards a mix that includes fewer registered nurses and greater numbers of unregulated and unqualified carers with minimal training, it is possible that gradual, incremental changes in response may not be noticed.

When medications are administered using primary routines—that is, when they are administered to the group of residents for whom nurses are responsible for the whole of a shift or a day—medication errors are fewer than when all medications are administered by one person over a large number of residents (Long 1992). As long ago as 1983, Garsnell identified a threshold number of eighteen medications which, when exceeded by any nurse, resulted in increasing error rates. In spite of these important research results, there are now fewer registered nurses in aged-care facilities, and these fewer nurses administer all medications—thus exceeding the threshold number of eighteen. Under these conditions, it is likely that medication error rates will increase unless special precautions are taken.

Modern administration aids, such as packages produced in a community pharmacy, might assist in self-administration, provided residents are able to demonstrate their ability to manage them. A suitable assessment format is available in the *Guidelines for Medication Management in Residential Aged-care Facilities* (Australian Pharmaceutical Advisory Council [APAC] 2002). The dynamic nature of the ageing process requires that this ability be re-demonstrated at regular intervals, as it can be expected to decline as people progress to older old age.

In residential settings where nurses administer medications, these packages, containing all the medications to be administered at certain times of day, are not without their problems. A professional responsibility of nurses is that they will know the medication they are administering, and know its functions, side-effects, interactions and adverse reactions. When medications are provided in mixed batches, identification of individual medicines for the purpose of withdrawal by nurses for any of a number of reasons might be impossible, particularly as many medications are available in various shapes and colours, depending on the trade version obtained.

If it is necessary for older persons to be admitted to hospital from extended-care settings, they will be further debilitated by their physiological crisis, and disorientated as they enter the new settings. When they are discharged back to their more familiar setting, another disruption occurs. Their movements in both directions are likely to prompt the need for changes in medication, and the resettling of aged people, including the readjustment of medications and dosages, can take some time. During these periods, extra vigilance is required with regard to response to medications.

Because residents of extended-care settings are not in constant contact with medical practitioners, it is usual for certain medications to be prescribed for administration 'PRN' (meaning 'as required'). Many of the medications prescribed in this way have a sedative effect, and nurses caring for the residents administer these medications according to their clinical judgement of the resident's condition. Although chemical restraint of residents is authorised only under very specific circumstances, a lack of other resources—such as staffing numbers or a physical environment that ensures physical safety—may force nurses to a decision to use PRN medications for the purpose of chemical restraint because, to them, the risks of chemical restraint are not as great as those of physical injury. Apart from the ethical issues, chemical restraint has its own physiological consequences, detracts from residents' quality of life and, in many cases, shortens their lives.

Strategies

Residents in extended-care settings are often admitted with a list of prescribed medications qualifying as polypharmacy. New residents in some nursing homes have a 'medication holiday' during which all medications are ceased, and then gradually re-introduced as the need for each of them is justified. This frequently results in the residents being prescribed a much smaller number of drugs than their pre-admission list. Where no 'medication holiday' occurs, all medications and the accompanying danger of polypharmacy are continued. Integrated Best Practice Model—Medication Management in Residential Aged Care requires regular medication review by a multidisciplinary team, which will certainly question situations suggestive of polypharmacy (APAC 2002).

In addition, nurses are introducing non-pharmaceutical therapies, such as massage, aromatherapy relaxation techniques and guided visualisation in extended-care settings. These therapies can enable health professionals to reduce the number of medications taken by residents, and thus contribute to their alertness and physical status. Australian anecdotal evidence suggests that residents who take fewer medications of all categories experience better mobility and balance and, consequently, a reduced incidence of falls and incontinence. Unfortunately, major barriers to the use of non-pharmaceutical therapies are lack of time, a dearth of staff members who are qualified to use the techniques, and a medically dominated culture that discourages their use.

Quality use of medicines

In 1992, the Australian Government formulated a policy on Quality Use of Medicines (QUM). The goal of the policy was: 'to optimise medicinal drug use (both prescription and over-the-counter) to improve health outcomes for all Australians' (Pharmaceutical Health And Rational Use Of Medicines Working Party 1992, p 15).

In the case of QUM, *quality* is defined as using medications in a manner that is:

- *safe*—minimising misuse, underuse or overuse, and providing the ability to solve medication-related problems such as adverse effects;
- *judicious*—defining the role of medications in treating illness and recognising that the management of many conditions lies in non-chemical therapies, such as lifestyle changes including diet, exercise and a wellness perspective—and alternative therapies; and
- *appropriate*—using the most effective medication under the circumstances, including those of the consumer's condition, risks, benefits and costs.

The policy was directed at all Australian citizens including consumers, the health professionals (who prescribe, dispense and administer medication and evaluate their effects), drug manufacturers and drug regulators (who decide on which medications will be available in Australia and how much the community will pay for them).

Educational programs for all stakeholders have been initiated, including 'Be Wise With Medicines' Week, plain-language consumer information enclosed in medication packaging, and increasing responsibility for consumer education by community pharmacists and medical practitioners. The policy is supported by generous research and education funding, which has resulted in a wide range of projects carried out by health professionals from many disciplines. The *Guidelines for Medication Management in Residential Aged-care Facilities* (APAC 2002) are an example of the outcomes of the QUM policy, and the commitment of the Australian Government to its implementation. However, despite many improvements as a result of QUM, there are still significant problems associated with the use of medications, including an estimated 80,000 hospital admissions per annum due to medication-related problems (Commonwealth of Australia 2002, p v).

CONCLUSION

Medication issues for the older person are many and varied—they overlap and form a complex web with factors from diverse sources, old and new, but the framework for addressing them exists in the QUM policy. The policy is supported morally, structurally and financially by successive governments, but it will change nothing unless the stakeholders—all Australians—are committed to its implementation.

VIGNETTE

Benzodiazepines and chemical restraint

Helen Baker

The issue of benzodiazepine use is a vexed one in aged-care settings. Their use is justified in many cases (although loneliness, sleeplessness and grief should not be seen as proper indications for their use). But despite this acknowledgement of their proper use in many cases, there is no doubt that benzodiazepines are overused and misused in aged-care facilities. Many factors contribute to this.

The proportion of residents with dementia in residential care is increasing. At the same time, funding imperatives have reduced numbers of staff. The number of registered nurses as a proportion of the staff has also been reduced. Many other carers, although they may have received training to enable them to carry out certain tasks, have little or no education about the nature of ageing or dementia.

Benzodiazepines are usually prescribed to treat a condition—as diagnosed by the attending medical officer. Where staff numbers and levels of insight into the reason for resident behaviours are low, there is a strong temptation for the drugs to be used to manage behaviours—that is, as chemical restraint. Unfortunately, alternative behaviour management requires larger numbers of staff with an understanding of the processes of ageing and dementia, and advanced skills in such techniques for behavioural management as meditation, guided visualisation, massage and aromatherapy. Private aged-care facilities must ultimately seek a profit, and government institutions are always trying to reduce costs, making it unlikely that these non-drug alternatives will be employed. In addition, the physical environments provided for residents in aged-care facilities are sometimes potentially dangerous. As one director of nursing observes: 'We have a freeway at the front and a river at the back. What do you want me to do, let them [the residents] wander?' In the absence of adequate, skilled staff, she resorts to chemical restraint—in the form of benzodiazepines that have been prescribed for a different purpose.

When benzodiazepines are prescribed, the orders give nurses and other staff discretion in their administration by allowing their use on a PRN basis. In aged-care facilities, the systems for drug tracking and recording are sometimes inefficient—and in some cases non-existent. Drugs are frequently provided in large numbers, even on the initial prescription, and no cessation date is specified. Under these conditions, persons for whom this class of medication has not been prescribed may also be given misappropriated drugs for the management of difficult behaviours. The short-term gain for the staff is a reduction of seemingly disruptive resident behaviour—and consequently, a reduced workload and a less stressful working environment. The long-term effects on residents (such as increased confusion, memory loss, incontinence, constipation and loss of mobility leading to injury) are dealt with as they arise—and rarely attributed to benzodiazepine use.

The means of reducing the use of this class of drugs by using alternative strategies is demonstrated by Gilbert et al (1993). However, this project was carried out before the advent of current funding and staffing arrangements. Under prevailing conditions, the underlying social and funding conditions are unlikely to be changed for the better, and the use of benzodiazepines for the management of behaviour is likely to continue, to the detriment of many residents of aged-care facilities.

References

Ali N 1992, Promoting safe use of multiple medications by elderly persons, *Geriatric Nursing*, 13(3), pp 157–9.

Australian Pharmaceutical Advisory Council (APAC) 2002, *Guidelines for Medication Management in Residential Aged-Care Facilities*, AGPS: Canberra.

Bird C 1990, Drug administration: a prescription for self-help, *Nursing Times*, 86(42), pp 52–5.

Bryant B, Knights K & Salerno E 2003, *Pharmacology for Health Professionals*, Mosby: Marrickville, NSW.

Caserta J 1987, It's a jumble ... no it's a maze ... no it's your client's medication shelf, *Home Healthcare Nurse*, 5, p 11.

Commonwealth of Australia 2002, Quality Use of Medicines—Statement of Priorities. Strategic and Action Plan 2001–2002, AGPS: Canberra.

Donovan J & Blake L 1992, Patient Non-compliance: deviance or reasoned decision-making? *Social Science and Medicine*, 34(5), pp 507–13.

Ebersole P & Hess P 1998, *Towards Healthy Aging* (5th edn), Mosby: St Louis.

Fielo S & Warren S 1993, Medication usage by the elderly, *Geriatric Nursing*, 14(1), pp 47–51.

Fremantle Hospital 1991, Readmissions to Fremantle Hospital (Parts 1 & 2), *Fremantle Hospital Drug Bulletin*, May, June & October, Fremantle, WA.

Garsnell R 1983, *The Relationship Between Interruptions During the Medication Procedure and the Occurrence of Medication Errors*, unpublished thesis (MN), Dalhousie University: Nova Scotia.

Gilbert A, Owen N, Innes J & Sansom L 1993, Trial of an intervention to reduce chronic benzodiazepine use among residents in aged-care accommodation, *Australian and New Zealand Journal of Medicine*, 23, pp 343–7.

Guerra HL, Firmo JO, Uchoa E & Lima-Costa MF 2001, The Bambui Health and Aging Study: factors associated with hospitalisation of the elderly, *Cad Saude Publica*, 17(6), pp 1345–56.

Holm S 1993, What is wrong with compliance? *Journal of Medical Ethics*, 19, pp 108–10.

Hopkins H 2000, 'Take as directed', whatever that means, *Australian Prescriber*, 23(5), pp 103–4.

Long T 1992, Pointing out medication errors, *American Journal of Nursing*, 92(2), pp 76–8.

Martin MT, Codina C, Tuset M, Carne X, Nogue S & Ribas J 2002, Drug-related problems as a cause of hospital admission, *Medicina Clinica Barcelona*, 118(6), pp 205–10.

Merkatz R & Couig M 1992, Helping America take its medicine, *American Journal of Nursing*, 92(8), pp 32–6.

Mowerson L 2002, Helping patients with vision impairment adhere to a medication regime, *Journal of Gerontological Nursing* 28(2), pp 15–18.

Myers S 2002, Interactions between complementary medicines and warfarin, *Australian Prescriber*, 25(3), pp 54–6.

National Health Strategy 1992, *National Health Strategy Paper No. 4*, Issues in pharmaceutical drug use in Australia, AGPS: Canberra.

Newby D 1999, Polypharmacy—how to minimise the risks, *Current Therapeutics* 40(10), pp 67–70.

Pearson A & Baker H 1992, Compliance or alliance? *Deakin Institute of Nursing Research Paper No. 9*, Deakin University: Victoria.

Pfister-Minogue K 1993, Enhancing patient compliance, *Geriatric Nursing*, 14(3), pp 124–32.

Pharmaceutical Health and Rational Use of Medicines Working Party 1992, *A Policy on the Quality Use of Medicines*, AGPS: Canberra.

Rossi S 2003, Compliance or concordance? *Australian Prescriber*, 20(5), p 105.

Sloane P, Zimmerman S, Brown L, Ives T & Walsh J 2002, Inappropriate medication prescribing in residential care/assisted living facilities, *Journal of the American Geriatrics Society*, 50, pp 1001–11.

Stoehr G, Ganguli M, Seaberg E, Echement D & Belle S 1997, Over-the-counter medication use in an older rural community: The Movies Project, *Journal of the American Geriatrics Society*, 45(2), pp 158–65.

CHAPTER 15

Physical restraints: can we free older people?

SUSAN KOCH

INTRODUCTION

As stated in the first edition of this book, the initiative to reduce restraint use is not new. However, increased public awareness and the innovation and availability of alternatives to restraint use have led to significant policy review both locally and internationally. In Australia in 1999, through the accreditation process for aged-care facilities, which includes the review of restraint-use policies and education of staff on minimising restraint use, a growing number of aged-care facilities are encouraging the minimal use of physical restraint on older people.

Studies undertaken by Evans & Strumpf (1989) proposed several ideas to explain the differences between those who advocate the use of restraint and those who do not: these included differences in philosophy and culture, differences in perception of the perceived legality of using restraint, and the availability of restraints. Studies examining why nurses use restraint as a therapeutic intervention consistently report client/staff safety as the most frequently cited reason for restraint use, yet there is no evidence of efficacy in using restraint to prevent injury (Koch 1994; Retsas 1997).

THE CURRENT SITUATION

Prevalence estimates of restraint use both locally and internationally have been the subject of extensive investigation. A number of Australian studies have revealed a high level of use of restraints in nursing homes, ranging from 23.6% in Queensland (Retsas & Crabbe 1997) to 26% in Western Australia (Retsas 1997) and Melbourne (Koch 1994). An Australia–wide study of restraint use found that 22.6% of patients were physically restrained (Woodward 1998). In its systematic review of patient injuries and physical restraint devices, the Joanna Briggs Institute (JBI) suggested that the proportion of residents in residential care who were restrained ranged from 12% to a maximum of 47% (JBI 2002). Similar prevalence (24%) was found in a Swedish study of nursing home restraint use (Karlsson et al 1996). However, comparisons of these estimates of prevalence may be confounded due to definitional differences. In a comparison of studies based on groups of residents with similar functional abilities and cognitive performance, Ljunggren et al (1997) described a low prevalence (less than 9%) of restraint use in Denmark, Iceland and Japan, 15–17% in France, Italy, Sweden and the United States, with Spain experiencing the highest prevalence, at almost 40%. Castle et al (1997) found that the prevalence of restraint use decreased from 36% in 1990 to 26% in 1993 after implementation of the *Omnibus Reconciliation Act 1987* (USA).

What constitutes restraint?

In the literature, what constitutes restraint varies. Some emphasise equipment, chemicals and other aids to restricting freedom of movement, while others focus more on intent. Sullivan-Marx (1994) referred to restraint as the limitation of voluntary movement through the application of devices in physical restraint or medications in chemical restraint, and Miles & Meyers (1994) defined restraint as a device attached or adjacent to the resident's body, which restricts freedom of movement or normal access to one's body. These may include the following devices:

- **posey vest**—a canvas harness that is placed on the person like a waistcoat. The vest crosses over at the back and can be secured to the chair by two long straps that can be tied. The device prevents the individual from standing and leaving their chair unaccompanied. The ties are long enough to be tied under the chair or behind the chair, thus ensuring that the restrained person cannot reach them to untie them.

- **geriatric chair**—a large lounge chair which has a tabletop attached. The tabletop can be removed as required. The tabletop is held in position by two prongs that slide into the arms of the chairs and is then tightened by wing nuts. The wing nuts are under the tabletop, making it difficult for the restrained person to release them without assistance. The person is unable to stand and cannot get out of the chair unsupervised.

Anecdotal evidence from practitioners suggests that staff sometimes use both devices—that is, the geriatric chair and posey vest—simultaneously, thus ensuring that the person is permanently seated until staff can release them. However, people have been known to slide beneath the table and have their head caught between the chair and the table (Evans & Strumpf 1987). There have also been suggestions that the person may be predisposed to strangulation by having their head caught and the vest sliding up around their neck.

Other restraints include:

- **cot sides/bedrails**—to some health-care workers, cot sides do not constitute restraint (Koch 1994; Nay & Koch 1999). However, if the reason for the use of cot sides is to restrict movement in order to prevent the person from getting out of bed, then it may be suggested that they are being used as a form of restraint. The cot sides or bedrails are attached to the sides of the beds and locked in position. The rails can be raised and lowered by an individual (such as a health-care worker) who is not lying in bed by releasing a catch, thus allowing the cot sides to collapse.

- **seat belts**—seat belts, or lap belts as they are sometimes called, are normally attached to wheelchairs, shower chairs and lounge chairs (Nay & Koch 1999). The seat belts are normally released like a normal seat belt in a car, although some staff prefer to have the release clasp outside the reach of the person restrained, perhaps at the back of the chair. The person cannot stand up or remove himself or herself from the chair without assistance.

- **other devices**—these include: **sheets** tied around the waist of the person to restrict movement; a **leg bag**, which looks like a sleeping bag in which the person is placed and the zipper closed to waist height, again restricting movement; and **mittens**, which prevent hand movements;
- **medications** (i.e. psychotropic drugs).

Strathen (1992) produced the following detailed definition:

Restraint should be seen in a broad context as embracing individual physical restraint on movement, physical restraint to circulation within and beyond a building, the use of certain drugs, excessive supervision and observation, some institutional. Professional and cultural attitudes, the allowing of situations to exist in which residents have insufficient money to afford reasonable mobility.

Strathen 1992, p 3

In 2002 the JBI undertook a systematic review of patient injuries and physical restraint devices, using as its definition:

any device, material or equipment attached to or near a person's body and which cannot be controlled or easily removed by the person and which deliberately prevents or is deliberately intended to prevent a person's free body movement to a position of choice and/or a person's normal access to their body.

Joanna Briggs Insititute 2002, p 2

Strumpf (1997) and Flicker (1996) see *intent* as integral to what is restraint. Nay & Koch (1999) in their report to the Commonwealth Department of Health and Aged Care reflect similar views to study participants, in that restraint is defined as:

any physical, chemical or environmental intervention used specifically to restrict the freedom of movement—or behaviour perceived by others to be antisocial—of a resident designated as receiving high or low care in an aged care facility. It does not refer to equipment requested by the individual for their safety, mobility or comfort. Neither does it refer to drugs used—with informed consent—to treat specific, appropriately diagnosed conditions where drug use is clinically indicated to be the most appropriate treatment. Thus restraint by definition may be seen to be a human rights rather than a medical issue.

Unpublished report to the Commonwealth Department of Health and Aged Care, p 4

The non-existence of a universal definition of restraint, descriptions of the devices used (both physical and chemical), the way they are used and the circumstances under which they are considered restraint rather than a treatment, cause confusion. Although researchers of the topic generally accept the definitions, in Australia there are different views from a legal and professional perspective. Until there is universal acceptance of what constitutes restraint, the confusion will continue, as will the practice. There is a need, in Australia, for a definition of restraint that is legally and professionally accepted (Koch 2002).

Chemical restraint

In Australia there has been limited research on the use of psychotropic drugs as chemical restraints in aged care (Clinnick 2000). Psychotropic drugs used as restraints have 'often been abused and can cause more harm and increase the level of confusion in an aged person' (Rovner et al 1996, p 7). Sloane et al (1991) suggest that 'pharmacological restraints are generally considered to be present when a neuroleptic, anxiolytic, sedative or hypnotic agent is used on a regular basis' (p 1278) and that a high percentage of elderly residents receive restraints in the form of psychotropic medication.

Research has found that behavioural symptoms are the most commonly cited reasons for prescribing psychotropic drugs (Sloane et al 1991; Nay & Koch 1999). Often the resident does not have a psychiatric condition that would benefit from these medications. As Buck noted:

> studies have led some to conclude that nursing homes do not administer psychotropic drugs therapeutically, but rather as a means to control behaviour and manage large institutional populations.
>
> Buck 1988, p 409

When these drugs are misused and mismanaged, the amount of care required to care for the resident may increase because of the side-effects these drugs can cause (Clinnick 2000).

Some researchers have suggested reasons why these medications are so widely administered to the aged (Clinnick 2000). One suggestion sees the increased number of residents who suffer from conditions such as dementia (Sloane et al 1991) as a reason because these conditions cause behaviours that may be seen as difficult or demanding to the carers. As Rovner et al state:

> more than 80 per cent of nursing home residents experience dementia, behaviour disorders, psychosis or depression, but fewer than 5 per cent receive mental health care.
>
> Rovner et al 1996, p 7

This suggests that residents who do have behavioural problems are not given adequate medical treatment and are often prescribed medication that may not help them (Clinnick 2000).

Another possible reason for the high use of psychotropic drugs as restraint is that the nursing homes are serving as psychiatric facilities and do not have adequate numbers of educated staff to cope with this increase of residents with behaviours of concern.[1] Rovner et al believe that:

> the high frequency of psychiatric symptoms of residents and the use of psychotropic drugs and physical restraint suggests that nursing homes serve as de facto mental institutions for older people.
>
> Rovner et al 1996, p 7

Sloane et al (1991, p 1278) suggest that nursing homes are becoming 'satellite psychiatric institutes', requiring specialist nurses. Nursing staff play a prominent role in this, and take responsibility for the decision to administer the chemical restraint. It has been suggested that staffing problems encourage the administration of psychotropic medications for behavioural problems, in preference to personnel interventions.

---

[1]Behavioural changes associated with dementia are usually described as challenging behaviours or behavioural problems. Alzheimer's Australia advocates instead using the term 'behaviours of concern'. This reflects a positive rather than negative connotation.

Risks of using restraint

The knowledge of nursing staff about the risks and potential ramifications of using restraints is generally considered to be poor. As might be expected, registered general nurses have been found to have a significantly higher level of awareness of the negative effects of restraints than nursing staff with a lower level of education (Murray & Cott 1998; Terpstra et al 1998). Nevertheless, a large number are still unable to identify physical injury, depression, skin trauma and humiliation as likely consequences of restraint (Molasiotis & Newell 1996). A large percentage of nursing aides are similarly unable to correctly identify critical safety issues concerning restraint usage (Neary et al 1991). Over 60% of respondents in the study by Neary et al (1991) did not see death as a potential hazard of restraint use. The findings of these overseas studies highlighting nurses' lack of knowledge about restraint use have been confirmed by recent Australian research (Retsas & Crabbe 1997), and Retsas (1997) found an unacceptably high level of restraint use in all Australian States, suggesting that nurses are either unaware of, or (in spite of research which suggests otherwise) indifferent to the physical, emotional and psychological consequences of restraint.

A lack of knowledge about the effects of restraint does not in itself explain the high levels of restraint usage. Murray & Cott (1998) surveyed 555 Canadian hospital nurses about their perceptions of restraint use. Even though most nurses were able to correctly identify the negative effects of restraints on patients' physical and emotional health, restraint usage remained high throughout the hospital.

There are numerous examples of restraints such as bedrails (Schnelle et al 1994; Miles 1996) or vests and straps (Miles & Irvine 1992) contributing to or causing death or serious injury. These instances are under-recognised and preventable clinical events (Parker & Miles 1997) which are involved in approximately 1 in 1000 nursing home deaths (Miles & Irvine 1992). Even when in the down position, bedrails make it more difficult to exit the bed (Ball et al 1997), thus increasing the risk of serious injury.

The forced immobilisation caused by mechanical restraint can cause physical problems such as the development of pressure sores (Strumpf 1997) and serious psychological stress. In the case of an older patient, such stress could lead ultimately to death (Robinson et al 1993). The psychosocial effects of restraint are no less significant than the physical and can lead to problems such as dependency and diminished quality of life (Mason et al 1995). These consequences are not limited to the patients alone—family members may also be psychologically adversely affected by seeing their loved ones restrained (Newbern & Lindsey 1994).

Although there is little doubt from the available research evidence that restraints have contributed to death or serious injury, the retrospective nature of most studies makes it difficult to determine the extent to which these consequences are directly due to restraint or the debilitated condition of the patients (Miles & Meyers 1994).

There are concerns also about the consequences of restraint removal. One of the main reasons for restraining patients is to prevent serious injury associated with falling (Koch 1994; Retsas & Crabbe 1997; Retsas 1997; De Santis et al 1997; Nay & Koch 1999), and there is a prevailing view that removal of restraints will lead to an increase in the number of falls. A number of studies, however, suggest that the removal of restraints does not lead to a significant increase in the number of falls or fall-related injuries (Bradley et al 1995; Capezuti et al 1996; Capezuti et al 1998; Dunn 2001).

Factors influencing the use of restraint

Caregiving staff frequently see few viable practical options available to them in lieu of restraint (Sundel et al 1994; Molasiotis 1995; Retsas & Crabbe 1997; Retsas 1997; Terpstra et al 1998; Nay & Koch 1999). The common belief that there are few, if any, alternatives to restraint may underpin the view that restraint remains an important intervention when caring for older patients (Terpstra et al 1998; Nay & Koch 1999; Koch 2002) and, moreover, may discourage caregivers from seeking alternatives. Over 60% of nurses surveyed by Murray & Cott (1998) felt uneasy about reducing the current levels of restraint use, even though they perceived the potential benefits to both the patient and their family in terms of greater happiness, independence, self-esteem and physical and psychological well-being. Although half the staff thought that a reduction in restraint use would create a better environment, the stronger belief was that this would result in more injuries. Despite the apparent lack of awareness about alternatives and the seeming desire to reduce the use of restraints, a South Australian study of staff concerning their educational needs rated restraints among the least-needed educational area (Coburn et al 1998).

Nurses are known to have a strong sense of duty of care and many feel legally obligated to use restraints for resident safety (Molasiotis 1995; Retsas & Crabbe 1997; Retsas 1997; Nay & Koch 1999; Koch 2002), even if the resident's dignity is compromised in the process (Neary et al 1991). Moreover, the unclear legal position in regard to restraint use (Flicker 1996; Nay & Koch 1999; Koch 2002) leaves many nurses feeling vulnerable to accusations of negligence should the resident be injured as a result of not being restrained (Murray & Cott 1998; Nay & Koch 1999). Nurses may therefore be reluctant to take responsibility for decisions not to restrain when that course of action is deemed to be risky for the resident and, in turn, for themselves (Nay & Koch 1999).

Many nurses see staffing as a critical issue in any endeavour to reduce restraint usage. A commonly held view is that a reduction in restraint use is not possible without an increase in the number of available staff (Molasiotis 1995; Molasiotis & Newell 1996; Nay & Koch 1999; Koch 2002), since restraint reduction is considered to be associated with more work and more stress (Murray & Cott 1998). In the absence of what is perceived as adequate staffing, restraint is considered to be the safest and most expedient option available (Nay & Koch 1999).

The use of restraints could also be based in part on the mix of staff and their varying knowledge and attitudes, especially as aged-care facilities are increasingly staffed by less-qualified personnel (Nay & Closs 1999; Nay & Pearson 2001). A study by Haber et al (1997) found that fewer registered nurses choose physical restraint to address difficult behaviour than do nursing aides—thus, the issue of restraint removal may become more problematic if less-qualified staff are providing care. This is supported by Murray & Cott (1998), who found that staff working in the long-term care setting do not perceive the effects of restraints as negatively as staff working in acute care. They suggest that this is related to the higher level of unskilled workers in aged care than in the acute-care setting.

The implication that staff working in long-term care may have a more tolerant attitude towards restraint use is given some credence by other research which indicates that aged-care nurses generally perceive fewer alternatives to restraint use (Neary et al

1991; Schnelle & Smith 1996; Retsas 1997). It is possible that nurses working in aged care see the sort of behaviour which precipitates restraint use as chronic and intractable, and therefore not amenable to other sorts of intervention (Lundervold et al 1993; Nay & Koch 1999). A less common but nevertheless significant carer attitude about restraint use is that people do not mind being restrained (Bradley et al 1995; Retsas & Crabbe 1997); some even ask for it (Molasiotis 1995).

ALTERNATIVES TO RESTRAINT

Nay & Koch (1999) identified a number of alternative means used. For example, some facilities had tried to adapt existing equipment (such as removing wheels from a bed to make it lower to the floor). Other means used were:

- hip-protectors;
- safety helmets;
- surveillance equipment for residents who tended to wander from the residence—for example, electronic tags worn by residents around their wrist or neck trigger a monitoring system if they walk through the front door or front gate. Other devices fitted to bedroom doorways detect movement (especially used at night), so if a resident leaves their bedroom or walks into another resident's room an alarm is activated.
- free access for residents to move from inside facilities to enclosed garden courtyards and meandering pathways;
- raised garden beds;
- a car for residents to wash;
- a chook shed (chicken coop);
- mailbox and bus shelter

(Nay & Koch 1999).

Taking care with or adapting the design of the facility was also seen as a means of minimising restraint (Nay & Koch 1999). Examples provided by participants included:

- the use of subdued colour to reduce stimulation and soothe those residents who had a tendency to be agitated;
- painting doors the same colour as walls to camouflage offices or rooms that residents were not to enter;
- the use of different patterns of tiling on floors to delineate one living space from another; and
- passages that connected, so residents could wander around, rather than a linear corridor that encouraged pacing up and down.

Facilities that had been purpose built and/or were relatively new reported greater ease in implementing restraint-minimisation policies than those which were ten or more years old (Nay & Koch 1999).

Sullivan-Marx (1995) considers it useful to reconceptualise the restrained person as a victim of trauma, rather than as a person in need of protection. The way an individual reacts to being restrained, she argues, depends on the subjective meaning that the experience holds for the person. This is perceived in turn to depend on any prior actual or symbolic trauma that that person may have previously experienced. Emotional responses to being routinely restrained—such as agitation, withdrawal, passivity and regression—are reported by Sullivan-Marx (1995) as all adaptive responses to avoid further restraint, or to adjust to their daily use. The routine use of restraints on individuals who have limited ability to process trauma effectively, it is attested, may increase the risk of them developing a post-traumatic stress syndrome or other mental health disorder.

Few studies have explored the impact of restraint from the viewpoint of the family. A survey by Dunbar et al (1997) indicated that the vast majority of families were in favour of restraint-free care. Wives of restrained elderly men interviewed by Newbern & Lindsey (1994) considered the use of restraints degrading as well as symbolic of their husbands' deteriorating health. The wives in this study resented the use of restraints and sought to have them removed when they were in attendance, or, if removal was not possible, they endeavoured to conceal the use of the restraint, 'covering it up with his shirt or lap robe or something' (Newbern & Lindsey 1994, p 137).

Making choices

Prior to living in aged-care agencies, older people have made autonomous choices during their lives. Making such choices would often have required a willingness to take risks. These choices and risks taken throughout life reflect the interests and values that make these people individuals. Older individuals may therefore have strong feelings about how they wish to live out the rest of their lives. However, those older people residing in aged-care agencies are often dependent on nursing staff to pursue their interests regarding respect, freedom and dignity. The responsibility of nurses to protect those in their care from harm includes protecting the autonomy of the individual.

It could be argued that regardless of the circumstances—and the form of restraint used—physical restraint always represents a major infringement on the interests of the individual being restrained. As noted previously, Evans & Strumpf (1987) have shown that the application of a physical restraint causes the individual who is being restrained to suffer a loss of autonomy. There is also evidence that the use of physical restraints may be hazardous to health. To allow informed decisions about restraint, nurses should provide the following information:

- the type of restraint being applied;
- the rationale for restraining;
- the rationale for the type of restraint chosen;
- the consequences of applying restraint;
- the duration of application; and
- the special care that will be provided when restraint is applied.

When a decision is made on behalf of the older individual, those making the decision should, as far as possible, be aware of the older individual's views on the use of physical restraint.

If the philosophy of nursing practice is based on the principle of autonomy, nurses must respect clients as autonomous beings. Part of being autonomous is being able to take risks. If nurses subscribe to the principle of autonomy, they are bound to reject the use of physical restraints, because such restraints have been shown to cause the restrained individual to suffer a loss of autonomy. Making morally sound decisions requires not just that clients be informed, but that nurses also be informed about the consequences of, and alternatives to, applying physical restraint.

Facilitating a restraint-free environment

A national study by Nay & Koch (1999) found that various organisations appeared to promote and implement a number of practices to minimise the use of restraints. These included diversional, social, physical, emotional and sensory therapies or activities. The study highlighted the fact that these were more effective if implemented within an organisational context which stated a clear restraint-free philosophy, had well-developed associated policies, implemented comprehensive client-focused assessments, and used a system of program evaluation. Best practice with regard to minimal restraint use was seen to be at its optimum when all staff were aware of organisational policy, liaison with families and interdisciplinary collaboration was promoted and a consistent system of practice evaluation was established. The need for ongoing resident and family education regarding restraint use was identified as necessary, with emphasis being placed on the importance of informing the resident and family members about the efficacy of restraint use and the emotional and physical impact it can have on an individual (Nay & Koch 1999).

Nay & Koch (1999) suggest that essential to creating a minimal restraint environment is a committed management director and team. Their report emphasised that the Director of Nursing had to support the idea in principle and in practice if it was to succeed.

In some situations, inappropriate equipment, such as the existence of non hi-low beds, was identified as being a hindrance in becoming 'minimal restraint'. New equipment or beds would be necessary, and many facilities could not absorb the cost of acquiring them (Nay & Koch 1999).

A major impediment to the implementation of restraint-free care is a lack of knowledge of the alternatives (Terpstra et al 1998; Nay & Koch 1999). This points to a fundamental problem in communication between the research and clinical communities, and in the application of research to improve practice. Research has yielded a variety of innovative approaches that enable a reduction in the need for restraints.

Central to these innovations is a paradigm shift from system-centred to patient-centred care (Brungardt 1994) and a philosophical shift from 'protection' to quality of life (Mason et al 1995). Most successful programs have the support of the administration: nursing administrators have a significant contribution to make in facilitating restraint-free care. They should be knowledgeable about restraint, willing to advocate for its implementation and able to lead and guide their facility through the change process (Dunbar et al 1997; Nay & Koch 1999). Because of the interrelationships between the conditions that lead to restraint, a multifaceted approach is required.

The types of programs which have been developed to reduce the use of restraints take the form of dedicated programs, dedicated people or dedicated units. *Dedicated programs* include education products such as videos, fact sheets, resource manuals and education programs (Nay & Koch 1999). Evaluation studies of the educational programs have found that the use of restraints has decreased during the program (Bradley et al 1995; Dunbar et al 1997); however, little information is available about whether this success is maintained after completion of the program.

Dedicated people refers to nursing specialist models of care, such as geriatric resource nurses (Lee & Burnett 1998) or clinical nurse specialists (Patterson et al 1995) who provide ongoing, informal, unit-based education and nursing consultation. These specialist nurses have expertise in assessing whether reduction of restraints is feasible and what alternatives are available, and they act as a resource for other staff who require guidance to improve individualised patient care. In the United States, gerontic nurse practitioners have been found also to improve care outcomes significantly (Wunderlich et al 1996).

Dedicated units are established to provide dedicated care in a particular area of practice. These special care units or nursing development units are repositories of specialist knowledge and skills which can help to improve patient outcomes (McCracken 1994). In an Italian study where special care units followed specifically designed care programs focusing on the environment and staff for the care of dementia patients, the data showed a reduction in the use of psychotropic drugs and physical restraints (Bellelli et al 1998).

Each of these approaches achieves its objectives though the implementation of best practice—that is, on the basis of the best available information, standard clinical practice is altered to achieve improved patient outcomes. The successful implementation of restraint-free practices depends too upon the attitudes of those charged with the care of elderly patients (Nay & Koch 1999). Given the known negative consequences of restraint usage, its prevalence has been justifiably referred to as a fundamental breach of human kindness (Frengley 1996). The more common view among paid caregivers, however, is that restraint is a necessary evil (Retsas & Crabbe 1997).

Assessment

Each resident's situation must be discussed with the individual and the family. If the resident cannot directly be involved in providing information, the family should be asked to provide a detailed history of the individual. Aspects of the history should include medical history, social history, personality, habits, coping skills and any other information considered relevant by the family.

Any family concerns regarding the removal of restraints must be addressed. In particular, the family may raise safety concerns. The nurse must ensure that the family is provided with information that will allow them to make a fully informed judgement regarding restraint removal. This information should include the consequences of an older adult being restrained, the right of the individual to take risks, the care that will be implemented to prevent injury, and the philosophy of the agency in providing quality care.

Removing the restraint may not be without cost because many of the residents may require alternative resources—including high–low beds, concave mattresses, bed poles, gym mats and improved lighting.

Assessment of the safety of the environment must also be undertaken prior to implementing a restraint-free environment. Matters to be considered include access to hazardous areas, and the presence of dangerous materials, such as cleaning products and medications. Some alterations to the facility may be required—incurring further costs.

Planning

On completion of a full assessment, the individual and/or the family should be in agreement with the staff regarding the implementation of individual strategies aimed at maintaining the safety of the individual. The strategies will depend on the information gained through the assessment process. Changes to the environment must also be implemented, as these may affect the safety of the individual.

Evaluation

Once the strategies have been implemented, an evaluation process should be organised—including staff and family—to discuss the outcomes. However, a major difficulty in evaluation of outcomes is that sometimes there is a lack of detailed documentation.

Documentation should indicate the strategies which have been implemented, and record any further falls after removal of restraint. Detailed information regarding other aspects of care should also be included. A lack of documentation regarding outcomes hinders the development of further strategies that can be used as an alternative to restraints. Without this information nurses are unable to provide evidence of best practice, and are unable to share their findings with colleagues.

Staff issues in implementing a restraint-free policy

Staff members may react negatively to the implementation of a restraint-free environment. They may become frustrated when certain strategies do not appear to work, and some staff members may advocate reverting to the old practices with which they have been familiar for many years. Unfortunately, staff members may pass on their negative views to the family, thus increasing family scepticism about the changes. However, full discussion of the care plan with the family, and with the person receiving care, may highlight aspects of care with which they are particularly pleased, and may provide them with the opportunity to raise outstanding issues that are continuing to give them cause for concern.

Discussions that include all carers, including the family, highlight the existence of a real partnership. For example, the family may indicate that their mother visits the toilet and has a bowel movement every day when they assist with her walking program. This may not be reflected in the notes because the family may not have considered it necessary to inform the staff. This may compromise the bowel-management program developed for the resident, because the staff may be under the impression that constipation is a problem for the woman in question. A positive outcome should reflect the fact that bowel management is now noted to be no longer an issue for this woman. The documentation would then record no further episodes of constipation since implementation of the initial strategies.

VIGNETTE

Falls management by nursing staff in a sub–acute setting

Daniel Olivieri and Dianne Johnson

A 78-year-old client with a diagnosis of reduced cognition, ataxia, restlessness and impulsive behaviour was admitted to a sub-acute hospital. The client had a history of a space-occupying lesion in the frontal lobe and repeated falls at a community home (supported residential service). The woman had no family.

On admission to the ward, a falls risk assessment was completed as part of the admission process, and a falls prevention program (documenting individual interventions required to reduce falls risk) was initiated by nursing staff.

The initial assessment of the client's falls revealed that on most occasions the falls occurred in the area of the client's chair, and sometimes from the bed at night.

Risk factors identified by the nurses included:

- toileting—continence assessment needed as staff at SRS reported increasing urinary incontinence;
- hearing loss—speech referral to assess level of hearing loss;
- footwear—podiatry referral to arrange orthotics/suitable footwear; and
- mobility—physiotherapy referral to advise most appropriate gait aid, mobility regimen and chair.

Strategies developed were outlined in the care plan:

- The client was accommodated in a room located near the nurses' station and with a toilet/bathroom nearby, to maximise staff supervision both during the day and at night.
- Non-slip continence mats were located near the client's chair within the room and dayroom.
- The client was seated in the dayroom nearest the nurses' station.
- Because of reduced cognition and impulsiveness, consistent staff response was provided to the client's questions. (It was difficult at times to reason with the client.)
- The client's mobility was poor, requiring (two) staff to help her to use a walking frame.
- The client's sit-to-stand was a difficult issue and required continued physio involvement to maintain strength in her quads and endurance, in order to assist her to mobilise from the room to the dayroom.
- The client often reached for items beyond her grasp, and so staff were required to leave appropriate items within reach for her use.
- The electric bed (high-lo) was kept in the low-low position, with no cot-sides.
- A fall-out chair (restraint) was used after discussion with the treating team.
- Following the voiding profile chart and bowel documentation and evaluation, three-hourly toileting was initiated by staff during the day and nocte urinary

incontinence experienced by the client was managed by continence pad use. Bowel management (diet and aperient) was required, as the client became restless when constipated; a non-slip continence mat was also used.

- The client's room was de-cluttered; a trial at night of a 'bed-fall mat' was unsuccessful.
- A walking program was developed by a physiotherapist, to help maintain the client's strength and endurance.
- The recreation officer was asked to assist with activities, but these were of limited success (cards in a group setting); the client participated for 20 minutes and then became restless. She enjoyed hand massages, but needed to move on to another activity. She showed no interest in books or magazines, but enjoyed the opportunity to go for wheelchair outings around the ward and the hospital.
- Discussion of the client took place in a weekly multidisciplinary team meeting, and the number of falls was reported.

The above measures helped to reduce the frequency of repeat falls and assisted the staff in approaching the patient's care proactively, ensuring that her needs were met and that her environment was safe.

CONCLUSION

Caring for residents without using restraints is not without cost. Many individuals may require alternative resources, such as beds that can be lowered to a minimal height, diversional activities that provide pleasure, and chairs that are comfortable without causing danger to the older individual.

Individuals and their families may require considerable support, especially if they have been informed that the use of physical restraint increases safety for the individual, but have not received the same depth of information regarding the adverse consequences of restraint use.

Staff may require further education in:

- developing alternative strategies to restraint;
- developing comprehensive assessment skills;
- acquiring knowledge of the consequences of applying restraint to an older individual;
- rehabilitation processes; and
- palliative care.

Getting nurses to fundamentally change their practice is never easy. For too long, the prevalent behaviour of nurses has been to use physical restraints as a reflexive measure, rather than as a last and limited resort. The prevailing presumption in favour of restraints must be reversed.

Eliminating the use of physical restraints will depend on altering attitudes and misconceptions concerning physical restraints and relative risks, and effectively persuading all those involved in health care to understand that thoughtful, selective replacement of restraint by other interventions will bring about an improvement in the quality of life for everyone involved in the provision and receipt of care (Kapp 1996).

References

Ball MC, Hanger HC & Thwaites JH 1997, Bed rails: a barrier to independence? *Clinical Rehabilitation*, 11(4), pp 347–9.

Bellelli G, Frisoni GB, Bianchetti A, Boffelli S, Guerrini GB, Scotuzzi A, Ranieri P, Ritondale G, Guglielmi L, Fusari A et al 1998, Special care units for demented patients: a multicenter study, *Gerontologist*, 38(4), pp 456–62.

Bradley L, Siddique CM & Dufton B 1995, Reducing the use of physical restraints in long-term care facilities, *Journal of Gerontological Nursing*, 21(9), pp 21–34.

Brungardt GS 1994, Patient restraints: new guidelines for a less restrictive approach, *Geriatrics*, 49(6), pp 43–4, 47–50.

Buck J 1988, Psychotropic drug practice in nursing homes, *Journal of the American Geriatrics Society*, 36, pp 409–18.

Capezuti E, Evans L, Strumpf N & Maislin G 1996, Physical restraint use and falls in nursing home residents, *Journal of the American Geriatrics Society*, 44(6), pp 627–33.

Capezuti E, Strumpf N, Evans L & Maislin G 1998, The relationship between physical restraint removal and falls and injuries among nursing home residents, *Journal of Gerontology*, 53A(1), M47–M52.

Castle NG, Fogel B & Mor V 1997, Risk factors for physical restraint use in nursing homes: pre- and post-implementation of the Nursing Home Reform Act, *Gerontologist*, 37(6), pp 737–47.

Clinnick L 2000, *Nurses' Perceptions of the Use of Psychotropic Medications as Chemical Restraint*, unpublished master's thesis, La Trobe University: Melbourne.

Coburn R, Tidswell R & Finucane P 1998, The educational needs of staff working in residential care facilities in South Australia, *Geriaction* 16(2), p 204.

DeSantis J, Engberg S & Rogers J 1997. Geropsychiatric Restraint Use, *Journal of the American Geriatrics Society*, 45(12), pp 1515–18.

Dunbar JM, Neufeld RR, Libow LS, Cohen CE & Foley WJ 1997, Taking charge: the role of nursing administrators in removing restraints, *Journal of Nursing Administration*, 27(3), pp 42–8.

Dunn KS 2001, The effect of physical restraints on fall rates in older adults who are institutionalised, *Journal of Gerontological Nursing*, 27(10), pp 40–8.

Evans L & Strumpf N 1987, Patterns of restraint: a cross cultural view. Editorial, 'Restrained in Canada—free in Britain'. In: Evans LK, *Restraint Use with the Elderly Patient*, paper presented at the First National Conference on Nursing Research and Clinical Management of Alzheimer's Disease, Minnesota: University of Minnesota, May 1988.

Evans LK & Strumpf NE 1989, Tying down the elderly: a review of the literature on physical restraint, *Journal of American Geriatric Society*, 87, pp 65–74.

Flicker L 1996, Australian Society for Geriatric Medicine position statement on physical restraint use in the elderly, *Australian Journal on Ageing*, 15(1), pp 8–10.

Frengley JD 1996, The use of physical restraints and the absence of kindness, *Journal of the American Geriatrics Society*, 44(9), pp 1125–7.

Haber LC, Fagan-Pryor EC & Allen M 1997, Comparison of registered nurses' and nursing assistants' choices of intervention for aggressive behaviours, *Issues in Mental Health Nursing*, 18, pp 125–38.

Joanna Briggs Institute 2002, *Physical Restraint, Part 1: Use in Acute and Residential Care Facilities*, Best Practice, 6(3), Blackwell Asia: Melbourne.

Kapp MB 1996, Physical restraint use in critical care, legal issues, *American Association of Critical Care Nurses*, 7(4), pp 579–84.

Karlsson S, Bucht G, Eriksson S & Sandman PO 1996, Physical restraints in geriatric care in Sweden: prevalence and patient characteristics, *Journal of the American Geriatrics Society*, 44(11), pp 1348–54.

Koch S 1994, Restraining nursing home residents, *Australian Journal of Advanced Nursing*, 11(2), pp 9–14.

Koch S 2002, *Tension Between Protective Custody and Human Rights*, unpublished doctoral thesis, La Trobe University: Melbourne.

Lee VK & Burnett E 1998, A case report: special needs of hospitalized elders, *Geriatric Nursing*, 19(4), pp 184–91.

Ljunggren G, Phillips CD & Sgadari A 1997, Comparisons of restraint use in nursing homes in eight countries, *Age and Ageing*, 26(S2), pp 43–7.

Lundervold DA, Young L & Jackson TH 1993, Factors influencing nurses' acceptability of treatments for problem behaviors of nursing home residents: initial results, *Clinical Gerontologist*, 12(3), pp 31–40.

McCracken AL 1994, Special care units: meeting the needs of cognitively impaired persons, *Journal of Gerontological Nursing*, 20(4), pp 41–6.

Mason R, O'Connor M & Kemble S 1995, Untying the elderly: response to quality of life issues, *Geriatric Nursing: American Journal of Care for the Aging*, 16(2), pp 68–72.

Miles SH 1996, A case of death by physical restraint: new lessons from a photograph, *Journal of the American Geriatrics Society*, 44(3), pp 291–2.

Miles S H & Irvine P 1992, Deaths caused by physical restraints, *Gerontologist*, 32(6), pp 762–6.

Miles SH & Meyers R 1994, Untying the elderly, *Clinics in Geriatric Medicine*, 10(3), pp 513–25.

Molasiotis A 1995, Use of physical restraints 1: consequences, *British Journal of Nursing*, 4(3), pp 155–7.

Molasiotis A & Newell R 1996, Nurses' Awareness of restraint use with elderly people in Greece and the UK: a cross-cultural pilot study, *International Journal of Nursing Studies*, 33(2), pp 201–11.

Murray J & Cott C 1998, nursing staff perceptions of the use and reduction in the use of physical restraints, *Perspectives*, 22(1), pp 2–10.

Nay R & Closs B 1999, *Recruitment and Retention of Qualified Nursing Staff in Long Term Care of Older People*, La Trobe University: Melbourne.

Nay R & Koch S 1999, La Trobe University, unpublished report for the Commonwealth Department of Health and Aged Care 2000. *A Restraint Free Environment. Barriers to Implementing a Restraint Free Environment in Aged Care Facilities*, Department of Health and Aged Care, Commonwealth of Australia.

Nay R & Pearson A 2001, Educating nurses to protect the past or to advance health care?: a polemic, *Australian Journal of Advanced Nursing*, 18(4), pp 37–41.

Neary MA, Kanski G, Janelli L, Scherer Y & North N 1991, Restraints as nurse's aides see them, *Geriatric Nursing: American Journal of Care for the Aging*, 12(4), pp 191–2.

Newbern VB & Lindsey IH 1994, Attitudes of wives toward having their elderly husbands restrained, *Geriatric Nursing: American Journal of Care for the Aging* 15(3), pp 135–8.

Omnibus Budget Reconciliation Act (US) 1987. In: Manias E (1998), Medication management in residents of aged care facilities, *Contemporary Nurse*, 7(2), pp 53–9.

Parker K & Miles SH 1997, Deaths caused by bedrails, *Journal of the American Geriatrics Society*, 45(7), pp 797–802.

Patterson JE, Strumpf NE & Evans LK 1995, Nursing consultation to reduce restraints in a nursing home, *Clinical Nurse Specialist*, 9(4), pp 231–5.

Retsas AP 1997, The use of physical restraints in Western Australian nursing homes, *Australian Journal of Advanced Nursing*, 14(3), pp 33–9.

Retsas AP & Crabbe H 1997, Use of physical restraints in nursing homes in Queensland, Australia, *Collegian*, 4(4), pp 14–21.

Robinson BE, Sucholeiki R & Schocken DD 1993, Sudden death and resisted mechanical restraint: a case report, *Journal of the American Geriatrics Society*, 41(4), 424–5.

Rovner BW, Steele CD, Shmuely Y & Folstein MF 1996, A randomised trial of dementia care in nursing homes, *Journal of the American Geriatrics Society*, 44(1), pp 7–13.

Schnelle JF & Smith RL 1996, To use physical restraints or not? *Journal of the American Geriatrics Society*, 44(6), pp 727–8.

Schnelle JF, Mac-Rae PG, Simmons SF, Uman G, Ouslander JG, Rosenquist LL & Chang B 1994, Safety assessment for the frail elderly: a comparison of restrained and unrestrained nursing home residents, *Journal of the American Geriatrics Society*, 42(6), pp 586–92.

Sloane PD, Mathew LJ, Scarborough M, Desai JR, Koch GG & Tangen C 1991, Physical and pharmacological restraint of nursing home patients with dementia, *Journal of the American Medical Association*, 265(10), pp 1278–82.

Strathen D 1992, *What if they Hurt Themselves?* Council and Care: London.

Strumpf N 1997, Royal College of Nursing Australia (1997) Conference—Restraint: Exploring the Pathway Between Risks and Rights, Canberra, February 13–14.

Sullivan-Marx EM 1995, Psychological responses to physical restraint use in older adults. *Journal of Psychosocial Nursing and Mental Health Services*, 33(6), pp 205, 401.

Sundel M, Garret RM & Horn RD 1994, restraint reduction in a nursing home and its impact on employee attitudes, *Journal of the American Geriatrics Society*, 42(4), pp 381–7.

Terpstra T, Terpstra TL & Van Doren E 1998, Reducing restraints: where to start, *Journal of Continuing Education in Nursing*, 29(1), pp 10–16.

Woodward M 1998, Physical restraint of older people: a study of Australian practices, *Australasian Journal on Ageing*, 17(4), pp 177–83.

Wunderlich G, Sloan F & Davis C 1996, *Nursing Staff in Hospitals and Nursing Homes—Is it Adequate?* National Academy Press: Washington, DC.

CHAPTER 16

Palliative care

JENNIFER ABBEY

INTRODUCTION

Palliative care for older people has been forced back onto the professional agenda of nurses by the technological revolution in health-care capabilities, increased public awareness of human rights issues, and a gradual change in the concept of well-being. In January 2003 draft guidelines for palliative care in residential aged-care facilities (RACFs) were posted on the Australian Palliative Aged Care (APAC) website (www.apacproject.org). These guidelines were developed by a team in Western Australia following a grant from the federal government to support the production of both an education program on palliative care and guidelines in relation to palliative care for staff working in RACFs. These guidelines and the education that will accompany them will be a major step forward in assisting nurses in the provision of palliative care for the older person. However, the dilemmas and difficulties posed by the introduction of palliative care for a person without a malignancy and/or known time trajectory of death will remain problematic and leave many nurses in a quandary over the right decision to make. This chapter suggests some ways of dealing with those dilemmas by focusing on problem identification, and also upon the issues to be debated, before discussing the introduction of palliative-care plans or pathways for clients in both residential settings and the community. Although there is a growing body of expert practice in this area, and although evidence-based work is developing, sadly there is as yet little evidence on which to base our practice.

WHAT IS PALLIATIVE CARE FOR OLDER PEOPLE?

The modern preoccupations of health care have been the prevention of death and the prolonging of life. There has been great success in extending life expectancy, but many people, and disproportionately those who are socioeconomically disadvantaged, will spend the last years of their longer life suffering from a chronic illness (Fries 2000). The prevalence of dementia is predicted to grow rapidly. By mid-century it is estimated that 580,000 Australians, which will be 2.3% of the population, will have dementia (Access Economics 2003). The commissioning by the federal government of the APAC study and, for example, the introduction of palliative-care legislation in Queensland, are illustrations of recent improvements in acknowledging the need for managed deaths and the preparations this change will require. There is also an increasing volume of literature relating to the particular difficulties of managing a good death for people with dementia (Panke & Volicer 2001; Volicer 2001; Blasi et al 2002; Hurley 2002).

However, for the public, euthanasia is often the only aspect of death and dying that is discussed and debated in the media, distorting the picture for the layperson. Any discussion or reporting of euthanasia tends to polarise opinion and cloud the other dimensions of care of the dying. This polarisation also results in confusion between *palliative care* and *euthanasia* when discussing practical solutions for the provision of palliative care for the older person. Also, palliation involves a kind of decision-making that is unfamiliar to most people. In discussing issues with older people the first point to make clear is that euthanasia is illegal and does not happen in Australia. There may be cases of physician-assisted suicide or voluntary euthanasia, but neither of these has any place in a discussion of palliative care.

The kind of assistance which older people, their family and their friends need will be individualised. All will feel vulnerable and probably confused. Studies still report that older people often feel powerless in the hands of health professionals. As Cameron found:

> The older persons felt conflict about their increasing dependence on health professionals. 'How do you tell a doctor that you think he was wrong?' a woman asked. 'I am afraid of offending him, and I really need him. I don't want him to be cross with me or think I am critical of his care.'
>
> Cameron 2002, p 544

From this it follows that the first set of skills we need to sharpen are those that promote open and easy dialogue about difficult issues. All attention must be on listening, supporting, explaining and assisting towards a plan of care that is recognised and accepted as suitable by the person who is dying, or their legitimate representatives.

DEATH AS A MANAGED PROCESS

Since the introduction of the aged care reforms of 1997–98, aged-care staff have been responsible for documenting and managing the death of those in their care in a systematic, planned fashion. When there is a clear prognosis and understood trajectory towards death—as is often the case with cancer—death can often, perhaps usually, be a straightforward, well-planned and managed process. The sick person will usually be aware of their choices and fully able to make them. Families can interrupt their own lives and rally round the person who is dying, with the communication being of obvious benefit to both parties. However, if death does not come gently and predictably—as is often the case with long-term chronic illnesses such as emphysema and dementia—clients, families, caregivers, doctors and nurses often come face to face with their values, hopes and limitations in a more complex, untidy and stressful process.

It is this confrontation with limitations and choices that underpins a discussion of palliative care for older people. A different framework from that provided by present aged-care routines, or by acute palliative-care service models, is needed—a framework that can be organised, planned and executed mainly by nurses, after due consultation and with the support and collaboration of other health professionals. This will involve an interdisciplinary approach using case conferences that include the client's friends and relatives, education for staff and supportive management structures (Froggatt & Hoult 2001).

The framework around which to build policies for palliative care for older people cannot be provided by mere sentimentality, or by an approach that says 'we do it anyway', without clarification of the issues. Planning for death needs to be a systematic process, with a well-defined purpose and a structure which is contextualised to suit the population in care, the carers themselves and the culture in which this care takes place.

PLANNING FOR LIVING AND PLANNING FOR DYING

Palliative-care principles espouse the same humanitarian approach which has guided health-care reformers for decades. Palliative care is about care, not cure.

The APAC team consider that there are three forms of palliative care for residents of RACFs and that it is important to distinguish between a palliative approach, specialised palliative-care service provision and end-of-life or terminal care.

- *A palliative approach*—this involves care planning, where the active treatment may be continued but consideration of comfort and holistic needs are paramount.

- *Specialised palliative service provision*—care planning benefits from advice from a palliative specialist where there is a need for treatment of complex symptoms or decision-making.

- *End-of-life terminal care*—in this approach, goals are focused on comfort and support for both the resident and their family and friends.

All of the above helpful distinctions can be subsumed in the term 'palliative care' for the purposes of this chapter, although it is acknowledged that palliative care for the older person may involve any one of these approaches at different times.

There has been little work undertaken on indicators that could trigger a move to palliation for the older person, so the nurse's intimate knowledge of the resident and their family is vitally important.

Palliative care planning can begin when an older person with a terminal illness expresses a clear wish not to have intervention that may increase the quantity of their life without increasing quality. The indicators for the introduction of palliative care for those with cognitive impairment are more complex, but the advanced wishes of the patient, and the present concerns of family and friends, are paramount. Covinsky et al (2003) undertook a study to characterise the functional trajectories during the last two years of life of patients with progressive frailty. It was found that for patients with and without cognitive impairment there was a prolonged, steady increase evident at least one year before death. There were no incidents or abrupt decline in function which signalled impending death. This is why a fine judgement, drawn from an intimate knowledge of the patient/resident, is the most important factor in timing the move to palliative care. Clients may make statements such as, 'Please help me die', or 'I'm no use to anyone any more'. It is often easier for carers who find it difficult to handle these questions to brush them aside with cheerful reassurances. But these kinds of comments from clients may arise from depression, or from coping with loss and grief, or they may indeed represent a genuine attempt to open up a dialogue about the process of dying. To differentiate the client's needs takes skill and an intimate relationship (Maynard 2003). We need to hold onto the close knowledge that develops when nurses care for clients every day. This kind of relationship will be needed if someone is wanting to talk about planning their dying. Offering the opportunity to discuss palliative care choices is one way of answering that need. It has been shown that the greatest concern of people is that they will not experience a peaceful, pain-free, dignified death. For example, Coyle & Layman-Goldstein quote one of their patients as saying:

> It is not dying that I'm afraid of—but how to get from A to D (alive to dead)—I don't want to suffer.
>
> Coyle & Layman-Goldstein 2001, p 363

Palliative-care planning cannot begin if the client expresses a clear preference for only curative intervention.

PLANNING PALLIATIVE CARE FOR OLDER PEOPLE

The authors of the draft palliative-care guidelines for RACFs clearly indicate that the interventions needed to address the complexity and number of issues that arise in caring for the older person dying from a non-malignant condition do not lend themselves easily to empirically based studies. This in turn hinders the development of evidence capable of guiding our practice. Nevertheless there is now a small but growing body of literature and expert opinion to assist the practitioner, and it will be imperative that those providing palliative care to the older person keep their knowledge base up to date. The transition from curative to palliative care is a fundamental shift in the most sensitive area of care of the older person, and palliative-care plans/pathways will need to be introduced, applied and documented with great care. These kinds of changes in nursing practice will not be easy to achieve or accept. However, it is time that professional, up-to-date nurse clinicians critically appraised their practice, philosophy and outcomes from the vantage point of what is appropriate for the client perceived as a whole person. Writing palliative-care protocols will take sensitivity, time, debate and caution. Every approach to the question of 'choice' is fraught with traps for the unwary. All planning for palliative care for older people will involve facing the assumptions, perceptions, beliefs and knowledge that make up the new construct of palliative care for older people. Dilemmas will arise during the planning process and the conflicts revealed may well be accompanied by a sense of cognitive dissonance, intellectual disquiet or ethical uncertainty. Since, by definition, a dilemma is 'a situation that requires a choice between options that are, or seem, equally unfavourable' (*American Heritage Dictionary* 1992) it is not surprising that discomfort will result. Choosing the most satisfactory alternative, and reducing the person's distress, will be necessary parts of the whole process.

Recognising the dilemmas of planning

Information from retrospective chart audits for a 12-month period before the death of residents in RACFs identified the most common symptoms during that time to be pain, dyspnoea, noisy breathing, delirium, dysphagia, fever and muscle spasm (Hall et al 2002).

The recognised stages of a terminal condition also involve weight loss, weakness, increasing fluid deficit, reduced peripheral circulation, possible electrolyte imbalance, probable lowering of blood volume and oxygen-carrying capacity, decreased urinary output and diminished skin turgor. The symptoms considered indicative of a 'terminal syndrome' by the APAC team include:

- requiring frequent intervention;
- being bed-bound;
- loss of appetite;
- profound weakness;
- trouble swallowing;
- dry mouth;
- weight loss;
- becoming semi-conscious with lapses into unconsciousness; and
- experiencing day-to-day deterioration that is not reversible (APAC Project 2003).

Many of these signs appear gradually in the older person, and skill is needed in determining whether such conditions as skin breakdown are a normal part of ageing or the beginning of terminal decline. In his study of older people, Fisher (2002) found that studies investigating the signs and symptoms of impending death and its recognition are few.

This puts much onus on the nurse to clearly record signs and symptoms of terminal decline. A palliative-care protocol needs to be based on the documentation and detailed assessment of these signs. Then the protocol can contain plans for managing expected critical events and for ongoing care. Some suggestions that could be important areas for consideration and planning follow.

General practitioners' visits

Without direction and documentation, there is a risk that nurses will not be sure whether they are to seek curative or relief measures when consulting with the client's GP. Reasons for nurses calling GPs to visit residents/clients include assistance in managing what is often loosely classified as the resident/patient being unwell, agitation, shortness of breath, or the results of a fall. In many cases, if relief rather than cure of suffering was the aim of the consultation, skilled nursing intervention may well have produced more comfort than could have been achieved by an ad hoc decision to request a visit from the GP.

Whether or not a GP is called often depends on the personality, clinical competence and religious or personal beliefs of the nurse on duty at the time (Abbey 1995). The outcome of the consultation depends on the same attributes in the GP (Hinkka et al 2002). Many decisions depend on the relationship among nurses, the client and the family rather than on the specific nature of the medical problem (Norberg et al 1994). Other variables which influence decisions—but which are often not recognised by those involved—have to do with the degree of congruence of the cultures of the family and the residential facility. In Cohen-Mansfield's study investigating medical decisions for troubled breathing in terminally ill nursing home residents, it was found that there was family involvement in only 45% of cases (Cohen-Mansfield 2002). It is therefore imperative for staff to fully realise the responsibility they carry for the 55% of patients/residents for whom they will possibly be the only advocate. Exposing and working through values to ensure constructive communication within an interdisciplinary team will be needed to reach mutually acceptable arrangements about clients' care. Once this has occurred, an agreed protocol for ongoing treatment, including agreed indicators of when a doctor's visit will be necessary, can be documented.

Use of analgesia

Paradoxically, despite having requested visits from clients' GPs and seeking medical solutions, nurses can often be reluctant to give prescribed medications in the recommended doses—including even analgesia—if the nurse(s) on duty at the time feel that the effect will cause the client to become less aware of their surroundings. The analgesia received by a client is too often dependent on a particular nurse's interpretation of the language of the ill person. Since pain and distress can often be interpreted only through body language, facial expression, screams or whimpers, judgements are often based on the observer's values and guesswork. It is not uncommon for treatment patterns to vary significantly across nursing shifts as a result of differences in these individual judgements and beliefs. Reports of under-treatment of pain for older people, especially those with cognitive impairment, have been numerous and spread over many years (Craig & Prkachin 1983; Ferrell et al 1990; Marzinski 1991; Huffman & Kunik 2000). Sadly, the present literature is reporting the same findings (Manfredi et al 2003; Amella 2003). Standardised techniques of pain assessment, regular timed doses of analgesics, and alternative therapies can all be considered in developing any palliative-care protocol. Pain assessment instruments help to systematise and eliminate some of the nurse's difficulties in deciding when and what form of pain relief is needed (Abbey 2003). The treatment of pain is an area in which providers will need to be increasingly vigilant. The extent of the provider's accountability for inadequate treatment of pain was illustrated recently by the guilty verdict handed down by a Californian court to a doctor judged not to have provided adequate pain relief to an 85-year-old dying man (Compassion in Dying Federation n.d.). Frank-Stromberg & Christensen make the point that in the past:

> the administration of excessive pain medications could lead to sanctions and even criminal penalties for nurses. Now nurses who administer inadequate pain medication can be investigated and disciplined as well.
>
> Frank-Stromberg & Christensen 2001, p 236

Treatment of infections

It has been shown that:

> aggressive medical treatment of infections does not affect the progressive course of dementia ... and has a limited effect on mortality rates.
>
> Hurley et al 1993, p 21

The comfort of the client may be far better served by administration of oxygen, sedation and narcotics. For example, in one study it is stated that the use of systemic antibiotics for patients with end-stage dementia may be contrary to good clinical practice (Evers et al 2002). Another critiques the high use of intravenous antibiotics and the large number of patients who were still receiving antibiotics at the time of death (Oneschuk et al 2002).

An additional consideration may be whether the routine administration of antibiotics contributes to the increase of resistant bacteria. Institutionalised residents have been described as 'biological amplifiers' of resistant strains of bacteria, bringing these with them when admitted into acute-care facilities (Gaynes et al 1985). These resistant strains can be carried into the community by staff and visitors. Concern is growing worldwide about the potentially devastating consequences of this resistance.

Any protocol of palliative care will require considered and documented decisions about the use of antibiotics most commonly used for chest or urinary tract infections. If antibiotics are not to be used, alternative comfort measures, such as the use of aspirin or regular sponging, can be planned.

Mobilisation and body maintenance

The practice of getting people out of bed, showering them and dressing them in day clothes has become the bedrock of care in most residential aged-care facilities. But is this practice directed at comfort and relief of suffering? The question cannot be avoided by reliance on custom and received wisdom. Getting clients out of bed helps to prevent pneumonia, reduce contractures, prevent pressure sores and—importantly—provide a sense of attentive caring for both staff and relatives. It is accepted orthodoxy that this normal procedure of 'getting up' during the day contributes to the valuing of the client as a person. These benefits are not without merit, but securing them may also contribute significantly to the client's distress.

Does the continuation of procedures such as these really show a valuing of the person as they are; or does it too often demonstrate an inability to calmly consider any alternatives? These clients are dying, but getting them up and dressed each day is treating them as if they are not. It is not unrealistic to ask whether the client is the principal beneficiary of such treatment, or merely the object of it. When palliation principles are applied, the routines of normal day-to-day life are replaced by routines that promote a dignified and comfortable death.

Supply of food and fluids

The possible withdrawal (or reduction) of food and fluids questions accepted nursing practice in a fundamental and most difficult way. Nourishing is basic to nursing and caring. The arguments about provision of food and fluid when a person is in the terminal stages of their illness, and indicating that they do not want or are not able to tolerate nutrition easily, range from one end of the spectrum to another. Hildebrand puts forward one point of view:

> When provision of food and water does not create excessive burdens (such as extreme pain and discomfort), and if the food and water can be digested and absorbed, denying such nourishment is immoral and unethical. Under these circumstances, this denial (by

commission or omission) is motivated by a real intention to cause death, whether or not that intention is explicitly recognized.

Hildebrand 2000

Ashby & Mendelson do not agree:

It is a normal part of the dying process for there to be a gradual reduction, and eventual cessation of oral intake. ... Clinical experience shows no basis for believing that patients receiving palliative care are experiencing symptoms of starvation and dehydration, which would be lessened or abolished by the routine provision by medical means of hydration and nutrition.

Ashby & Mendelson 2003, p 264

Young (2002) indicates that the introduction of an artificial means of feeding is increasing and in some cases becoming a routine procedure for people with dementia. She sets out ethical arguments for and against prolonging the supply of nutrition and hydration but is clear about the lack of evidence to show that artificial feeding is a benefit to the patient.

Convention and instinct tell us that feeding is synonymous with the act of healing. However, it is arguable that feeding a client who, for example, has advanced dementia, is equivalent to keeping a person alive on a life-support machine. There is a fine line between deliberately withdrawing food and water, and being neglectful to the extent that the person suffers from hunger and thirst. Eating has an important symbolic place in our lives, but many people reject food as they approach death, and that may be a message we should hear—a 'decision' we should respect.

The effects of fasting can produce a sense of euphoria. Hunger ceases (Keenan 1992; Mandela 1994). Dehydration in the terminally ill can have positive effects:

- Pulmonary secretions decrease and there is less coughing and shortness of breath.
- Nausea, vomiting and abdominal pain are all reduced.
- Urinary output decreases, resulting in fewer linen changes, and therefore less disturbance for the client (McAulay 2001).

The client may suffer from a dry mouth, which can be treated with mouth care or by giving ice chips to suck. The person may sometimes suffer from electrolyte imbalances, which can lead to muscle spasms and an altered level of consciousness. If the effects of electrolyte imbalance are causing unnecessary suffering, rehydration may be needed. Alternatively, the person can be treated palliatively with antispasmodics or sedation.

PALLIATIVE CARE FOR RESIDENTS SUFFERING FROM DEMENTIA

Where these approaches are most difficult in practice is in illnesses such as Alzheimer's disease (AD). Although there are now some treatments for AD, a cure is not possible (Lahiri et al 2000; Kmietowicz 2001; Luine et al 2002; O'Neil 2002; Walker & Perks 2002). When people are aware that they have an incurable cancer they may or may not choose such intervention as palliative radiation. They may instead choose only relief of pain and suffering as palliation. Alzheimer's disease does not 'kill' in the orderly, easily measured and well-researched way that cancer does.

However, this semantic distinction unduly privileges a specific approach to health care and, from a holistic perspective and nursing perspective, hinders understanding. Cancer cells cause organs to stop functioning, but so too do the plaques and tangles of AD and the thromboses of multi-infarct dementias. The plaques and tangles of AD invade the brain with consequences as damaging as invasive cancer cells, but in a much slower and more insidious form. They do not of themselves 'kill'. They do not affect the mechanical apparatus that keeps the heart pumping and the lungs exchanging oxygen. It is other complications of the disease process, such as immobility, or the iatrogenic consequences of institutionalisation, that result in the physical, as distinct from the spiritual, death of people with dementia.

Although the use of advance directives/living wills is important for all the population, it is especially important for people diagnosed with dementia.

Early diagnosis and assessment of dementia provides an opportunity for primary health-care workers, the persons with dementia and their caregivers to collaborate in setting goals and making decisions regarding care. One of the major issues that needs to be addressed at this stage is the option of documenting an enduring power of attorney, not just for financial affairs but for health-care decisions as well. New generic documentation planned for residential care facilities (Department of Health and Ageing 2002) and for community services (Owen & Eagar 2003) includes details to be recorded about advance directives. However, many older people do not have close family near them to act as advocates or do not feel confident to sign these forms. The responsibility of decisions relating to palliative care is then left to the health professionals, and the issues are often blurry and complex. Hurley's advice is that health-care workers should:

> assist patients with AD and their loved ones through the terminal phases of the illness by preparing them for the relentless progression of the disease and by supporting them through the intellectual and emotional conflicts accompanying the end of life.
>
> Hurley 2002, pp 23–24

All members of the interdisciplinary team need to be educated and aware of the need for this preparation. We know the progression of the diseases such as Alzheimer's, in much the same way that we know about cancer, but death will be slower and accompanied by much difficulty. It is fair that we supply everyone involved with information about the process of death, and encourage choices to be documented while capacity is still present.

THE REALITIES OF CHOICE

In recent times, government policy has moved to a 'user-pays' health system, indicative of its widely supported maxim that individual choice is an important moral focus in modern Australian society. However, political economy repeatedly reminds us that the individual's choice is limited by socioeconomic factors, access to public goods and services, and the culture which structures the environment. Restriction of choice by any or all of these factors may limit the older person's control over their destiny. Providing opportunities for collaborative planning of nursing care—before death approaches—empowers older people. There are many examples of living wills, advance directives, and life-value statements to assist people to document their wishes, and to experience the 'good death' for which they hope. Most States now have a *pro forma* where these wishes can be recorded. Information about advance directives can be accessed at:

- http://www.medicineau.net.au/clinical/palliativecare/palliativec1256.html (Medicine Australia 2003); and

- http://www.mja.com.au/public/issues/172_11_050600/biegler/biegler.html (Biegler et al 2000).

At the moment, the use of living wills and the documentation of advanced wishes is rare, although a 'good death' is sometimes produced by understanding those wishes through the process of intimacy and knowledge developed over time in the caring relationship.

The following vignette tells about a well-managed death, where a palliative-care nurse consultant and a sympathetic and involved GP contributed to assisting the older person to get her needs met. Increasingly, this is the kind of management choice that needs to be offered to those who conclude that their life is becoming intolerable.

VIGNETTE

The value of care planning

Karen Glaetzer

Emilia was an 86-year-old divorced woman from the Ukraine. Her only son lived in America and she had no other surviving relatives. She had been a resident in a low-level residential aged-care facility for the past five years. Her GP noted a neck mass on a routine visit and she was transferred to a public hospital for further investigation. A CT scan was performed, and showed an extensive infiltrating mass, originating from the thyroid. A biopsy confirmed a high-grade non-Hodgkin's lymphoma. Surgery was excluded as a treatment option, due to the mass being adjacent to the carotid artery. Emilia was offered chemotherapy and/or radiotherapy, but declined treatment when the expected side-effects were explained. She requested to be transferred back 'home' to her aged-care facility. Prior to hospital discharge, she was reviewed by the palliative-care consulting team and a referral was made to the regional palliative-care service. This is when I first became involved in Emilia's care.

I arranged to visit her at the low-care facility. At my initial consultation I found a frail elderly lady who was well adjusted to her cancer diagnosis. She spoke openly about her life, the good and the bad times. Her one request was that she be allowed to die without pain in her own bed. Her current symptoms included weakness, anorexia and mild stridor as a result of the enlarging neck mass. I suggested we arrange a case conference with her GP and facility staff, so a plan of care for future management could be documented. The facility supported 'ageing-in-place' so her request to die in her own bed was possible. The main concern was the issue of respiratory compromise, due to the possibility of the neck mass causing airway obstruction. A care plan was drawn up with clear guidelines and sufficient medication orders to manage episodes of acute respiratory distress, if they occurred. The staff were encouraged to approach the situation confidently and calmly and the GP offered her home phone number if needed outside normal working hours. The after-hours number for the palliative-care service was also provided.

Emilia's general condition continued to deteriorate over the next week. Her respiratory status was becoming increasingly compromised. A small dose of subcutaneous morphine (2.5 mg) was administered via an intima catheter four-hourly, to ease her respiratory distress. The staff spent as much time as possible sitting with her and providing personal care as needed. On the day before her death, it was decided that a respite nurse would be arranged overnight, funded by The Cancer Council, to ensure that she did not die alone. Emilia died peacefully in her own bed, as she had requested.

Planning a good death

The fact that each of us is a unique individual means that the nature of death may be very different for each person. In many cases, managing a good death is fraught by clashes of values, differences of professional opinion and opposing demands from relatives and clients. These all contribute to tension, frustration, low work productivity and low morale in some facilities. Planning and documentation can reduce these difficulties. The *Guidelines for Good Palliative Care Orders* (Maddocks et al 1997) is a useful document to assist in this process. Research shows that people do want to have their end-of-life wishes honoured, and that the use of advance directives/living wills is increasing (Cartwright 1995).

Organisational philosophy and values clarification

The first step in coping with the issues of rights and choices is to undertake a values-clarification exercise. Staff may not be able to cope with the dilemmas posed by the changes in practices involved in the introduction of palliative care—or be able to act on documentation setting out palliative-care protocols—until processes and procedures have been raised, discussed and clarified.

Tackling the difficulties of day-to-day care through values clarification may sound like an academic and tangential exercise, but the process involves much more than injunctions to allow people a choice as long as it does not cause harm to anyone else (Conley 2001). Wisdom is needed to understand the personal torment of another. Wisdom rests on having the opportunity, skills and encouragement to reflect on the experience of oneself and others.

Before staff can undertake values clarification to assist them in transforming their experience into understanding, the philosophy of the employing organisation within which their action is to be taken will need to be clearly set out. Staff will need education and practice in working out their own value position *vis-a-vis* their work responsibilities. In some organisations, the philosophy of care of the dying may be clearly spelt out by the cultural or religious group of clients catered for in that environment. Staff will have contracted to work within that framework and will have to clarify their value position within the expected care protocols. At the other end of the spectrum are organisations where clear moral frameworks may have to be created out of an inchoate jumble of implicit assumptions and habit. Without an agreed moral structure, different practices will emerge which, because of their inconsistency, can cause unnecessary suffering for the client. Once a values-clarification process has laid comfortable foundations for the implementation of a palliative-care proto-col, education about handling the care of the dying can commence.

DOCUMENTATION FOR END-STAGE CARE

As stated previously, The National Model Care Documentation system for Residential Aged Care, which is at present in draft form, and the community care documentation, which is presently being trialled, will set the guidelines for comprehensive documentation in the near future. However, some areas that may need particular attention in the case of palliative care are as follows.

ASSESSMENT AND GOALS

Outcome: a dignified, pain-free death.

Pain

Goal: To control the pain to a level nominated by the client (identify a pain level as per a score on a pain scale).

Description: (client's own words) Aggravating factors, relieving factors, interference with ADLs, response to current therapies, associated symptoms (nausea, anxiety, dyspnoea). Monitor condition for deterioration, inability to perform ADLs, sleep deprivation (non-verbal signs). Other (specify).

Respiratory

Dyspnoea

Goal: To relieve the dyspnoea without adding other problems.

Cough

Goal: To relieve stress related to the cough. Type: dry and non-productive, wet and productive, wet and non-productive. Monitor for difficulty with breathing.

Respiratory secretions (terminal phase)

Goal: To provide reassurance to family and carers. To ensure client's breathing is not made difficult.

Weakness/Fatigue

Goal: To minimise levels of weakness and fatigue. Provide comfort as weakness and fatigue increase.

Skin integrity

Wound management

Goal: To identify and implement a realistic treatment option. Palliative care of wounds rather than attempting to cure.

Prevention

Goal: To prevent pressure area development. Assess for risk of pressure area development. Balance the need for prevention of pressure area development with need for comfort.

Culture, religion/spirituality

Goal: To understand and respect individual's background. To identify any religious, spiritual or cultural needs.

Sexuality, body image

Goal: To identify any sexual needs. Identify any specific cultural, religious or spiritual needs (specify).

Be aware that any unresolved issue may heighten other symptoms such as pain and anxiety.

Oral hygiene

Goal: To maintain the integrity of the mucous membrane (mouth: thrush, dryness, stomatitis, taste impairment, halitosis, denture problems). To relieve dry mouth due to cessation of food and fluids.

Nausea and vomiting

Goal: To minimise nausea and vomiting. Identify vomiting mechanism(s).

Nutrition

Goal: To monitor nutritional intake and provide only what is tolerated comfortably. Monitor tolerance to various food items. Monitor appetite levels. Provide comfort for weakness arising from anorexia, decreased fluid/food intake.

Constipation/elimination/continence

Goal: To monitor bladder and bowel function. To prevent constipation. To prevent or control incontinence.

Emotional state/anxiety

Goal: To control anxiety levels. To ensure that family, friends and patient have information and a chance to express their wishes and needs.

Depression

Goal: To monitor for signs of depression and refer appropriately. Watch for signs of worthlessness, hopelessness, guilt or suicidal ideation. Other (specify).

Dementia

Goal: To provide a safe environment, comfort and dignity. Ensure there are enough opportunities for family and friends to be involved in care. Ensure advocacy if no supports available.

Carer strain

Goal: To relieve high levels of carer strain. Identify whether any social supports are required for carer. Determine current health status of carer. Consider any special needs the carer may have.

Adapted from Department of Veterans' Affairs 2000

Apart from assessment and refining the goals for the client, case conferencing will be imperative. Many residential and community organisations undertake case conferences, but keeping a record of what is said, and especially what is decided, within these case conferences is often not handled well.

The case conference structure is as important to the introduction of palliative-care protocols as the process of assessment set out above, values clarification, the education of staff and an understanding of how to manage the different paradigm of care. Changes to Medicare refunds and the introduction of new Enhanced Primary Care Medicare Benefit Schedule (EPC MBS) items have made it possible to assist GPs in their role in case conferencing. The Department of Health and Ageing reports that:

> The aim of these new EPC MBS items is to strengthen the role of general practitioners in residential aged care services through integration and linkages with other primary health providers, and deliver improved health for residents.

> The delivery of quality care in residential care needs to be a partnership between providers, families, the Government and professionals, such as GPs. These new Medicare items will encourage GPs to involve themselves more fully in the delivery of care in residential aged care services.

> GPs are now able to contribute to a multidisciplinary care plan for a care recipient in a residential aged care facility …

> As with the corresponding EPC MBS items in the community setting, this item is available to residents with a chronic medical condition and multidisciplinary care needs. (A chronic condition is defined as a medical condition that has been, or is expected to be, present for 6 months or longer, or that is terminal.)

> The GP's involvement in care planning for a person receiving care in a residential aged care facility must be at the request of the facility in question. The contribution made by the GP should be documented in the multidisciplinary care plan maintained by the RACF, and recorded in the resident's medical record. GPs are not able to organise a multidisciplinary care plan for people receiving care in a residential aged care facility, as care plans are already required to be prepared by the facility.

> GPs are also now able to organise and coordinate, or participate in, multidisciplinary case conferences for people receiving care in all residential aged care facilities. These items, similar to those practised in the community setting, are available to residents with a chronic condition and multiple care needs. The items are time-tiered, ranging from case conferences lasting at least 15 minutes to conferences lasting at least 45 minutes. The GP must give a record of the conference (or a record of his/her participation in the conference) to the residential aged care facility, place a copy in the resident's medical records and offer a copy to the resident.

> Department of Health and Ageing 2000

It is essential that information from the case conference be transferred to the nursing care plan. Decisions made at the conference will need to be spelt out in nursing actions in a clear manner. The comfort of the patient depends on consistency. The need for well managed interdisciplinary case management is well proven (Sowell & Meadows 1994; Smyth et al 2001; Shannon 2002).

CONCLUSION

The patterns of social change discussed above, and new moral assumptions about the importance of choice for palliative care for older people, are well advanced. The wishes of those who do not want to suffer, who do not want their life prolonged if they are suffering from a debilitating terminal illness, cannot be left unmanaged. Relatives will increasingly demand that they not be left unmanaged. Best practice in modern aged care means offering a choice of a 'managed death' which is dignified and personalised. Organisation of this task will be the most important role for gerontic nurses in the next decade.

References

Abbey J 1995, *Death and Late-Stage Dementia in Institutions: A Cultural Analysis*, unpublished PhD thesis, Deakin University: Victoria.

Abbey J 2003, Ageing, dementia and palliative care, In: Aranda S & O'Connor M (eds), *Palliative Care Nursing—A Guide to Practice* (2nd edn), Ausmed: Melbourne.

Access Economics 2003, The dementia epidemic: economic impact and positive solutions for Australia, March, Canberra.

Amella EJ 2003, Geriatrics and palliative care, *Journal of Hospice & Palliative Nursing*, 5, p 40.

APAC Project 2003, *Palliative Care Guidelines for Residential Aged Care Facilities*, draft, 13 January 2003, funded by The Commonwealth Department of Health and Ageing.

Ashby M & Mendelson D 2003, Natural death in 2003: Are we slipping backwards? *Journal of Law and Medicine*, 10, pp 260–4.

Biegler P, Stewart C, Savulescu J & Skene L 2000, Determining the validity of advance directives, *Medical Journal of Australia*, 172, pp 545–8.

Blasi Z H, Hurley AC, & Volicer L 2002, End-of-life care in dementia: a review of problems, prospects, and solutions in practice, *Journal of the American Medical Directors Association*, 3(2), pp 57–65.

Cartwright CS 1995, Decision-making in terminal care: older people seek more involvement, *Social Alternatives*, 14, p 7.

Cameron ME 2002, Older persons' ethical problems involving their health, *Nursing Ethics*, 9(5), pp 537–51.

Cohen-Mansfield JL 2002, Medical decisions for troubled breathing in nursing home residents, *International Journal of Nursing Studies*, 39(5), pp 557–61.

Compassion in Dying Federation (n.d.), Tomlinson Case Summary. Online: http://www.compassionindying.org/tomlinson/casesummary.php, accessed 12 January 2004.

Conley V 2001, *The Role of Values in Caregiver Information-seeking Behavior*, doctoral dissertation, University of South Florida, p 170.

Covinsky KE, Eng C, Lui LY, Sands LP & Yaffe K 2003, The last two years of life: functional trajectories of frail older people, *Journal of the American Geriatrics Society*, 51(4), pp 492–8.

Coyle N & Layman-Goldstein M 2001, Pain assessment and management in palliative care. In: Matzo ML & Sherman DW (eds), *Palliative Care Nursing*, Springer: New York, pp 362–486.

Craig K & Prkachin K 1983, Nonverbal measures of pain. In: Melzack R (ed), *Pain Measurement and Assessment*, Raven Press: New York.

Department of Health and Ageing 2000, Primary Care Initiatives, Enhanced Primary Care Package. Fact Sheet: Changes to the Federal Government's Enhanced Primary MBS items. New MBS Items. Online: www.health.gov.au/hsdd/primcare/enhancpr/mbsitems.htm, accessed 2 November 2003.

Department of Health and Ageing, Aged Care Division 2002, Draft National Model Care Documentation Systems for Residential Aged Care. Online: http://www.health.gov.au/acc/reports/modeldoc.htm

Department of Veterans' Affairs 2000, Palliative Care Clinical Pathway. Online: http://www.dva.gov.au/health/provider/community%20nursing/pathways/pallcare.htm

Evers M, Dushyant P, Daniel K, Khalid M & Deborah B 2002, Palliative and aggressive end-of-life care for patients with dementia. *Psychiatric Services* (American Psychiatric Association) 53(5), pp 609–13.

Ferell BA, Ferrell BR & Osterweil D 1990, Pain in the nursing home, *Journal of the American Geriatrics Society*, 38, pp 409–14.

Fisher RJ 2002, End-of-life care for seniors: public and professional awareness, *Educational Gerontology*, 28, p 353.

Frank-Stromberg M & Christensen A 2001, A serious look at the undertreatment of pain, *Clinical Journal of Oncology Nursing*, 5(5), pp 235–6.

Fries JF 2000, Compression of morbidity in the elderly, *Vaccine*, 18(16), pp 1584–9.

Froggatt K & Hoult L 2002, The provision of palliative care in nursing homes and residential care homes: a survey of clinical nurse specialist work. *Palliative Medicine*, 16(6), pp 481–7.

Gaynes R, Weinstein R, Chamberlain W & Kabins S 1985, Antibiotic-resistant flora in nursing-home patients admitted to the hospital, *Archives of Internal Medicine*, 145, pp 1804–7.

Hall PS, Schroder C & Weaver L 2002, The last 48 hours of life in long-term care: a focused chart audit, *Journal of the American Geriatrics Society*, 50(3), pp 501–6.

Hildebrand AJ 2000, Masked intentions: the masquerade of killing thoughts used to justify dehydrating and starving people in a 'persistent vegetative state' and people with other profound neurological impairments, *Issues in Law and Medicine*, 16(2), pp 143–65.

Hinkka HK, Kosunen E, Metsänoja R, Lammi UK & Kellokumpu-Lehtinen P 2002, Factors affecting physicians' decisions to forgo life-sustaining treatments in terminal care, *Journal of Medical Ethics*, 28(2), pp 109–14.

Huffman J & Kunik M 2000, Assessment and understanding of pain in patients with dementia. *The Gerontologist*, 49(5), pp 574–81.

Hurley AC 2002, Alzheimer disease: 'It's okay, Mama, if you want to go, it's okay', *Journal of the American Medical Association*, 288, p 2324.

Hurley A, Volicer B, Mahoney M & Volicer L 1993, Palliative fever management in Alzheimer patients: quality plus fiscal responsibility, *Advances in Nursing Science*, 16(1), pp 21–32.

Keenan B 1992, *An Evil Cradling*, Vintage: London.

Kmietowicz Z 2001, NICE approves drugs for Alzheimer's Disease, *British Medical Journal*, 322, p 190.

Lahiri DK, Farlow MR, Hintz N, Utsuki T & Greig NH 2000, Cholinesterase inhibitors, ß-amyloid precursor protein and amyloid ß-peptides in Alzheimer's Disease, *Acta Neurologica Scandinavica*, 176(Suppl), pp 60–7.

Luine VN, Mohan G, Tu Z & Efange SM 2002, Chromaproline and chromaperidine, nicotine agonists, and donepezil, cholinesterase inhibitor, enhance performance of memory tasks in ovariectomized rats, *Pharmacology, Biochemistry and Behavior*, 74(1), pp 213–20.

Maddocks I, Abbey J, Beck K, Debellis A, Glaetzer K, McLeod A, Parker D & Pickhaver A 1997, *Palliative Care in Nursing Homes*, Educational Resource Package, Palliative Care Unit, The Flinders University of South Australia: Adelaide.

Mandela N 1994, *Long Walk to Freedom*, Abacus: London.

Manfredi P, Breuer B, Meier D & Libow L 2003, Pain assessment in elderly patients with severe dementia. *Journal of Pain and Symptom Management,* 25(1), pp 48–52.

Marzinski L 1991, The tragedy of dementia: clinically assessing pain in the confused, nonverbal elderly, *Journal of Gerontological Nursing*, 17, pp 25–8.

Maynard C 2003, Differentiate depression from dementia, *Nurse Practitioner: American Journal of Primary Health Care*, 28(3), p 18.

Medicine Australia 2003, Palliative Care and Advance Directives. Online: http://www.medicineau.net.au/clinical/palliativecare/palliativec1256.html

Norberg A, Hirschsfeld M, Davidson B, Davis A, Lauri S, Lin JY, Phillips L, Pittman E, Vander Laan R & Ziv L 1994, Ethical reasoning concerning the feeding of severely demented patients: an international perspective, *Nursing Ethics*, 1(1), pp 3–13.

O'Neil J 2002, Testing medicine and memory, *New York Times*, 151, F7.

Oneschuk D, Fainsinger R & Demoissac D 2002, Antibiotic use in the last week of life in three different palliative care settings, *Journal of Palliative Care*, 18(1), pp 25–8.

Owen Q & Eagar K 2003, *Ongoing Needs Identification in Queensland Community Care: How and Why*, Centre for Health Service Development, University of Wollongong, Queensland Health, Brisbane.

Panke J & Volicer L 2001, Caring for persons with dementia: a palliative approach, *Journal of Hospice and Palliative Nursing*, 4, p 143.

Shannon E 2002, The devil is in the detail: lessons for multi-disciplinary care teams from a local evaluation of coordinated care, *Australian Health Review*, 25(2), pp 87–94.

Smyth C, Dubbins S, Restrepo A, Nueva-Espana H & Capezuti E 2001, Creating order out of chaos: models of GNP practice with hospitalized older adults, *Clinical Excellence for Nurse Practitioners*, 5(2), pp 88–95.

Sowell RL & Meadows TM 1994, An integrated case management model: developing standards, evaluation, and outcome criteria, *Nursing Administration Quarterly*, 18(2), pp 53–64.

Volicer L 2001, Care at the end of life, *Alzheimer's Care Quarterly*, 2(3), pp 59–66.

Walker C & Perks D 2002, Do you know about donepezil and succinylcholine? *Anaesthesia*, 57(10), p 1041.

Young J 2002, Artificial nutrition in older people with dementia: moral and ethical dilemmas, *Nursing Older People*, 14, p 19.

CHAPTER 17

Sexuality and older people

RHONDA NAY

INTRODUCTION

An older lady with dementia—let's call her Mrs Jackson—was a resident in a long-term care facility. She had a regular male visitor who had been her 'boyfriend' many years before. Staff were certain that his visits involved sexual activity but as Mrs Jackson was very capable of indicating robustly when she was unhappy and she always seemed delighted and relaxed after his visits, they did not interfere. On one occasion her son, who had not been seen for a very long time, 'caught' the older couple in the act. He was furious and advised staff that this man was never to visit his mother again. Staff did his bidding and banned the old man. After that, Mrs Jackson had no visitors—her 'boyfriend' was not allowed to visit and her son didn't bother. Whose interests were served? Did the son have the right to vet his mother's activities in this way? Did staff do the right thing in respecting his wishes and apparently ignoring the wishes of Mrs Jackson?

These types of situations challenge staff not infrequently but there is little by way of guidance to them in how they might resolve such dilemmas. Sexuality and older people largely remain mutually exclusive topics. This chapter is one attempt to bring sexuality out in the open, dispel some of the myths and at least generate debate on the sexual rights of older people.

DEFINING SEXUALITY

The World Health Organization (WHO) defines sexuality as:

> the integration of the romantic, emotional, intellectual and social aspects of sexual beings in ways that are positively enriching and that enhance personality, communication and love.
>
> WHO, cited in Woods 1984, p 117

This definition is fairly limited and ignores the social construction of sexuality and the use of sexuality to dominate, control, manipulate, cause pain and humiliation, and so on. In previous work I have defined sexuality as:

> referring to the socially constructed roles, behaviours, identities and processes—prescribed and prohibited, enacted and avoided, admitted and denied, valued and devalued, relational and non-relational—associated with female and male eroticism, reproduction, sex acts, thoughts, feelings, beliefs and attitudes. It refers specifically to those aspects of sensual, psychosocial and physical stimuli and responses associated with the pleasures and pains, fulfilments and humiliations of the person in the name of sex. It is broader than, but includes, the acts of sex and being female or male.
>
> Nay 1993, p 199

In a small Melbourne study (Nay et al 1997) the following definitions of sexuality emerged from the older residents of a long-term facility:

- looking nice;
- spending time with the opposite sex;
- being able to cuddle up in bed with a partner through masturbation; and
- intercourse with a long-time partner and relieving one's frustrations with a sex worker.

In terms of what they associated with feeling and acting sexual, the following were identified:

- getting dressed up and feeling pampered;
- being complimented was still important;
- spending time in mixed-sex groups;
- looking one's best;
- enjoying sexually stimulating/explicit media—magazines, TV, videos;
- talking 'dirty';
- going to bed with a partner and cuddling;
- kissing and 'having sex'; and
- masturbating and being with a sex worker.

Over the years in lectures on this topic I have asked hundreds of students, from school-leavers to mature-age, to identify how they define sexuality and what makes them feel and act sexual. Invariably their responses are consistent with what these older residents said.

For the purposes of this chapter, references to sexuality exclude any form of abuse of rights. Like all ethical dilemmas, it is not always easy to determine if or when this is occurring; but recognising the significance of sexuality and at least beginning to discuss the issues will reduce the likelihood of abuse that may be more subtle but is pervasive in a world of ignorance and taboo.

SEXUALITY AND IDENTITY

Sexuality is described in the literature as central to identity (Ansuini et al 1996). Caplan asserted that:

> in modern western society, one's sexual orientation is a very important part of one's identity, [and] people are encouraged to see themselves in terms of their sexuality which is interpreted as the core of the self [whereby] through sexual liberation comes personal liberation.

Caplan 1987, p 6

Further, Weeks argued that:

> through our sex we are expected to find ourselves and our place in the world. Through it we experience ourselves as real people; it gives us our identities, our sense of self, men and

women, as heterosexual and homosexual … Sex has become, as … Foucault famously put it, 'the truth of our being'.

Weeks 1986, p 13

And, more recently, Pangman & Seguire note that:

In the literature sexuality has been described as one of the most natural and basic aspects of life that affects an individual's identity as a human being. Sexuality provides the opportunity to express affection, admiration, and affirmation of one's body and its functioning. It not only encompasses the whole individual, but it serves as a reference frame in relation to others. In addition, sexual health is an essential component of overall wellness during one's developmental lifespan.

Pangman & Seguire 2000, p 49

Despite the recognition that sexuality is central to identity and essential to well-being, it has been, and continues to be, assumed by many that sexuality is the preserve of the young, and that older people are asexual. Ask almost anyone if their parents still 'have sex' and the response is a unanimous look of disbelief, if not disgust.

SEXUALITY, OLDER PEOPLE, IMAGE AND ATTITUDES

In general, although sex has been talked about, glamourised and publicised, this has occurred on a superficial level. Sex is still a subject which parents find difficult to discuss with their children, which health professionals avoid with their clients, and about which many individuals have little informed knowledge (Booth 1990; Foucault 1976; Nay 1993; Satran 1986). Kaplan (1996), among others, has written of the negative attitudes towards the sexuality of the elderly. These range from disbelief (that the aged could have sex), to ridicule or outright disgust. Butler & Lewis (1982) identified five common attitudes:

- Elderly people do not have sexual desires.
- They are not able to make love even if they wanted to.
- They are too fragile and might hurt themselves if they attempted to engage in sexual relations.
- They are physically unattractive and therefore sexually undesirable.
- The whole notion of older people engaging in sex is shameful and perverse.

These attitudes are reflected in or led by the media. In a study of the sexuality of older people in films, Bildtgard (2000) studied all feature films released in Sweden between 1990 and 1995. Of the 2000 films, only nine had older people in starring roles. He searched these to discover what rules governed representations of older people and sexuality. He found the following:

- Sexual relationships have to be affectionate.
- Elderly people who are sexually active have to be 'well preserved'.
- Elderly people who are sexually active have to be lively.
- Elderly people who are sexually active have to conform to gendered expectations.

- Sexually active elderly people have to be single.

(Bildtgard 2000, pp 173–6)

Trying to explain these 'rules', Bildtgard suggested that they may be based on the assumptions that young = beautiful = healthy and, conversely, old = ugly = sick. Furthermore, he suggested that as female sexuality has been associated with reproduction, elderly female sexuality is 'out of place'. Although men are 'allowed' to be sexual for longer than women, if they display sexual interest in older age they are at risk of being defined as 'dirty old men'. There is no similar term for older women, probably because they hide their sexuality more effectively and/or the asexual definition has been so successfully internalised by the societal psyche that even when they do exhibit sexual interest, it is misinterpreted.

Such attitudes reflect societal denial of sexuality in older age, but more importantly they translate into behaviours that create barriers to older people fully and freely expressing their sexuality (Pangman & Seguire 2000).

THE REALITIES OF SEXUALITY IN OLDER AGE

The image of asexuality in older age is not supported by the evidence. Indeed, research demonstrates that older people generally maintain sexual interest into very old age and many continue to be sexually active into the ninth decade and/or until illness, disability or death make it impossible (Trudel et al 2000). The research has to be read bearing in mind the reluctance of the current older generation to discuss their sexuality openly. Still, it is clear that sexuality remains very important to a significant number. McCracken (1988) found a number of consistent themes in relation to sexuality and the aged:

- With reasonable health, and a partner, sexual relations are possible into the ninth decade of life.
- Sexual drive varies with each person, and in each person, from time to time.
- Despite a decline in sexual interest as people age, sexuality continues to hold an important place in most older personalities.
- Sexual patterns persist throughout a person's lifetime, and maintenance of capacity and sexual activity are dependent upon opportunity for expression.

Although sexuality has been associated with coitus and heterosexuality, many aged people define sexuality more broadly and include things such as touching, hugging, getting roses, comfort, warmth or being dressed up (Smith & Schmall 1983). Golan & Chong (1992) suggest that sexuality in later life is more concerned with intimacy than with the sexual act, and with recreation than with procreation—emphasising companionship, physical nearness and intimate communication, as well as pleasure-seeking physical relationships. Touch becomes more important as sensory loss reduces other pleasures (Ragno 1996). This is not to say that older people lose interest in sexual intercourse.

Hillman (2000, pp 23–4) reported that sexual intercourse occurred at least once a month among: 96% of 19–24 year olds, 92% for 30–34, 83% for 50–54, 57% for 65–69 and 27% for those over 75. Although the average for the over-75s was 27%, the oldest-old in this group reported sexual intercourse on average three times per month. Diokno et al (1991) reported from a study of over-60 year olds: 74% of married men were sexually active compared with 31% unmarried, and 56% of married women were sexually active compared with 5% of unmarried. The Archives of Sexual Behaviour report that among 80–102 year olds:

- 30% of females and 63% of males have intercourse;
- 10% of females and 29% of males have intercourse 'often';
- 71% of females and 88% of males have fantasised in the past year;
- 40% of females and 72% of males masturbate;
- 14% of females are married and 25% have regular sex partners; and
- 29% of males are married and 53% have regular sex partners

(Bretschneider & McCoy 1988, pp 109–29).

While most evidence indicates that men are more sexually interested and active than women, Marsiglio & Donnelly (1991) surveyed 807 over-60 year olds and found no gender differences. Starr & Weiner (1981) reported that 75% of elderly respondents said sex was the same or better with age (a relief for those of us who are rapidly ageing!). Hillman (2000) suggests that sexuality in later life may be linked to a desire to:

- foster emotional intimacy;
- experience and enjoy physical pleasure;
- satisfy continuing biological urges;
- assert independence and experiment with new things;
- feel youthful;
- challenge societal myths and stereotypes;
- re-establish sexual identity;
- heighten bodily awareness; and
- engender comfort and familiarity with a changing body (p 18).

Certainly ageing brings with it changes to sexual function, as it does in most areas of function. In general there is a slowing down, a reduced response, and it takes more stimulation to arouse a response. Nevertheless, again as with other areas of function, the experience, reduced stressors and confidence that come with age often leave older people enjoying their sexuality more than they did when they were young. Some research suggests that men are more active and interested in sex in old age than are women. Other work indicates that our attitudes and behaviours in old age reflect a continuation of our attitudes and behaviours throughout our lives: if we were sexually active and interested as younger people this is likely to continue; if we never liked sex, it is unlikely that we will become lusty old folk!

BARRIERS TO SEXUAL EXPRESSION

Of course at any age there are barriers to expressing and enjoying sexuality. Masters & Johnson (cited in Kay & Neelley 1982, p 40) listed some of the known barriers to active and enjoyable sexuality:

- the monotony of a 'repetitious sexual relationship';
- preoccupation with career or economic pursuits;
- mental or physical fatigue;
- over-indulgence in food or drink;
- physical or mental infirmities; and
- fear of failure.

It takes little consideration to realise that these barriers can affect us at any age. Many factors that reduce sexual satisfaction in older age are related to lack of a partner, lack of privacy, illness, disability, psychological factors, and ageist medical and nursing practices.

Perhaps because of ageist attitudes, an older person's sexual history/desires are rarely addressed by health professionals, and the impact of illness or treatment rarely discussed. Some of the changes, illnesses and disabilities that have been reported to have a negative impact on sexual function include: arthritis, chronic pain generally, depression, incontinence, orthopaedic surgery, hysterectomy, prostatectomy, hernia repair, retroverted uterus, haemorrhoids, hormonal changes, stroke, diabetes, myocardial infarction (MI) and cancer (Cheung 2002; Hoznek & Abbou 2001; Ambler et al 2001; Trudel et al 2000; Gelfand 2000; Hillman 2000). It is not clear what proportion of consequences relate to the treatment as such and what to the psychological affects and fears related to the treatment. It does seem that education regarding retrograde ejaculation reduces post-prostatectomy impotence and preoperative counselling reduces post-hysterectomy and post-MI sexual problems. Recognising that older people are sexual will also encourage health professionals to investigate and treat more appropriately any presenting condition.

In addition, many medications adversely affect sexual interest and activity. The most common include: antipsychotics, antihypertensives, tricyclic-antidepressants, and anti-Parkinsonian drugs (Trudel et al 2000; Gelfand 2000; Hillman 2000). All patients, including older people, should be advised of the risks of any medication they take, so they can make an informed choice. Ageist attitudes preclude doctors from giving this advice to older people in relation to drugs that reduce their sexual satisfaction.

Older people who enter residential care face major problems in expressing their sexuality. The two biggest problems are lack of privacy and staff/family attitudes. A number of studies have identified staff intolerance of sexual behaviours. In particular they are affronted by 'inappropriate' removal of clothing, masturbation, touching staff 'private parts', and making lewd remarks (Ragno 1996; Nay et al 1997; Ehrenfeld et al 1999; Bonifazi 2000). Education is required to alert staff to the fact that all these behaviours are common in society; the difference is that people in residential care are not provided the privacy that most of us enjoy. So otherwise 'normal' behaviours are stigmatised and the victim blamed, when the real problem is created by the resident not being afforded privacy. Educational programs can improve the attitudes of staff, families and residents (Walker & Harrington 2002; Inch 1992; Goldstein & Runyon 1993; Katzman 1990; Ooijen 1996; Steinke 1997).

The literature is unanimous in suggesting that the expression of sexuality is a continuing human need that should be consciously addressed in long-term care (Ehrenfeld et al 1999; Lewis 1993; Lyder 1991, 1994; Tunstull & Henry 1996; Wallace 1992). Most writers agree that organisational policies and staff practices should recognise the expression of sexuality as a right, and should promote healthy sexual functioning among residents (Berger 2000; Campbell & Huff 1995; Lewis 1993). In the United States, federal law has required each State to institute a bill of rights—that includes issues of sexuality—for older adults living in nursing homes. This bill provides for the assured rights of spouses to privacy or, if both are patients, the sharing of a room unless medically inadvisable (Campbell & Huff 1995). In Australia, regulations and standards for long-term care institutions that emphasise the rights of residents to dignity, respect and treatment as individuals provide a broad policy framework. However, they do not explicitly address issues of sexuality (Branzelle 1987; Commonwealth Department of Health and Aged Care 2001; Sargeant 1992). Quoting a spokesperson from one facility in the United States, Bonifazi writes:

> It's not about our views ... but about their civil rights ... we're here to create an environment that allows grown-ups to do what grown-ups do.
>
> Bonifazi 2000, p 24

VIGNETTE

'Will I never sleep with my husband again?'

Helen Page

As Director of Nursing, how does one respond to the question: 'Will I never be able to sleep with my husband again?'.

By the time a person is admitted to a nursing home, the number of losses they have endured is enormous. No matter how well intentioned we may be, as nurses working in the field there is often little we can do to mend these losses—or the pain they cause. We see the sadness in the eyes of husbands and wives who visit daily and, when they leave after their visit, we see the confusion and distress in the eyes of residents left behind with their new 'family'.

Mrs C would come daily to visit her husband. She was a ground-floor resident of our hostel, her husband being a first-floor resident. She would arrive soon after breakfast. They commandeered a couch together and we arranged for her meals to be sent up—lunch and dinner—which she ate with her husband. When it was time for Mr C to go to bed, Mrs C would kiss him goodbye and go back downstairs to her single room in the hostel.

Mr C's dependency was largely a physical one, and Mrs C's of a cognitive nature. It was obvious to us that their frailties had balanced them as a couple, and that, when they were together, there was a synergy that didn't exist when they were separated. They had had over fifty years to perfect this synergy but, because of a system which separates couples according to their care needs, they had been parted.

In response to the couple's desire to sleep together, I invited Mrs C to transfer to the Nursing Home—accepting a much lower level of funding for her than would normally be tolerated.

Mr and Mrs C preferred a double bed, rather than two singles. Some resistance from nursing staff was expected. Most have trained and worked using a 'hospital' model of care. The concept of providing nursing care for two people in the same bed was alien to them. The main concerns raised were of a practical occupational health and safety nature—which were easily overcome by the use of technology. I was able to have a bed specially made—queen size, with electric high-low and individual head-raising capacity. I also invested in some slide-transfer sheets.

By the time the new bed had arrived, all in the nursing home were happily anticipating its installation. Mr and Mrs C had become celebrities—even the ABC's *7.30 Report* had been to interview them.

There has been some speculation as to the sexual nature of Mr and Mrs C's relationship—now that they once again share the same bed. To me, this is irrelevant—and is nobody's business but their own. The fact that they are able to continue their relationship in a way that is meaningful to them is what really matters.

My hope is that, in the future, funding models and facility design will allow this form of 'ageing-in-place' to be the norm, and that people's intimate lives will be respected and accommodated. I also hope that similar accommodation is offered, not only to married couples of over 50 years' duration, but to all people who require this level of care, and who wish to continue their intimate relationships.

DEMENTIA AND SEXUALITY

Perhaps the area of sexuality that creates the greatest dilemma for staff and families is when one or both people engaging in sexual activity have cognitive impairment. Staff and family want to 'protect' the person and can become very angry at what they see as abuse of a vulnerable resident (Ehrenfeld et al 1999; Walker & Ephross 1999). The issue of consent concerns them and, more recently, sexually transmitted diseases (STDs) have been mentioned as a reason to 'protect' residents. Families may argue that Mum or Dad would never have behaved that way before and so it is important to maintain their pre-dementing morals. Berger (2000) questions whether it is appropriate to assume that only the pre-dementing self is authentic. We have recognised in many other ways the value of validating the dementing person's feelings and behaviours. Why should sexuality be different—perhaps dementia has liberated them from previous inhibitions? It may also be a way of expressing an unmet need for attention and touch that could be addressed by massage, dancing and other less sexually explicit interventions. Zeiss & Kasl-Godley (2001) draw attention to guidelines developed by Lichtenberg & Strzepek for assessing the competency of a person with dementia to participate in a sexual relationship—these guidelines explore awareness of the relationship, ability to avoid exploitation and awareness of risk (p. 23). As staff assess numerous times every day what a person with dementia wants or doesn't want, likes or dislikes, and will or will not do, I question why a special case is made for sexuality. No such concern appears to exist regarding a person's consent to take medications, eat, have a shower and the like. Individualised care and 'knowing' the resident will usually alert staff to whether the activity is pleasurable or being resisted. At times a spouse will need to be counselled either in relation to their own now unrecognised, unwanted advances or a new relationship that the resident spouse is enjoying. Some families, with education and support, come to accept that the new relationship is bringing happiness, and understand that it is not a rejection of them. Pre-empting the surprise by ensuring that all families are aware of this possibility can reduce stress in the eventuality. Most people with dementia do not engage in 'inappropriate' sexual behaviour, and regular assessment, attention to boredom, loneliness, the need for touch and to feel worthwhile will reduce sexual 'acting out'. In older age, love appears to be experienced more strongly; perhaps the realisation of potential loss is more imminent (Ehrenfeld et al 1999, p 144).

Ehrenfeld et al (1999) observed institutionalised older people with dementia and categorised manifestations of sexuality as follows:

- love and caring—strong affection, a feeling of attraction or desire for someone, support time together;
- romance—the basis of emotion and a dynamic mental experience of love with the scope of emotions tending to idealise the object of one's affection;
- hand-in hand, flattery, cheek kiss—nothing intimate; and
- eroticism—sexual excitement or desire, touching breasts, genitals. Only in a minority of cases did sexual behaviour occur between resident and staff (16%; elderly male residents and female staff) (p 146).

Berger (2000, p 310) suggests that residents should, however, have access to such supports as private space, condoms, vibrators, lubricant and Viagra. He also notes that masturbation is the least disruptive sexual act and if facilitated it may reduce sexual behaviours that involve other people.

A SEXUAL RIGHTS POLICY

Being in residential care does not remove human rights from the resident; nor should the resident's rights result in the abuse of the rights of others. Staff are not the moral gatekeepers of residents, and families' rights should not take precedence over the residents'. Although most care is guided by organisational policy and/or protocol, staff are usually left without guidance when it comes to sexuality. In an effort to address this gap the Melbourne study (Nay et al 1997) developed, through action research and participation of all interested stakeholders, a sexual rights policy which was supported by management, could be used to educate and inform staff, residents and families, and provide a guide to practice. The Policy is reproduced below.

The North West Hospital Policy on rights and responsibilities related to sexuality of clients affirms the following principles, notwithstanding that if there is any conflict with relevant legislation the law will always override these principles:

- Clients can expect their maleness, femaleness, sexual orientation and preference to be respected and supported by management and staff.
- Where a staff member feels their own morals are compromised in relation to a client's sexual behaviour the staff member has a responsibility to refer the matter to their Supervisor and the right to be exempted from care that is felt to be morally compromising.

- Wherever possible, clients will be provided opportunities to enable their choice of sexual expression provided such expression does not impinge upon the rights of others.

- Where sexual behaviour is seen to impinge upon the rights of others or threaten professional practice, staff and/or clients will be expected to refer the situation to the relevant Department Head and appropriate boundaries will be negotiated and discussed with all parties concerned —if a resolution is not reached, the Department Head will seek advice from their line manager.

- In situations related to sexuality where a client is cognitively impaired and/or they request family/guardian involvement, the family/guardian will be consulted. However if the family's wishes appear to conflict with the interests of the client, appropriate (e.g. depending on circumstance this may be a religious minister, counsellor, legal advisor, etc.) mediation will be sought.

- Clients can expect staff to treat their sexuality confidentially—discussion with other health professionals should only occur with the permission of the client or if behaviour impinges on the rights of others and requires staff intervention.

- Clients are entitled to be provided with maximum privacy, recognising structural constraints, to enable sexual expression.

- Clients are entitled to the same assistance with hygiene surrounding sexual activity as is given in relation to other activities of daily living —e.g. ensuring cleanliness before and/or after sexual activity should be treated no differently than occurs in regard to meals, toileting, incontinence and so on.

- Staff should not assist clients directly with intimate sexual activity as this may compromise the staff member and constitute abuse of the client.

- Staff should respect a client's right to access sex support services, and senior staff may assist access by, for example, providing a telephone or making a call for the client if they feel comfortable doing so.

- Management will promote and staff will maintain sensitive, positive language and behaviour toward the sexual expression of clients.

- Staff and management will provide information for clients to assist with informed choice relating to consent, fertility and disease.

- Chemical or physical restraint will not be used to control sexual expression except in crisis situations and/or when every possible supportive intervention has been tried, failed and the client remains a threat to others.

Staff, relatives and clients are entitled to education and support to assist in the implementation of this policy.

CONCLUSION

Sexuality is central to identity and well-being. Contemporary practice frequently ignores the sexual needs, interests and rights—and thus the identity and well-being—of older people. This is especially prevalent in residential care but also occurs whenever medications or treatments are commenced that adversely affect sexuality without the older person being fully informed. The special needs of people with dementia and their families require consideration and support. If health professionals are to support the human rights of older people they too must be educated and supported by organisational policy.

Acknowledgements

Acknowledgement is given to Don Gorman for his assistance in preparing the first edition version of this chapter.

This chapter draws upon research funded by La Trobe University and North West Hospital, and the authors acknowledge members of the Steering Committee: Clare Hetzel, Cathy Barrett, Barbara Hayes, Margaret Hartley, Jenny Gough and Judy Brown. Also, Chris Bigby and Cally Berryman are acknowledged for their assistance with data collection.

References

Ambler N, Williams A, Hill P, Gunary R & Cratchley G 2001, Sexual difficulties of chronic pain patients, *Clinical Journal of Pain*, 17, pp 138–45.

Ansuini C, Fiddler-Woite J & Woite R 1996, The source, accuracy, and impact of initial sexuality information on lifetime wellness, *Adolescence*, 31(122), pp 283–9.

Berger J 2000, Sexuality and intimacy in the nursing home: a romantic couple of mixed cognitive capacities, *Journal of Clinical Ethics*, 11(4), pp 309–13.

Bildtgard T 2000, The sexuality of elderly people on film—visual limitations, *Journal of Ageing and Identity*, 5(3), pp 169–83.

Bonifazi W 2000, Somebody to love, *Contemporary Long Term Care*, April, pp 22–8.

Booth B 1990, Does it really matter at that age?, *Nursing Times*, 86(3), pp 50–2.

Branzelle J 1987, Legal currents—ensuring residents' rights to sexual desire and expression, *Provider*, pp 30–3.

Bretschneider J & McCoy N 1988, Sexual interest and behavior in healthy 82–102 year olds, *Archives of Sexual Behavior*, 17, pp 109–29.

Butler RN & Lewis MI 1982, Special concerns—racism, sexism, retirement, crime, alcoholism, deafness, blindness and sexuality. In: Bowen D (ed), *Aging and Mental Health—Positive, Psychosocial and Biomedical Approaches* (3rd edn), Mosby: St Louis.

Campbell J & Huff M 1995, Sexuality in the older woman, *Gerontology & Geriatrics Education*, 16(1), pp 71–81.

Caplan E 1987, *The Cultural Construction of Sexuality*, Tavistock: London.

Cheung R 2002, Sexual functioning in Chinese stroke patients with mild or no disability, *Cerebrovascular Diseases*, 14, pp 122–8.

Commonwealth Department of Health and Aged Care 2001, Standards and Guidelines for Residential Aged Care Services Manual.

Diokno A, Brown M & Herzog AR 1990, Sexual function in the elderly, *Archives of Internal Medicine*, 150, pp 197–200.

Ehrenfeld M, Bronner G, Tabak N, Alpert R & Bergman R 1999, Sexuality among institutionalized elderly patients with dementia, *Nursing Ethics*, 6(2), pp 144–50.

Foucault M 1976, *The History of Sexuality—An Introduction*, trans. Robert Hurley, Penguin: Middlesex.

Gelfand M 2000, Sexuality among older women, *Journal of Women's Health and Gender-Based Medicine*, 9(1), pp S15–S20.

Golan O & Chong B 1992, Sexuality and Ageing: Some Physical Aspects, *Geriaction*, 11(4), pp 10–11.

Goldstein H & Runyon C 1993, An occupational therapy educational module to increase sensitivity about geriatric sexuality, *Physical and Occupational Therapy in Geriatrics*, 11(2), pp 57–76.

Hillman J 2000, *Clinical Perspectives on Elderly Sexuality*, Kluwer Academic/Plenum Publishers: New York.

Hoznek A & Abbou C-C 2001, Impact of interventional therapy for benign prostatic hyperplasis on quality of life and sexual function, *Current Urology Reports* 2(4), pp 311–17.

Inch B 1992, The pleasure of old age, *New Zealand Nursing Journal*, pp 18–20.

Kaplan L 1996, Sexual and institutional issues when one spouse resides in the community and the other lives in a nursing home, *Sexuality and Disability*, 14(4), pp 281–93.

Katzman E 1990, Education for sexual-health care, *Journal of Nursing Education*, 29(3), pp 141–2.

Kay B & Neelley J 1982, Sexuality and aging: a review of the current literature. *Sexuality and Disability*, 5(1), pp 38–46.

Lewis K 1993, Sexual rights policies emphasize freedom, privacy, respect for all, *Provider*, 19(12), pp 35–6.

Lyder CH 1991, Examining sexuality in long-term care, *The Journal of Practical Nursing*, 41(4), pp 25–7.

Lyder CH 1994, The role of the nurse practitioner in promoting sexuality in the institutionalized elderly, *Journal of the American Academy of Nurse Practitioners*, 6(2), pp 61–3.

McCracken AL 1988, Sexual practice by elders: the forgotten aspect of functional health, *Journal of Gerontological Nursing*, 14(10), pp 13–18.

Marsiglio W & Donnelly D 1991, Sexual relations in later life: a national study of married life, *Journal of Gerontology*, 46(6), pp 338–44.

Nay R 1993, *Benevolent Oppression—Lived Experiences of Nursing Home Life*, School of Sociology, University of New South Wales: Sydney.

Nay R, Barrett C, Gorman D & Berryman C 1997, *Developing a Sexual Health Policy for Long-Term Facilities*, Gerontic Nursing Professorial Unit, La Trobe University: Melbourne.

Ooijen V 1996, Learning to approach patients' sexuality as part of holistic care, *Nursing Times*, 92(36), pp 44–5.

Pangman V & Seguire M 2000, Sexuality and the chronically ill older adult: a social justice issue, *Sexuality and Disability*, 18(1), pp 49–59.

Ragno JG 1996, Successful redirection of the sexually disruptive resident. In: *The Abusive Elder*, pp 37–42, Haworth Press.

Sargeant D 1992, Sexual behaviour and persons with acquired brain damage, *SBRC Review*, 6(2), pp 1–2.

Satran M 1986, Prejudice clouds sex among elderly, *Wisconsin State Journal*, July 1986, pp 129–30.

Smith MM & Schmall VL 1983, Knowledge and attitudes toward sexuality and sex education of a select group of older people, *Gerontology and Geriatrics Education*, 3(4), pp 259–69.

Starr B & Weiner M 1981, *On Sex and Sexuality in the Mature Years*, Stein and Day: New York.

Steinke E 1997, Sexuality in aging: implications for nursing facility staff, *The Journal of Continuing Education in Nursing*, 28(2), pp 59–63.

Trudel G, Turgeon L & Piche L 2000, Marital and sexual aspects of old age, *Sexual and Relationship Therapy*, 15(4), pp 381–406.

Tunstull P & Henry ME 1996, Approaches to resident sexuality, *Journal of Gerontological Nursing*, 22(6), pp 37–42.

Walker B & Ephross P 1999, Knowledge and attitudes toward sexuality of a group of elderly, *Journal of Gerontological Social Work*, 31(1/2), pp 85–107.

Walker B & Harrington D 2002, Effects of staff training on staff knowledge and attitudes about sexuality, *Educational Gerontology*, 28, pp 639–54.

Wallace M 1992, Management of sexual relationships among elderly residents of long-term care facilities, *Geriatric Nursing*, 13(6), pp 308–11.

Weeks J 1986, Sexuality. In: Hamilton E (ed), *Key Ideas*, Ellis Horwood/Tavistock Publications: Sussex/London.

Woods N 1984, *Human Sexuality*, Mosby: St Louis.

Zeiss A & Kasl-Godley J 2001, Sexuality in older adults, *Generations*, Summer, pp 18–25.

CHAPTER 18

Contemporary care planning

BILL KOCH

INTRODUCTION

The potential benefits of computerised care planning have been discussed in nursing literature for many decades, with early proponents such as Cook (1982) and Watt (1987) predicting substantial time savings and improvements in documentation standards. More recently, Corkhill (2001) remains optimistic about the benefits and efficiencies that computerisation may bring. Despite this, many aged-care facilities continue to use paper-based resident record and care-planning systems. One reason for this apparent lack of progress may be the paucity of substantive data to underpin the variety of claims made by proponents of computerisation. In the absence of such data, derived from implementation and evaluation of computerised care-planning systems within aged care, many clinicians may remain sceptical about the claimed benefits to be derived from computerising this area of their practice. In addition, where computerised systems have been implemented, the failure to involve potential end-users in design and implementation phases of computerisation can impede both the usability and acceptability of such systems (Darbyshire 2000).

This chapter provides evaluation data from a number of aged-care sites where nurses have replaced their paper-based care plans with a computer-based alternative. It outlines the developmental processes which were followed, from the initial paper-based model which led to an earlier PC-based version, through to the current internet-based care-planning system. While the focus is on one longitudinal project, the underlying design strategies and lessons learned along the way can be applied more broadly by readers seeking to implement computerised care-planning solutions within aged-care facilities.

CLINICAL DECISION-MAKING

Parallel to the professional discussion of computerisation there has also been growing interest in clinical decision-making within health care since the early 1980s. One reason for this interest has been the recognition that the information available to clinicians has the potential to outstrip the human capacity to store and process it (Fineberg 1981; Chittaro 2001). Several authors have also reported the complexities which specifically faced nurses when they attempted to process clinical data in a variety of nursing specialities such as medical–surgical nursing (Prescott et al 1991), psychiatric nursing (Regan-Kubinski 1991) and critical care nursing (Fisher & Fonteyn 1991). More recently, in the context of gerontic nursing in Australia, Koch (1997, 1999) identified both the large volume of data and the complicated nature of these data, which emerged when nurses undertook resident assessments. In addition, gerontic nurses commonly report the lengthy processes involved in manually examining these data in order to develop individualised plans of care for residents. Further pressure is placed on Australian gerontic nurses by the links between documentation of care provision and funding levels (Pelletier et al 2002).

A POSSIBLE EXPERT SYSTEM SOLUTION

The research project described in this chapter sought to address these issues of data complexity and care planning as follows. A type of artificial intelligence application called an *expert system* was thought by the author to offer a promising approach to both computerised care planning and provision of decision support to gerontic nurses. An expert system is a computer program which models the expertise and rules used by such experts (Benfer et al 1991; Webopedia 2003), and also acts as an expert interpreter of data within a narrowly focused domain—in this instance, care planning.

The term 'artificial intelligence' (AI) was first coined in 1956 by John McCarthy, and while this may still conjure up visions of science fiction and seem remote from the realities of clinical practice, this chapter outlines an ongoing application of AI within gerontic nursing. Radosevich (1999), in a computer science context, pointed out that interest in expert systems peaked in the 1980s but then waned after the initial hype and expectation was not met by subsequent delivery of useable products. A search of nursing literature also reveals a parallel trend of activity then diminished interest in this area, for much the same reasons. Radosevich also claimed that the term 'artificial intelligence' had become so sullied by this failure to deliver that software developers became reluctant to use the term to describe their product, preferring instead such alternatives as 'knowledge management' or 'computational intelligence tools'. While these concerns were recognised it was nonetheless felt that the expert system approach held promise if applied to care planning, for the following reasons.

Previously Koch & McGovern (1993) had demonstrated that it was logistically possible to model the rules used to reach nursing diagnoses within an expert system used for care planning. Rules could be articulated as follows:

IF the resident has *a* ... OR the resident has *b* ... THEN *x* may be concluded, where *a* or *b* represent defining characteristics of the resident, and *x* represents the nursing diagnostic conclusion which can be reached.

In this way a large number of data relations can be modelled within the expert system. This set of IF ... THEN rules is commonly referred to as the knowledge base of the program. Importantly, it should be stressed that this data processing model did not embrace a reductionist approach but rather sought to create a tool which used both the strengths of the computer software and the individual nurse's experience or intuition. The software was able to rapidly process large volumes of data and suggest nursing diagnostic conclusions to use within a care plan. Nurses, however, maintained full control as they could accept these nursing diagnoses or reject them if they felt that they did not apply to the resident under consideration. Chou (1995) evaluated an earlier prototype of this expert system that contained only a limited data set, to test the acceptability of the approach. Encouraged by the generally positive responses of gerontic nurses to this prototype, the author began work on constructing a more extensive expert system designed to run on the Microsoft Windows™ operating system.

BUILDING THE EXPERT SYSTEM

When completed, the extended version contained approximately 1000 possible descriptors of residents and 120 nursing diagnostic conclusions. It was constructed as follows. Registered nurses ($n = 5$) considered to be representative of the likely users of the expert system were invited to contribute to this design phase, when general design principles and functionality were implemented. The importance of involving potential end-users at the earliest possible stage of software development is stressed in order to maximise a common understanding of the system between end-users and developer (Agresti 1986; Koch 1999).

Despite never having worked with an expert system, these nurses were able to specify aspects of functionality which they felt would be vital to its acceptability. This included minimisation of repetitive data entry such as resident name, and special needs or allergies. They also wished the resultant care plan to automatically show the date and time of production, in order to clearly identify the last time that the resident's case had been reviewed. In related quality assurance issues, these nurses also stressed that care plans should also show the nurse(s) responsible for the resident care, and contain a section for nurses to comment on progress toward achievement of resident goals.

The general overarching concept articulated by these nurses was that, in order to be an acceptable tool, the program should allow quality care plans to be generated in less time than it took to produce these manually, and generally be easy to use, without the need for on-site support from information technology staff. As additional requests were added to this 'wish list' it was interesting to note that some directly mirrored the nursing literature from the mid-1980s. For example, nurses also wanted the program to be able to explain how diagnostic conclusions were reached. This had been recommended many years previously by Bennett (1986) and Hyslop (1987), who both stated that an expert system used for nursing diagnosis should have the ability to teach neophytes how diagnostic conclusions were reached.

Nurses wanted the program to not only print a care plan that showed resident goals and nursing interventions, but also allow them to customise all aspects of this care plan. They also wished to produce individual resident summaries that showed only the defining characteristics for a specific resident. This latter feature was requested for use at case conferences, whereby defining characteristics that were no longer relevant could be removed, or new data added.

During the design phase, dialogue with these nurses was conducted mainly on a one-to-one basis, with less frequent group meetings where issues of consensus had to be established, such as the order of items within the program interface, and the layout of the completed care plan. This regular communication ensured not only that a common vision of development was maintained within the group but also that those nurses involved were provided with direct control over the functionality and appearance of the software as it evolved and 'a tangible partnership' with the system developer as advocated by Darbyshire (2000). His interpretative study using focus groups demonstrated that acceptance of computerised information systems within the clinical area is not merely dependent on overcoming technical or literacy issues but involves a whole gamut of underlying social and political issues. It is evident from participants' responses that some felt that such systems were 'dumped' on them by management, or that they were merely operationalising someone else's agenda, suggesting that they were still a 'dependent profession' or treated like 'IT soldier ants' who simply entered data for others who dictated what data was collected and how it was used.

The importance of involving end-users is also highlighted by the Standish Group (1995), who indicated that 31.1% of all software projects are cancelled before they are completed, and 52.7% of projects cost nearly twice their original costing. Two key themes are central to these data. The single largest contributing factor to successful projects was user involvement, and the two major factors in project failure were incomplete functionality and lack of user involvement. Despite the common-sense nature of this advice, anecdotal evidence from nurses continues to suggest that many developers still fail to liaise with the clinicians who will eventually be expected to use the system, resulting in negative attitudes towards the proposed system, resistance and lack of commitment to its use. Nurse managers ignore this reality at their peril.

As mentioned earlier, at the heart of this expert system lay the knowledge base which suggested possible diagnostic conclusions for data entered by nurses. Using literature developed by the North American Nursing Diagnosis Association (NANDA), this project developed an expert system to provide decision support for nurses responsible for diagnosis in aged-care settings. This strategy of using literature was recommended by Durkin (1994) and overcame the problems traditionally associated with acquiring relevant knowledge from experts, due to their common inability to articulate the knowledge or expertise used in problem solving. NANDA literature, however, represented a formally agreed-upon explication of knowledge within this specific domain, and provided the means of creating the knowledge base at the heart of the expert system. The acceptability of this taxonomic approach to care planning to Australian gerontic nurses has been demonstrated by Koch (1999).

The reliability of diagnostic conclusions suggested by the expert system was established by inputting real case data and checking the diagnostic conclusion against the literature from which they had been derived. The validity of the diagnostic conclusions of the resultant expert system was then established by comparison with the diagnoses proposed by a panel of experts ($n = 8$) for the same case data. In the course of these phases of development, changes were made to the knowledge base to increase the diagnostic accuracy of the expert system, resulting in 95% convergence with this panel of experts. Once a validated knowledge base was in place, the expert system was implemented. It should be noted that in addition to this level of convergence with the panel the program could identify substantially more correct diagnoses for possible inclusion in the care plan than any individual expert was able to achieve from the same data.

Once this validated version of the software was ready it was implemented in ten aged-care sites. In return for agreement to implement the expert system in their clinical area, responsibility for the following undertakings was assumed by the author. The expert system was provided free of charge to each site, along with staff training in its use, plus on-site technical support for the duration of the project, in return for written evaluation of the program by registered nurses. Nine sites in the Melbourne metropolitan area and one in Vancouver Island, BC, Canada, agreed to participate, resulting in a sample of forty registered nurses.

THE PROGRAM–USER INTERFACE

Because a range in the level of users' computer skills was anticipated, a key goal from the onset of this project was also to make the program interface as simple as possible, in order to increase acceptance of the software. Thus the challenge for developers was to provide a program interface that would accommodate a variety of skills levels in users, and also be functionally transparent to the user. An early advocate of this approach, Norman (1988) contended that in the best computer programs, the computer itself 'disappears', and clear pathways to complete the task are obvious, giving a sense of a transparency to computer involvement in the task. Although computer operating systems change over time, the basic principles which are likely to achieve transparency remain similar. More recent accounts of how this may achieved are provided by Hackos & Redish (1998) and Galitz (2002), who emphasise the importance of building systems which reflect both user computer literacy levels and the tasks to be undertaken.

In the initial PC version this meant sticking as closely as possible to the look and feel of a typical Windows™-based program, which integrated into nurses' workflow as follows. By default the program operated in a novice mode whereby users were automatically taken to the next relevant step in the care-planning process by clicking on the 'Continue' button. As users became more familiar with the program they could exit this mode and determine their own path through the program.

After completing a resident assessment, nurses entered the data that best described the resident. At the heart of the program was the expert system, which:

- identified *all* the possible nursing diagnoses that can be reached from these resident data;
- provided the specific resident data that supports each diagnosis;
- suggested resident goals and interventions that can be modified for individual residents; and
- rapidly produced comprehensive printed care plans that can also be easily modified.

Importantly, one can see how the application of an expert system approach to care planning provides not just the replication of a paper-based task, but a transformation of the task. It is important to make this distinction, as using the expert system approach, the nurse can not only produce a legible care plan, in which fields can be made mandatory to prevent omissions, but is also exposed to the reasoning used by expert clinicians, as the program can articulate the reasoning used by its underlying knowledge base to reach specific diagnostic conclusions. Using their own professional judgement, nurses can retain full control over what is included in the final care plan, which emphasises a facilitative, as opposed to prescriptive, approach. This also helps the nurse produce care plans that reflect individual resident's needs, rather than being generic and impersonal. In addition, each time a care plan was printed, the program automatically recorded the nursing diagnoses that were included in the care plan, so at any point a nurse could see the emerging profile of all diagnoses for that facility.

USER FEEDBACK

Different methods of evaluation were used at different phases of this software development. In this earlier PC-based phase, a technique known as MultiAttribute Utility Theory (MAUT) was used to structure written user feedback. The main focus of this approach is to determine the *value*, *worth* or *utility* of a complex evaluation object that possesses multiple attributes, in this case an expert system for care planning. It is not possible to present a detailed explanation of this technique here; however, readers who are interested in MAUT are referred to Edwards & Newman (1982), which would be considered both the logical starting point and a seminal work in the area. The underlying logic of the MAUT approach is fundamentally straightforward. It allows users to first consider groups of attributes, then individual attributes of a software package, and list these in order of importance—thus, some users may rate a feature such as time spent on care planning, or ability to modify the care plan, as being more important than ease of use, or feedback on why program errors occur, and so forth. Logically, attributes that are rated as being of greater importance contribute more weight to the final evaluation score.

After completing this ranking process, the various attributes of the program are then considered individually, and this time given a performance score ranging from zero to ten. Using these two pieces of data, an overall score is derived for the software and its individual components by multiplying the initial attribute weighting by the subsequent performance score. In this way a program feature may be rated as highly important, and weighted accordingly. However, if it was be deemed to have been poorly implemented, this would have the effect of dragging the score down. Conversely, an attribute which was deemed to be highly important and weighted accordingly, and which was also thought to perform well, would increase the overall score.

In this way MAUT allows subjective ratings of evaluation objects to be transposed into numerical scores, which may then be subject to quantitative analysis. This expert system for care planning, like any multifaceted evaluation object, may therefore be conceptually decomposed into individual components that contribute to an overall score. This process subsequently allowed the identification of program parameters that are functionally acceptable to users, and those which require attention.

The original PC-based version obtained an overall utility score of 0.73 (on a possible range of 0 to 1.0), indicating the acceptability of this care-planning approach to nurses in the study. Users indicated that the main strengths of the software, in order, were as follows:

- The program increased the standards of documentation by preventing omissions and illegible handwriting, and provided an aesthetically pleasing format to the resulting care plan.

- All goals and interventions for individual residents were easily modifiable. This is an important issue as, anecdotally, computerised care plans appear to have gained a reputation for being generic and thus not reflective of individual resident's needs. Nurses clearly recognised the value of the editing systems built into the program. While the program suggested goals and interventions related to diagnostic conclusions, nurses could override these by editing, deleting or adding new goals and interventions on individual residents' care plans.

- They could also make similar amendments to the program's default goals and interventions using a global editor. Using this latter tool, the next time a specific diagnosis was concluded from resident data, these new defaults would be suggested for the care plan. In this way nurses at individual sites enhanced the program as they integrated local protocols, or new evidence from practice.

- A very low level of computer keyboard skills was required to use the program. Because it was anticipated that users would vary greatly in their keyboard skills, the need for such skills was deliberately minimised by making most user interactions mouse-based.

- The program provided justification for funding claims made via resident classification scales. This was unique to the Australian nurses in the study as, in Australia, at the time of writing, funding for care provision is directly linked to the documentary evidence which can be provided to substantiate the dependency level claimed for an individual resident.

- The program increases nurses' confidence in their own diagnostic reasoning. Nurses reported that since the program explained what data were used to reach nursing diagnoses, they extended the range of diagnostic conclusions they could reach when they next encountered a resident with these presenting features. Although this had not been anticipated or an intended focus of the evaluation, nurses indicated that a vicarious educational process was experienced when using the expert system.

- The time spent on care planning was reduced. It is also interesting to note that this outcome was only rated sixth, yet the need to accomplish this goal was commonly mentioned in the design discussions, but was superseded by what may be considered more professional issues, as noted above. Specifically, some nurses reported up to a 50% reduction in the time taken to produce a care plan relative to undertaking the task manually. Individual managers can do their own projections of local time and cost savings based on these data.

Nominal variables such as site, area of practice, country, self-reported levels of competence using nursing diagnosis, computer skills and educational level were all compared with utility scores using Kruskall-Wallis tests. No significant differences were detected. Finally, the length of experience nurses had in using nursing diagnosis was compared with utility scores. This was the only bivariate comparison to reveal significant differences. A Mann-Whitney U test was undertaken by recoding years of experience to ordinal level data, whereby 1–8 years' experience was recoded as 1, and 9–16 years' experience as 2. These data were then compared to utility scores. This yielded $z = -2.259$ and $p = 0.023$, which demonstrated a statistically significant difference between the two groups. This meant that the nurses with more experience in using nursing diagnoses perceived greater utility in using the expert system. Because of the small sample size and distribution of utility scores it was not possible to split the groups any further than these two in an attempt to further investigate differences between these two variables.

The expert system was modelling expertise in the very narrowly focused domain of nursing diagnosis, and providing decision support by identifying all diagnoses which it was possible to conclude from resident data. Thus users required some basis for accepting or rejecting these suggestions. This suggested that users do need to have some domain-specific expertise to be able to use the decision-support output provided by the expert system and discriminate between appropriate and inappropriate conclusions.

Web-enabling the software

This most recent phase of the program development was undertaken to build on the positive feedback from the nurses at the ten evaluation sites, and to use the emerging approach of web-enabling. The term 'web-enabling' means converting the software to a version that will run on the internet. The new web-enabled version built on the existing program strengths and also allowed the program to be used on any internet-connected PC with appropriate access rights. As Eder (2000) and Dahanayake & Waltraud (2002) point out, there are many inherent strengths in this approach, as data may be shared by many users, passed between and used by different applications, and accessed from multiple locations. This in turn results in a more cost-effective and streamlined method of data management.

In the case of the care-planning software, this means that the key functions run on a central computer (or server), where the resulting care plan data is also processed and stored. Users see all data displayed within an internet browser in the same way that they would see typical web pages. Nurses can update the resident data from any internet-connected PC, and GPs can update records from their practice or the aged-care facility. This also resolves the previous need to keep multiple copies of resident records at different sites. Data can also be passed between modules within the program. For example, once a Resident Classification Scale (RCS) calculation for an individual resident has been undertaken, this result can be passed on to the finance module.

Focus groups

During this web-enabling phase of the software development, end-users were again heavily involved in the system redevelopment and evaluation of emergent iterative versions. This time the ongoing evaluation was undertaken via focus groups at individual sites or at regular regional meetings with users. These focus groups have enabled users to identify any issues of concern and collectively agree on the means of resolution within the group, as outlined by Wilkinson (1998).

This was successful in resolving a variety of issues, such as how much retrospective access should be given when writing progress notes. Additional issues such as establishing levels of user access to resident data and program functionality were also readily resolved within these groups. All nurses involved in the care-planning process were given access to their residents' data, and could therefore modify progress notes and care plans, but they asked for only one person at each site to be assigned administrative rights, which allow that person to add new users and adjust default goals or interventions for care plans. The only restriction imposed on the groups has been the need to reach consensus on program functionality, as it was not feasible to support the development of features and versions specific to individual sites.

In consultation with these user groups, program functionality was extended to include progress notes, which may be accessed and appended by GPs, physiotherapists, podiatrists and other health-care professionals. In addition, in response to user group discussion, progress notes and an RCS calculation tool were added, as well as a form-building tool that allows nurses to replicate existing assessment forms such as mobility, communication or bladder management.

The focus group phase involved four aged-care facilities in Victoria and Tasmania, with bed numbers ranging from 45 to 600, and representing approximately 1100 beds overall. It also included a mix of high-care and low-care provision. One facility was privately owned, and the others were owned by church or charitable groups. The following information is an amalgamation of viewpoints and decisions from these focus groups. These groups consisted of forty registered and enrolled nurses, with some of the former also holding the position of Director of Nursing in the facilities.

Operational risks

Embarking on a process of computerising care plans must be recognised as presenting an element of risk to facility owners and managers. Operational risks included the expenditure necessary to buy PCs or reallocate existing PCs to relevant locations to facilitate access by nurses. There was also the possibility of increased staffing costs if the system created more work or if there was lack of uptake of the new system by staff.

A Director of Nursing at one site noted that they had recently implemented another computerised documentation system that was now largely redundant as it had failed to meet requirements, which made her reluctant to consider adopting another computer solution. This provided an example of how one computerised system that had failed had the potential to generally give the approach a bad reputation.

Some facilities that had agreed to evaluate the software for a trial period were also about to go through accreditation, which presented additional concurrent pressures for the nurses involved. Against this backdrop the four aged-care facilities entered the evaluation of the web-enabled version of the software.

IT literacy

Nurses conceded that initially they were hesitant about using the program, because of the feeling that they had been planning care manually for so long that there was no need to change this. Also, many had never accessed the internet, and there was limited access to computers at the workplace, so some issues of comfort with using computers had to be addressed.

With this in mind, training in the use of the program started with low-level issues such as: 'What is a mouse and how is it used?'. Where possible, nurses were trained individually rather than in large groups, to maximise interaction and to satisfy the trainer that the nurse concerned had grasped key objectives. These sessions used real resident data, which resulted in at least the kernel of a resident's care plan at the end of the session, as opposed to using hypothetical data which would be of limited value after the training sessions. Around a week later, follow-up training was provided to clear up any issues which had resulted from using the program. Nurses with internet access from home were also encouraged to use the program in this way. In addition, an animated tutorial was created for the program using Macromedia Flash™. This was provided to any user who wanted a copy. Rather than consulting a paper-based manual to review functionality, users could simply run this program, which demonstrated via animated sequences how to use all aspects of the program. They could then simply replicate what they had seen in this demonstration to the care plan they were currently creating.

In this way the initial hurdle of basic computer skills was addressed largely through individual training. The time taken per nurse ranged from 1.2 to 1.6 hours, with group training taking around 2.5 hours. At the end of these sessions and with personal practice, around 80% of users indicated that their initial concerns with IT were now alleviated. Some remaining users seemed to lack confidence and tended not to seek help when unable to log in, or stated their fear of losing data. These issues were addressed with some additional support from their more confident colleagues and the software developers.

Education and professional development

Using the program and seeing the care plans generated by colleagues allowed staff to build on their existing knowledge base, a phenomenon also reported by nurses using the PC version (Koch 1999). Other developmental examples included seeing suggested interventions or nursing diagnoses not previously considered. Some staff indicated that they had become more analytical in their care planning, and one facility indicated a desire to use the collected data to engage staff in local research of resident care needs.

Some unexpected comments were also made. Some staff felt that being part of a large project that required their input generated better communication between geographically distant nursing homes. They also reported a sense of better communication with management and senior staff as a result of using the same care-planning system.

As mentioned earlier, the initial concerns of Directors of Nursing included the operational risks involved in adopting a computerised care-planning solution, whereas other nurses were more focused on the day-to-day issues of whether or not the program would assist them in undertaking care planning. It is interesting to note that directors reported that nursing staff uptake and support of the software gave them confidence in the viability of the approach.

Time savings

Based on a guestimated eight-hour creation time for a typical care plan, nurses felt that time savings were in the vicinity of 60% or 4.8 hours, which roughly mirrored what users of the antecedent PC version of the software had reported. Again, nurse managers are invited to extrapolate these potential time savings to their individual facilities. As Pelletier et al (2002) point out, Australian studies addressing time spent on documentation are sorely missing, but estimates from the United States suggest that nurses spend as much as 60% of their time undertaking manual documentation (Windle 1994). It is recognised that documentation could potentially incorporate recording other resident data in addition to care planning, but the issue remains that these processes do take up a substantial amount of nursing time.

Terminology

Terminology used within the defining characteristics section of the program required more clarification than previously anticipated or encountered. In some aged-care facilities, registered nurses who had attended training sessions subsequently showed personal care attendants how to use the planning software, and this latter group reported difficulties with the professional language used—examples include tachycardia, rhonchi and nocturia. The terminology in the web-enabled version was exactly the same as the PC version which preceded it. This observation gave rise to some spirited debate within groups about who should be involved in the care-planning process. One means of resolution suggested by the focus groups was to provide pop-up definitions of terms as the mouse is moved over the term, a facility which can be switched on or off as required. This technique is fairly commonly used within program interfaces to inform users of what clicking on various interface icons and buttons will achieve.

With the advent of computerised nursing documentation and care-planning systems it has also become increasingly apparent that these processes of sharing or examining data can be hampered in the absence of common nomenclature. Unfortunately, because of differences in nomenclature it is often difficult to collate data and map terms from one taxonomy to another, which in turn limits the ability of nurses to compare data with colleagues using another taxonomic approach. The Systematized Nomenclature of Medicine Clinical Terms, better known as SNOMED CT®, is an example of an attempt to provide a common language within health care. It is currently purported by SNOMED International to be in use in 28 countries worldwide. The taxonomy used within this care-planning development was that developed by NANDA, which is SNOMED-approved. It is interesting to note that in the course of both the PC and web-enabled implementation phases described in this chapter, various versions of the software have been used in around twenty Australian aged-care facilities, and no registered nurse at any of these sites has reported any difficulty in understanding the terminology used or applying the NANDA taxonomy within an aged-care environment.

Dialogue with other international nursing colleagues involved in language development and/or similar software development also underlines the need for nursing to assume a more convergent position on language development than is currently the case.

Data quality

Nurses reported that using the program led to more frequent collection of data, and customisation of care to suit individual residents. In addition, fewer errors and better quality of data in general were thought to result. Most nurses also felt that they were in control of the care plan.

Data mining and knowledge discovery

While the feedback from nurses using the web-enabled software remains encouraging, the potential to stockpile a large volume of data is clearly evident. As Chen et al (2002) point out, such volumes of data tend to overwhelm the abilities of manual processes to undertake analyses. However, use of a web-enabled software model provides opportunities for data mining and knowledge discovery. These authors make important distinctions between these terms. *Data mining* refers to the process of applying search algorithms to data in order to extract patterns from these data. *Knowledge discovery* refers to the additional steps of considering these patterns of data in the context of prior knowledge.

Nurses using a web-enabled care-planning tool should then give consideration to the types of data which can be automatically extracted from care plans. This may include—provided sites agree to do so, and existing privacy legislation is adhered to—data from multiple sites aggregated to show:

- the most common nursing diagnoses across sites;
- the most common nursing problems encountered;
- the most commonly resolved and unresolved resident problems; and
- timeframes to resolution of problems.

In this way substantive data can be presented for individual sites, regions or States. This information can be directly extracted from the care plans by means of automated background reporting tools, which are transparent to the user. Although manual processes could also achieve these reporting outcomes, they would be extremely time consuming and tedious.

THE FUTURE OF PAPER-BASED RECORDS

Because the demise of paper-based methods of recording resident care has been predicted for around thirty years it would seem foolhardy to now predict their imminent demise. However, the data gathered in this project is convergent with that from several others. In Canada, Romanow (2002) indicated that paper records clearly impose certain limitations on the flow of information, impede the integration of health care delivery, create barriers to research, and limit the information available for administration and decision-making

The term 'evidence-based practice' is also frequently used and nurses are encouraged to use this to guide their practice. While this stance is applauded, the volume of data in favour of computerised care planning and record systems from many countries must surely now require ongoing advocates of paper-based systems to provide substantive data to legitimate this proposed practice.

VIGNETTE

Computerised care planning: the clinician's perspective

Steve Demeye

It is a generally accepted notion that effective and efficient care planning is the lynchpin to the provision of holistic resident-centred care. Achieving consistency of outcomes that are both positive and meaningful for those charged to our care should be actively pursued and appropriately documented. Until recently there have been few options for staff working in aged care to explore anything other than conventional paper-based systems when considering the formulation of resident care plans. Recent advances in technology have made possible the efficient collection, collation and reporting of clinical data from the bedside. Clinical data collection in this format lends itself to the formulation of a full electronic resident medical record, including the resident care plan. Clinical data collection at the bedside has been taken one step further still, with the ability of those systems to be application service provider (ASP) based, with staff using secure connections across the world wide web to send and receive clinical data specific to individual residents. It was with the introduction of these advances that this facility sought to ultimately take the plunge into relatively unknown waters.

One of the most significant steps in the process was making the initial decision and commitment to implement a new clinical information system that on the one hand emulated current practices, but on the other was widely divergent from current processes. The decision to move forward was based on a clear understanding that while there were many benefits to be gained, there were also significant barriers to be overcome.

The benefits included:

- more efficient documentation practices;
- collection of a richer source of documentation in terms of quality and quantity of clinical information;
- increased ability to collate and report on clinical information; and
- the potential for improved clinical decision-making because of the availability of increased levels of clinical information.

The major barriers included:

- the widely ranging IT skills of staff;
- staff being firmly ensconced in paper-based systems and not necessarily wanting or seeing any benefit in moving from those systems;
- staff fearing IT and computers in general; and
- residents' and their families' concerns regarding issues of privacy.

Despite this, and subsequent to a review of the proposed IT system, it was clear that successful implementation would create a number of efficiencies. One area that was particularly exciting was the introduction of an 'expert system' for the purposes of producing resident care plans. Implementation of this aspect of the system alone had the potential to save significant time and effort by care staff in the process of generating and reviewing resident care plans. It was interesting to note that even in the early stages of exposing staff to the care-planning software through staff training exercises, staff very quickly picked up on the ability of the system to propose individual care deficits and associated interventions, which were sometimes overlooked using more conventional systems. This made the job of change management much easier to facilitate and was certainly a catalyst in the movement to full implementation of the system.

In order to implement the system with a minimum of resistance, a number of strategies were employed. Structuring the rollout of the system in a planned and staged manner was a key to getting staff to take up the new technology and associated processes. Gradually exposing staff to the advent of technology in the workplace, where virtually none had existed before, allowed them time to assimilate and consolidate knowledge gradually, rather than in a rush.

Early in the implementation phase it was decided that, rather than introducing equipment and processes that were completely unfamiliar to most staff, the introduction of more mainstream computing hardware (desktop computers) would be preferable to start with. Once the staff were comfortable with the feel, use and interface of the various software modules using the desktop computer, introduction of palm computers or personal digital assistants (PDAs) would be simply an extension of the principles already learned. While the software application was ASP based, with the advent of broadband internet connectivity, staff were ostensibly oblivious to the fact that they were transacting clinical information across the world wide web. Using a mouse, initiating the application was a simple point-and-double-click exercise. On loading, the web page was clear and uncluttered, offering the user easy navigation to their chosen destination. The various software modules offer the user an easy step-by-step approach to completing the various tasks required. The software applications were extremely user friendly and once started, users were easily engaged. This ease of user engagement was pivotal in enabling users to move freely through the system, experiment with the various options and produce an outcome that was both professional and polished.

Staff first had access to the system through hands-on training exercises. Initially staff were invited to attend training sessions, where they would pair up and work through a one-hour facilitated training session. This was augmented by staff having access to a software-training package that emulated the training session. Staff could run the training package at home or within the workplace. Further to this, as the application was internet-based, staff with home-based internet connections could, at their leisure, log onto the website and work through the principles learned in the training session. Feedback from staff at the training sessions was universally positive, with many subsequently reporting that they had accessed the software through their home-based internet connection.

Throughout the training sessions it was noted that a number of staff were very enthusiastic about the system and its capabilities. Those staff were asked to form a focus group with the objective of taking a closer look at the system and identifying strategies for successful implementation. They were given the job of designing new processes that involved other staff using the new hardware and software in their daily activities. The focus group identified a number of strategies, including:

- initially rolling out the system to a small, defined number of beds and practising with these first before embarking on full inclusion of all beds;
- placing appropriate discreet signage around the workplace to remind staff about the use of the hardware and associated software;
- in collaboration with staff, redeveloping duty lists that included the use of the new system;
- commencing a journal within the workplace that staff could access in order to jot down any issues or experiences they had with the system;
- sitting down with staff on a one-to-one basis to take them through the system; and
- concentrating on one aspect of the system at a time, ensuring that staff had full knowledge and were comfortable with its use and application. This meant initially using the electronic progress notes, then the care-planning software, and finally the RCS funding module.

Throughout the process, the focus group were gently steered in the required direction, and were given extra time outside their clinical workload to work with the system and develop the associated processes required for full rollout of the system and take-up by staff. Full support was offered through the software vendor, with the vendor acting on many of the staff comments, ideas and embellishments to make the system even more functional. Staff reacted well to this, as it promoted their perceived level of ownership.

In relation to concerns voiced by the resident/family group, an information session was conducted and individual residents and family members were invited to attend. Initially, the rollout of the system was conducted as a trial in which a small number of beds were targeted for inclusion on the new system. For residents who were initially included on the system, a consent form was drawn up, allowing them to withdraw from the trial if they so desired. It provided amongst other things a guarantee of privacy for information being transacted across the world wide web. It was anticipated that, following a successful and positive implementation across a trial group, full rollout and implementation to all beds would be facilitated using the trial group's experience as a springboard for others.

The whole process lasted approximately six months, from the initial decision to the final rollout and take-up by staff. There were many keys to the successful implementation of the system and these are best summarised as follows:

- involvement of staff at the very early stages and then continued involvement throughout the whole process;
- staging the implementation in small bite-sized pieces and ensuring that each piece was 'digested' before moving on to the next;
- identifying enthusiastic and willing users (champions) of the system early and giving them additional time, rights and ownership to drive the remaining staff group;
- recognising the wide variation in staff experience and comfort levels with IT and the associated processes, and targeting training and support at the lowest denominator;
- use of a journal for staff to record their experiences with the system;
- staff being able to access the system at home or in the workplace to build on skills learned in the training sessions; and
- involving the resident and relative group individually and giving them an opportunity to ask questions and make comments.

Without doubt, the implementation phase of the new clinical information system was an extremely positive one. Staff absorption of the new processes was better than anticipated. Although it is still too early to judge whether all the anticipated efficiencies have been achieved, early indications suggest that we are on the right track. We anticipate that while staff continue to use the system, their level of competence will also continue to expand. We look forward fervently to the new horizons to be uncovered as we continue to develop and work with this new and exciting technology.

CONCLUSION

Over the six years since the onset of this care-planning development, several key lessons have been learnt. First, it is critical to involve the end-users in product development if work flow and processes are to be modelled appropriately. Once the core functionality of the software had been established and evaluated, user focus groups worked as a method of determining the ongoing direction of development, because consensus was necessary before adding a new feature to the program.

It is also critical to get the software interface correct. If the use of the computer can be made as transparent as possible to the user, this allows them to focus on the task at hand—in this case care planning—and not be hindered by the additional task of interacting with the computer.

Even when every attempt is made to achieve transparency, some users will require extra assistance to gain confidence in using computerised care-planning systems. In this project this assistance was mainly provided in two ways: first by the program developers in the form of regular site visits to deal with user issues, and secondly by identifying competent and confident users in each facility who could provide support for their peers during the implementation phases.

Getting to the stage of the existing web-enabled version has taken many thousands of hours of development time and discussion. Those involved in computerising nursing documentation will no doubt be acutely aware of how time consuming and therefore how costly these developments are. Given this reality, it seems logical to build on what has been established as working, rather than continually attempting to build new systems from scratch.

When replacing paper-based systems it is important to think of how the computer solution will transform, and not simply replicate, a paper-based record. Currently available data aggregation and automatic reporting tools make it possible to automatically extract data produced for the primary purpose of care planning and present these for additional purposes such as staff or resource allocation, processes which would require substantial amounts of time if using paper-based tools.

Although some of these issues may appear to be of more pressing importance to software developers, it is crucial that gerontic nurses are also aware of these issues in order to empower them in discussions with developers, facility IT staff and other health-care professionals, and also to avoid having computer solutions imposed on them without consideration of their needs.

References

Agresti W 1986, New paradigms for software engineering, *IEEE Computer Society Meeting Paper*, IEEE: Washington.

Benfer R, Brent E & Furbee L 1991, *Expert Systems*, SAGE: London.

Bennett MJ 1986, Nursing Diagnosis—ramifications for nursing practice … In the Beginning, paper presented at Phillip Institute of Technology, *Proceedings of Nursing Diagnosis Seminar*, July 1986, Melbourne.

Chen M, Yu P & Liu B 2002, *Advances in knowledge discovery and data mining*. Proceedings of 6th Pacific-Asia Conference, PAKDD 2002, Taipei, Taiwan, May 6–8 2002, Springer: Berlin.

Chittaro L 2001, Information visualization and its application to medicine, *Artificial Intelligence in Medicine*, 22, pp 81–8.

Chou SC 1995, *Evaluation of an Expert System's Utility for Nursing Diagnosis*, unpublished minor thesis, RMIT, Melbourne.

Cook M 1982, Using computers to enhance professional practice, *Nursing Times*, 78(33), pp 1542–5.

Corkhill M 2001, Keeping track: electronic health records, *Collegian (Lifescape)*, 8(4).

Dahanayake A & Waltraud G 2002, *Web-enabled Systems Integration: Practice and Challenges*, Idea Group Publishing: Hershey, PA.

Darbyshire P 2000, The practice politics of computerised information systems: a focus group study. *Nurse Researcher*, 8(2), pp 4–17.

Durkin J 1994, *Expert Systems: Design and Development*, Macmillan: New York.

Eder L 2000, *Managing Healthcare Information Systems with Web-Enabled Technologies*, Idea Group Publishing: London.

Edwards W & Newman JR 1982, *Multiattribute Evaluation*, SAGE: Newbury Park.

Fineberg HV 1981, Medical decision making and the future of medical practice, *Medical Decision Making*, 1, pp 4–6.

Fisher AA & Fonteyn ME 1991, The nature of nursing experience. In: Grobe S & Pluyter-Wenting ESP (eds), *Nursing Informatics: An International Overview For Nursing in a Technological Era*, Elsevier: Amsterdam.

Galitz W 2002, *The Essential Guide to User Interface Design: An Introduction to GUI Design Principles and Techniques*, John Wiley: New York.

Hackos J & Redish J 1998, *User and Task Analysis for Interface Design*, Wiley: Sydney.

Hyslop A 1987, Are programs intelligent? *Nursing Times*, 83(8), pp 56–8.

Koch B 1997, Expert nurse: a PC-based expert system to provide decision support for nursing diagnosis in aged care, *Informatics in Healthcare Australia*, 6(1), pp 23–7.

Koch B 1999, *Development, Validation, and Evaluation of an Expert System to Provide Decision Support for Nursing Diagnosis in Aged Care*, unpublished PhD thesis, RMIT: Melbourne.

Koch B & McGovern J 1993, EXTEND: a prototype expert system to teach nursing diagnosis, *Computers in Nursing*, 11(1), pp 35–41.

Norman DA 1988, *The Psychology of Everyday Things*, Basic Books: New York.

Pelletier D, Duffield C, Gietzelt D, Larkin P & Franks H 2002, Global aging. The complexities of documenting clinical information in long-term care settings in Australia, *Journal of Gerontological Nursing*, 28(5), pp 8–12.

Prescott PA, Ryan JW, Soeken KL, Castorr AH, Thompson KO & Phillips CY 1991, The patient intensity for nursing index: a validity assessment, *Research in Nursing and Health*, 14(3), pp 213–21.

Radosevich L 1999, AI wises up, *Infoworld*, 20(31), pp 1–6.

Regan-Kubinski MJ 1991, A model of clinical judgement processes in psychiatric nursing, *Archives of Psychiatric Nursing*, 5, pp 262–70.

Romanow R 2002, Building on values; the future of health care in Canada, *Commission on the Future of Health Care in Canada Final Report*, Saskatoon.

Standish Group 1995, The Chaos Report. Online: http://www.pm2go.com/sample_research/chaos_1994_1.php, retrieved 8 July 2003.

Watt S 1987, Applications of computers in nurse management. In: Koch B & Rankin J (eds), *Computers and Their Application in Nursing*, pp 1–16, Harper and Row: London.

Webopedia 2003. Online: http://www.webopedia.com/TERM/e/expert_system.html, retrieved 1 July 2003.

Wilkinson S 1998, Focus group methodology: a review, *International Journal of Social Research Methodology, Theory and Practice*, 1(3), pp 22–37.

Windle P 1994, Critical pathways: an integrated documentation tool, *Nurse Management*, 25(9), 80F–80L, 80P.

Part 3

Research issues and innovations

CHAPTER 19

Evidence-based nursing: quality through research

ALAN PEARSON

INTRODUCTION

This chapter examines the link between quality improvement and the use of research findings in practice. The findings of research are a central source of *evidence* for practice and the need for an evidence-based approach is increasingly being advocated in aged care. This chapter discusses how nurses who practise in this specialist field can improve quality through incorporating the most up-to-date evidence into the care process. The focus is essentially on residential care, but this can be applied to the care of older people in their own homes and other non-residential-care settings.

APPLYING RESEARCH IN AGED-CARE PRACTICE

What research there is on the practices which occur in aged-care settings suggests that the main focus is on the maintenance of traditional patterns of care and compliance with managerial dictates, rather than on research-based activity and intervention (Pearson 1989; Pearson et al 1990; Pincombe et al 1996; Nay 1993; Retsas 1997).

The successful residential-care facilities of the future will be those that pay attention to the constant search for information needed to guide care practices, and everyday practice will change as a result of this.

The provision of residential care for the aged and vulnerable has been subject to considerable public criticism and reform in Australia since Federation. This pressure on governments to reform aged care has increased since the late 1970s because of the ageing of the population. A major, highly sequenced and planned aged-care reform process commenced in 1985 and a new wave of reform commenced in 1996–97 following the election of a new federal government.

Because of the high costs of aged care on the one hand, and the demands of the community for common standards of care on the other, governments are politically bound to improve care at minimal cost. In the 1996–97 Budget, the incoming coalition government announced its plans to engage in far-reaching reform of residential aged care to ensure dignity, comfort and security for older Australians.

When the *Aged Care Bill 1997* passed through Parliament, a new framework for reform was rapidly developed. Central to the reforms was the introduction of a system of accreditation of the aged-care industry. Although this system of accreditation continues to be largely based on management, systems and outcome audits, evidence-based practice is included as an element of the process. The accreditation process involves the assessment of a residential aged-care facility in five broad areas:

- the quality of care and services;
- the quality of accommodation;
- the management of accommodation bonds;
- the ratio of residents who are exempt from the payment of accommodation bonds to those who are not; and
- consumer protection.

The first of these—the quality of care and services—consists of four major factors:

- management systems, staffing and organisation development;
- health and personal care;
- residential lifestyle; and
- physical environment and safe systems.

Within each of these factors are subsets of specific standards. Most of these sub-sets relate to resident needs and the practices that aim to meet those needs, but which have virtually no research foundation. Many of these practices are based solely on custom and practice, or on the knowledge nurses gain from experience. This is not to say that all of these practices are inappropriate. However, were nurses asked to defend their practices, they would often be unable to do so.

A recent search of the international literature revealed that only a small proportion of references to aged care were the result of any form of systematic research. Of these, none involved the study of aged-care practices in terms of their effectiveness. A similar search, which concentrated on the use of research findings or evidence, revealed even fewer papers that mentioned this, and none reported a regular reliance on best available evidence within the aged-care sector internationally.

It seems clear that changing practice so that it has a growing reliance on evidence is an important goal for the aged-care sector, and that current reforms will increasingly demand that this occurs.

BASING PRACTICE ON THE BEST AVAILABLE EVIDENCE

Evidence-based nursing, although a new term, is a much older concept. Nurses have been talking about, and encouraged to engage in, 'research-based practice'. Evidence-based nursing is the same thing as research-based practice in nursing. As more knowledge is generated through research, and as the ability to transmit information via such media as the internet or direct broadcast increases, all professionals in all fields will come under increasing pressure to show that they are abreast of current knowledge, and that they exhibit this through delivering services which are in line with the most recent and rigorous evidence.

Evidence of use to nursing can be derived from a variety of sources. Although the results of scientific, experimental research can be an excellent source of evidence on which to base those areas of practice that relate to definable interventions, much of nursing is subjective and not amenable to measurement and experiment. Other sources of evidence which can underpin the nursing of older people include:

- research that focuses on qualitative issues and data;
- expert, consensus opinion; and
- the collective experiences and stories of older people and their carers.

Evidence-based nursing is nursing which draws on the most up-to-date evidence in the planning and delivery of care. It is frequently confused with basing practice on the results of research into effectiveness.

RESEARCH INTO EFFECTIVENESS AND EVIDENCE-BASED PRACTICE

By definition, research into effectiveness refers directly to the relationship between a cause and an effect. It is concerned with such questions as: *If X is given/applied/carried out, what effect will it have on Y?* The worldwide evidence-based medicine (EBM) movement—now often referred to as evidence-based health practice—is essentially concerned with evidence on effectiveness (see below).

A wide range of care practices in aged care can be guided by this kind of evidence. For example, the prevention and treatment of pressure ulcers (Joanna Briggs Institute [JBI] 1997b,c), and the management of leg ulcers (Roe et al 1994; Cullum 1994), are common problems in aged care, and interventions which are not based on the best available quantitative evidence are clearly inappropriate.

VIGNETTE

Evidence-based practice in action: wound care

Bart O'Brien

Current wisdom in wound management stresses the benefits of moist wound healing over dry options. In a recent education session with staff of an aged-care facility, the discussion turned to the success they had been having with the use of simple, non-occlusive dry dressings for skin tears. Staff observed that using moist occlusive dressings seemed to extend wound-healing times, and that there was frequently accumulation of pus under these dressings even if the wound did not become infected.

The anecdotal impressions presented by the staff sounded contrary to the expectations of contemporary wound management theory. It came as a pleasant surprise to read, a few weeks later, of an Australian study which supported the observations of staff in this facility that skin tears respond better to non-occlusive dressings.

Edwards et al (1998) had demonstrated, in a controlled pilot study of four dressing types, that the non-occlusive option led to faster healing, lower rates of wound breakdown/infection, and potential cost advantages. Although cautious about the small numbers in their study, the researchers had thus lent some support to the clinical observations of staff, who now have the published evidence of Edwards et al (1998) to substantiate their personal anecdotal observations.

However, a systematic review of all rigorous research on skin tears is required to provide stronger evidence to justify practice. Such a review may demonstrate that further original research is required to settle the issue. Although Edwards et al (1998) have pointed in a certain direction, it would be premature to assume that theirs is the last word on the subject.

This brief vignette highlights a number of matters:

- the importance of staff being observant in their professional experience and being prepared to critically examine accepted practice;
- the value of evidence-based research in providing guidance to rational and effective nursing practice; and
- the need for ongoing, thorough research to confirm (or deny) anecdotal clinical experience and initial research findings.

EVIDENCE FOR PRACTICE IN AGED CARE

The term 'evidence' is generally used to mean substantiation or confirmation of an issue. When used in relation to clinical practice, health professionals seek evidence to substantiate the worth of a very wide range of activities and interventions, and thus the type of evidence needed depends on the nature of the activity and its purpose.

Evidence of effectiveness

Effectiveness is the extent to which an intervention, when used appropriately, achieves the intended effect. Clinical effectiveness is about the relationship between an intervention and clinical or health outcomes. Thus, when one is seeking evidence of effectiveness, the focus is on the objective measurement of the effect of an intervention on specific outcomes. An example of evidence of effectiveness is the measurement of wound healing rates when a dry dressing is applied. To establish the effectiveness of this intervention on the outcome (healing rates), the intervention must be administered in the same way for all the subjects and the outcomes must also be measured in the same way. The most reliable approach to generating evidence of effectiveness is the conduct of a controlled clinical trial where residents are randomised to a treatment group; as many of the variables as possible are controlled so that only the effects of the intervention are likely to have led to the outcome, and quantitative measurements are compared using statistical techniques.

Evidence of appropriateness and meaningfulness

Appropriateness is the extent to which an intervention or activity *fits with* or is *apt in* a situation. Meaningfulness is about how an activity or intervention relates to the context in which care is given and the personal experience, opinions, values, thoughts, beliefs and interpretations of residents or clients. In the example of the effectiveness of the use of dry dressings on wounds, we may well find that it is less effective in achieving the outcome of increased healing compared to moist applications, but if we were interested in how appropriate or meaningful such an intervention is for the resident, we would be seeking the residents' accounts of their own experience, and the evidence from this perspective may not be as positive as the evidence of effectiveness. Evidence of appropriateness and meaningfulness is best generated through the rigorous conduct of interpretative research with residents.

Evidence of feasibility

Feasibility is the extent to which an activity is practical. Clinical feasibility is about whether or not an activity or intervention is physically, culturally or financially practical or possible within a given context. In our wound healing example, although moist dressings may be more effective and may even be appropriate and meaningful, in low socioeconomic populations it may not be feasible because of its cost.

The evidence-based practice movement focuses largely on *evidence of effectiveness*. Pearson, in arguing that evidence-based practice should include an interest in research into clinical effectiveness but is not confined to this interest, says:

> randomised trials are the gold standard for phenomena that we are interested in studying from a cause and effect perspective, but clearly they are not the gold standard if we are interested in how patients and nurses relate to each other, or if we are interested in how patients live through the experience of radiotherapy when they have a life threatening illness. We have yet to work out how to assess the quality of alternative approaches to research other than the RCT.
>
> Pearson 1998

Pearson goes on to suggest that 'evidence-based practice is not exclusively about effectiveness; it is about basing practice on the best available evidence'.

The diverse origins of problems in aged care require a diversity of research methodologies. Thus, methodological approaches in this area need to be eclectic enough to incorporate both classical, medical and scientific designs and the emerging qualitative and action-oriented approaches from the humanities and the social and behavioural sciences. The development of interdisciplinary research and a greater understanding of the relationship between medical, nursing and allied health interventions are also fundamental to the emergence of research methodologies which are relevant and sensitive to the health needs of consumers.

The nature of evidence

In general terms, *evidence* refers to data or information used to decide whether or not a claim or view should be trusted. In aged care, practitioners, residents and their families make numerous decisions and, in doing so, draw on numerous sources of information and weigh it up before taking action. Although an obvious source of evidence are the results of well-designed research, they are by no means the only data used in everyday practice; the resident and her or his relevant others, the practitioners' own experiences, and the nature and norms of the setting and culture within which care is being delivered, are all rich sources of evidence to draw on in making clinical decisions.

RESEARCH

Research is essentially the systematic search for truth or knowledge. Such a fundamental enterprise is, of necessity, the subject of much scrutiny, debate and opinion. There are therefore a wide range of views and perspectives on what constitutes 'good' research, how varying research approaches can be classified, and how the research process can best be understood and communicated.

Since the emergence of modern science in the eighteenth century, health professionals have pursued a number of different pathways to develop their work (clinical practice) and to generate knowledge (medical, nursing and health science). Science is systematically developed knowledge and is advancing rapidly internationally as health professionals increasingly engage in research from both a qualitative and a quantitative perspective.

- *Qualitative data* is collected in order to derive understanding of phenomena from a subjective perspective. The focus is on description, understanding and empowerment. Theory can be developed through a process of inductive reasoning, grounded in reality as it is perceived and experienced by the participants.

- Conversely, *quantitative data* is collected in order to control phenomena. The focus is on theory testing, prediction and control. Theory derived from previous research is used to formulate a hypothesis or testable idea. Based on the process of deduction, the hypothesis is then tested using objective methods.

The relative merits of both these forms of data are the subject of much heated debate in the health-care system. On the one hand, qualitative methods are seen to most certainly increase understanding but they are often criticised as 'biased' and subjected to the question, 'Well, now that we understand, so what?'. On the other hand, quantitative methods are seen to give an apparently unbiased, objective picture of a situation or phenomenon, but they are often criticised as being 'only half the story' or of being overly concerned with numbers and statistics.

DEVELOPMENTS IN USING RESEARCH IN AGED CARE IN AUSTRALASIA

The Joanna Briggs Institute (JBI) and The Australian Centre for Evidence Based Aged Care (ACEBAC) are contributing significantly to the summarising of international evidence to support research utilisation and evidence-based practice in aged care.

The Joanna Briggs Institute

The Joanna Briggs Institute (JBI) is an international research collaboration established in 1996. The headquarters of JBI, located at Royal Adelaide Hospital, South Australia, coordinates collaborating centres in nursing in all Australian States and Territories, New Zealand, England, Thailand, Spain and Hong Kong; in physiotherapy, occupational therapy, medical radiation in Adelaide; in nutrition and dietetics in Newcastle, New South Wales; in Rural Health in Queensland; and in aged care in Melbourne. The aims of the collaboration are to improve the effectiveness of health-care practice and health-care outcomes by:

- conducting systematic reviews and analyses of the research literature;
- collaborating with expert researchers and clinicians to facilitate the development of practice-information sheets based on the systematic review of research;

- participating in the dissemination and implementation of practice information sheets and evaluating their impact on practice;
- initiating randomised clinical trials and other primary research when indicated by the findings of the systematic review; and
- contributing to cost-effective health care through the promotion of evidence-based practice.

The JBI has the feasibility, appropriateness, meaningfulness and effectiveness of health-care practices as its central focus and regards the results of well-designed research studies grounded in any methodological position as providing more rigorous evidence than do anecdotes or personal opinion. The approach which the JBI takes to evaluate evidence is tailored to the specific focus of the review, and all types of evidence are included. The development and peer review of a protocol is fundamental to the JBI approach to reviews (JBI 1997a).

In conducting systematic reviews, the JBI follows the process developed by the Cochrane Collaboration. However, unlike the Cochrane Collaboration, the JBI does not establish review groups which engage in ongoing reviews and continuous updates. Based on the approach of the NHS Centre for Reviews and Dissemination at the University of York (University of York 1996), a JBI review is undertaken by a consultant who works to a review panel, and the review process is confined to a period of six months. Updates of reviews are undertaken when required, as identified at annual strategic-planning meetings.

Every systematic review conducted by the JBI is managed and supervised by a review panel consisting of staff from the Adelaide headquarters, expert nursing clinicians, expert clinicians from related fields (where appropriate), a nursing researcher, a nursing manager, and representatives of special-interest groups where appropriate.

When a draft review report and practice-information sheet is complete, both are distributed to at least one expert in the field associated with every JBI centre for comment and feedback. When agreement is reached by all centres, the review report is written up as a Best-Practice Information Sheet. These are widely distributed as free inserts in Australian, New Zealand, Irish and Hong Kong nursing journals. Every practice-information sheet published is evaluated in terms of its effect on practice variability.

The Institute conducts workshops designed to teach nurses about evidence-based nursing, and to encourage its implementation. The JBI also offers support to organisations and individuals who become members of the Institute.

The Australian Centre for Evidence Based Aged Care

The Australian Centre for Evidence Based Aged Care (ACEBAC) is a collaborating centre of JBI and is located at Bundoora Extended Care Centre (BECC) and is a part of La Trobe University, Melbourne. It aims to improve service delivery in aged care through research programs that focus on:

- the conduct of systematic reviews and analysis of the literature in areas such as continuous quality improvement in aged care, the development of innovative models of care delivery, and clinical effectiveness in aged care;

- developing and evaluating guidelines for best practice in service delivery and organisation in aged care, based on the systematic review of research findings;
- conducting international, multisite programs to implement best practice guidelines; and
- evaluating the impact of the implementation of best practice guidelines on health and social outcomes in aged care.

EVIDENCE THAT GUIDES AGED-CARE PRACTICE

The JBI has established an evidence review program specifically for aged care, as part of the JBI Clinical Information Service. The JBI Clinical Information Service conducts evidence reviews on clinical practice topics to support the development of evidence-based policy and practice manuals for corporate members. An evidence review involves the initial review of current research literature on a wide range of topics and a subsequent review update each year. The evidence review process consists of a systematic search of published literature, the critical appraisal of studies retrieved, and the development of an evidence summary and recommendations for practice. The quality of the evidence is rated following the standard approach of:

- **Level I:** Evidence obtained from a systematic review of all relevant randomised controlled trials.
- **Level II:** Evidence obtained from at least one properly designed randomised controlled trial.
- **Level III:** Evidence obtained from well-designed controlled trials without randomisation, or evidence obtained from well-designed cohort or case control analytic studies, preferably from more than one centre or research group. Or evidence obtained from multiple time series with or without the intervention.
- **Level IV:** Opinions of respected authorities, based on clinical experience, descriptive studies or reports of expert committees. Or evidence obtained from descriptive studies of provider practices, patient behaviours, knowledge or attitudes or a systematic review of descriptive studies.

THE JBI CLINICAL INFORMATION DATABASE

The JBI Clinical Information Database consists of standardised summaries on a wide range of health-care interventions and activities identified by corporate members. Each year, every existing entry is updated and new entries are added in response to requests from corporate members.

The standardised format for each entry is:

Intervention/activity

Equipment/materials needed

Recommended practice

Narrative summary of the evidence review

Level of evidence

References/further reading.

An evidence review follows an Evidence Review Protocol:

Topic

Objectives

Criteria for considering studies for this review

Key words for identification of studies

Selecting studies for inclusion

Date review to commence

Date review to complete

Date for review update

'Alert' strategy for continuous update

Critical appraisal and strategies of summarising the retrieved papers follow the standardised JBI approach. Examples of evidence reviews in aged care include:

- admission to residential aged-care facilities
- nasoenteric feeding management
- restraint
- external urethral drainage (condom drainage).

Admission to residential aged-care facilities: the evidence

(Joanna Briggs Institute 2003)

This evidence review relates to the development of patient-focused care plans and the role of welcoming patients to reduce personal anxiety. The review identifies the following evidence points for practice:

- Admission to a residential-care facility should be seen as part of the process of care, not a procedure (Price 1983).
- The relationship between nurse and resident begins with the opportunity for the nurse to help new clients feel respected, understood and empowered through the provision of information (Bender et al 1994).
- The initial greeting is part of a continuum of care, which for the resident began before admission and may extend beyond discharge (Price 1983). It is, in effect, an acknowledgement that people have social, psychological and physical needs.
- This holistic perspective may be enhanced by the development of service-oriented corporate vision statements (Price 1983).
- Resident assessment is recognised throughout the literature as the defining phase that determines nursing care for the resident (Holt 1995; Wright 1992; Young-Meyer 1992; James & Reaby 1987).

- The relationship between effective nursing practice and quality, outcomes-based care in aged-care facilities has been described as a series of planning stages. The focus is on identifying needs and problem-solving strategies with the residents and their significant others within the social community (Department of Health and Aged Care 1998). In developing care plans for older adults, the nursing process is used to identify the individual's capabilities, needs and problems—actual and potential.

- Ensuring the older adult is significantly involved in making informed choices about accommodation is identified as significant in producing a positive long-term outcome (Nolan et al 1996).

Nasoenteric feeding management: the evidence

(Joanna Briggs Institute 2003)

Nasoenteric feeding is indicated to be the method of choice for patients with functional gastrointestinal tracts (Arrowsmith 1993). The advantages of enteral feeding identified by Ziccardi et al (1993) include low cost, simplicity of administration, the ability to deliver large quantities of nutrients and a low incidence of complications. The ability to tailor feeds to the individual's metabolic requirements, the maintenance of the enteral mucosa, and enhanced immunocompetence are also reported. The review identifies the following evidence points for practice.

Risk factors

The literature recommends identification of patients at high risk for complications prior to the commencement of feeding. Risk factors for aspiration include pregnancy, peptic ulcer disease, obesity, extreme age, hiatal hernia and neurological impairment (Huerta & Puri 2000). Eisenberg (1994) stated that patients with neurological deficits and/or reduced gag reflex should be considered at high risk for complications related to gastric feeding.

Nursing care

- Nursing staff are the most significant care providers in the assessment, prevention and recognition of complications associated with nasoenteric feeding (Arrowsmith 1993). Nursing care associated with nasoenteric tubes includes promotion of patient comfort, patient safety and tube maintenance. Patient comfort has been associated with improved compliance and tolerance of nasoenteric tube maintenance and a decreased risk of complications arising from nasal tube placement (Reilly 1998).

- Residual checks, listening for bowel sounds, observation for abdominal distension and investigation of any references made by the patient regarding bloating, 'fullness' or associated problems is reported to reduce the risk and severity of aspiration (Eisenberg 1994).

- Continuous feeds increase the risk of aspiration as the oesophageal sphincter remains open; nursing the patient at a minimum of 30° elevation and jejunal tube placement are reported to reduce the risk (Eisenberg 1994).

- The value of general observation for nasal erosion, encrustation and oral hygiene is also emphasised.

- The literature indicated that nasal care should include daily changing of tape adhering to the nose and cleansing of the nose to remove oils and build-up of adhesives from the tape on the nose (Reilly 1998).

- Weekly or twice-weekly weighing of the patient is thought to be more effective than daily weighing as this reduces the influence of daily variations in fluid balance (Arrowsmith 1993).

- Extended periods of fasting prior to commencement of nasoenteric feeds increases the risk of 'refeeding syndrome'. This is characterised by significant shifts in fluid balance and altered metabolic functioning.

- Accurate recording of fluid input and output, particularly in vulnerable patient groups such as the neurologically impaired and in the presence of renal failure, is a key process in the detection of refeeding syndrome (Arrowsmith 1993).

- Patient safety issues identified in the literature on nasoenteric feeding relate to ongoing verification of tube position, tube patency and the risk of aspiration. Measurement and documentation of limiting marks is recommended as a method of determining whether the tube has slipped (Arrowsmith 1993; Reilly 1998). Eisenberg (1994) recommended checking the tube length after initial insertion, prior to each feed and once per shift in continuous feeds. However, measurement of tube length does not indicate whether internal migration of the tube has occurred. Migration has been reported to occur downward into the duodenum or jejunum as well as upward into the oropharynx or lungs (Rakel et al 1994).

- Severe vomiting or coughing may displace some tubes and radiographs may be required to verify tube position (American Gastroenterological Association 1994). Methods of monitoring should then have the capability of determining with precision all possible outcomes of migration.

- Air auscultations, altered phonation, visualisation of aspirate, and pH testing of aspirate have been reported as unreliable indicators of placement (Arrowsmith 1993; Rakel et al 1994).

- Tube patency is important for maintaining nutritional and fluid balance requirements. Nasoenteric tubes are susceptible to occlusion following interruptions to the feeding regimen, gastric aspiration and medication administration (Arrowsmith 1993).

The use of restraint: the evidence

(Joanna Briggs Institute 2003)

The systematic review conducted by JBI suggests that 12% to a maximum of 47% of residents are restrained, while 32% of residents are restrained for at least 20 days each month in the residential-care sector. These findings suggested that a large number of residents are subjected to physical restraint. There is great variability in practice in terms of the devices used, the proportion of people restrained and the period of restraint (Evans et al 2002).

Findings of the systematic review suggest that within the residential care setting, restraint is more common for the frail elderly, and factors such as incontinence and inability to independently perform activities of daily living increase the likelihood of restraint (Evans et al 2002). Restraint within a residential-care setting is associated with a number of adverse outcomes such as a decline in social behaviour, cognition and mobility and an increase in disorientation, development of pressure sores and bladder or bowel incontinence. Based on limited evidence, the risk of injury is greater for residents who were subjected to continuous restraint and the discontinuation of restraint appeared to reduce the risk of falls-related injuries (Evans et al 2002).

The systematic review also evaluated research that discussed the use of restraint-minimisation programs. There was scant research found and only one randomised controlled trial (evaluating the impact of restraint education programs within a residential-care setting) was found.

Education is identified as an integral component of a restraint minimisation program. However, there is little evidence regarding the optimal format, timing and duration (Evans et al 2002).

A number of recommendations for practice were reported in the review:

- Organisations and health-care providers should adopt a standardised approach to the use of physical restraint devices.
- Physical restraint should only be used as a last resort, and when the potential benefits are greater than the potential harm secondary to the enforced immobility caused by the restraint.
- Only the minimal level of restraint that ensures the safety of the person should be used.
- The need for restraint should be reviewed regularly.

The systematic review acknowledged that limited evidence existed on many of the issues related to the use of physical restraint devices. Despite this, several suggestions for practice were made based on the findings of a number of different studies and investigations to minimise the risk of injury. These included:

- ensuring correct application of the restraint device;
- maintaining appropriate observation during the period of time a person is restrained; and
- providing staff orientation and in-service education on the correct use of physical restraint devices.

CONCLUSION

The diverse problems in aged-care practices require a diversity of research methodologies—and a great deal of current nursing research is grounded in approaches which value qualitative data and the use of interpretation. The emphasis on randomised controlled trials in the evidence-based practice movement has been criticised by many nurses, although little of this criticism is evident in the literature. From a nursing perspective, the selection of research studies for systematic review needs to be eclectic enough to incorporate both classical medical/scientific designs, and the emerging qualitative/action–orientated approaches from the humanities and the social and behavioural sciences.

Evidence-based practice in health care has become well established and it is likely that the Australian aged-care reforms will put an increasing emphasis on the need for practices to be based on the best available evidence. Nurses practising in aged care will need to consider how they can become full participants in the evidence-based practice agenda.

VIGNETTE

A reflection on evidence–based practice

Bart O'Brien

Evidence-based practice (EBP) can be seen as yet another imposition on already stretched resources. Alternatively, it can be viewed as a boon for busy practitioners and managers, especially with the assistance of such bodies as the Cochrane Collaboration and the Joanna Briggs Institute for Evidence Based Nursing (JBI), who are increasingly doing the hard work of reviewing the enormous research output related to aged-care nursing.

Aged-care organisations and individual practitioners can adopt EBP in two ways: by responding to EBP, or by initiating EBP. Those who are responsive will integrate themselves with the range of resources from which guides to EBP can be obtained. Those who show initiative will, in addition to accessing this available material, demonstrate a commitment to upgrading the levels of evidence currently available.

For both groups, there is the initial requirement to develop a clear understanding of what EBP is and how it affects clinical practice. As noted previously in this chapter, EBP is a movement towards increasing 'effectiveness' in clinical practice. Different levels of evidence are used to confirm the effectiveness of clinical interventions such that clinicians using EBP can be increasingly sure that their practice is justifiable in a given context. The Cochrane Collaboration and the JBI define and confirm different levels of evidence, and undertake the task of rigorously evaluating the increasing mass of clinical research. Nurses can now increasingly refer to these bodies for summaries of best practice, thus reducing the need to continuously review the published literature, and the need to choose which studies are relevant, and which are rigorous enough, to incorporate into procedures and clinical practice.

Responding to EBP

Health agencies that subscribe to the JBI receive:

- open access to all practice-information sheets through the Institute's web page;
- a bound, customised EBP manual;
- copies of all practice information sheets and binders for each ward or full-time equivalent (FTE) community nurse;
- opportunities to participate in practice-variability studies; and
- copies of the Institute's bimonthly bulletin.

Subscribing to one of the contemporary Australian nursing journals will also help clinical nurses to stay in touch. Practice information sheets, produced by the JBI, are regularly disseminated through these journals, and they also publish articles about EBP.

Initiating EBP

Aged care has a respectable history in the development of best practice and EBP. Examples of this initiative are the two nursing development units (NDUs) which were established at Julia Farr Centre in 1991 for the specific purpose of researching and developing aged-care and extended-care nursing (O'Brien 1996; O'Brien & Pope 1994). Among the work undertaken by these NDUs has been research into therapeutic regimens for topical steroids and antifungals, best practice in long-term tracheostomy care, and gastrostomy management. These projects were developed from literature searches which revealed that there was very little published research in these fields. Work done in the NDUs was used to write procedures and treatment protocols for the organisation as a whole.

Initiatives such as journal clubs, which encourage participants to develop skills in critical review of relevant published material, and specialist working parties, can also help organisations to decide whether there is available evidence to support existing practice. Where there is little supporting evidence, the organisation has to justify current practice. One emerging option is the use of the increasing number of post-graduate students. By developing working links with local universities, aged-care organisations may well be able to tap into a group of committed researchers who are possibly looking for research topics, who are bound by the university's ethical and research requirements, and who are supported by its supervisory capacity.

Conclusion

For nurses practising in the field of aged care, the emergence and development of EBP is both a blessing and an opportunity. The burgeoning mass of published research is increasingly being critically reviewed and summarised by resources to which individuals and aged-care organisations are unlikely to have had access in the past. In addition, the principles of research critique, and the accepted guides to various levels of evidence, make individual review possible.

Whether organisations and individuals choose to take advantage of the increasing volume of published EBP guidelines, or whether they initiate research into unexplored aspects of aged care, the result can only be for the benefit of Australia's ageing population.

References

American Gastroenterological Association 1994, Medical position statement: *Guidelines for the Use of Enteral Nutrition.*

Arrowsmith H 1993, Nursing management of patients receiving a nasogastric feed, *British Journal of Nursing*, 2(21), pp 1053–8.

Bender M, Joslin G & Mitchell C 1994, Welcoming patients—an underrated necessity, *Nursing Times*, 90(49), pp 36–7.

Cochrane AL 1979, 1931–1971: A critical review, with particular reference to the medical profession. In: *Medicines for the Year 2000*, pp 1–11, Office of Health Economics: London.

Commonwealth Department of Health and Family Services 1997, *Living In Nursing Homes: Outcome Standards*, AGPS: Canberra.

Cullum NA 1994, *The Nursing Management of Leg Ulcers in the Community: A Critical Review of Research*, Report to the Department of Health from the Department of Nursing, University of Liverpool: UK.

Department of Health and Aged Care, Aged and Community Care Division 1998, *Documentation and Accountability Manual*, Commonwealth Department of Health and Aged Care, Canberra.

Edwards H, Gaskill D & Nash R 1998, Treating skin tears in nursing-home residents: a pilot study comparing four types of dressings, *International Journal of Nursing Practice*, 4(1), pp 25–32.

Eisenberg P 1994, Nasoenteral tubes, *RN*, 57(10), pp 62–9.

Evans D, Wood J, Lambert L & Fitzgerald M 2002, *Physical Restraint in Acute and Residential Care: A Systematic Review*, No. 22, The Joanna Briggs Institute, Adelaide.

Holt P 1995, Role of questioning skills in patient assessment, *British Journal of Nursing*, 4(19), pp 1145–8.

Huerta G & Puri VK 2000, Nasoenteric feeding tubes in critically ill patients (fluoroscopy versus blind), *Nutrition*, 16(4), pp 264–7.

James J & Reaby L 1987, physical assessment, skills for RNs? *The Australian Nurses Journal*, 17(1), pp 39–41.

Joanna Briggs Institute for Evidence Based Nursing (JBI) 1997a, *Administrative Guidelines*, JBI: Adelaide.

Joanna Briggs Institute for Evidence Based Nursing (JBI) 1997b, *Pressure Sores—Part 1: Prevention of Pressure-related Damage*, Best-Practice Information Sheet 1: 1, Blackwell Science: Melbourne.

Joanna Briggs Institute for Evidence Based Nursing (JBI) 1997c, *Pressure Sores—Part II: Management of Pressure-related Damage*, Best-Practice Information Sheet 1: 2, Blackwell Science: Melbourne.

Nay R 1993, *Benevolent Oppression*, unpublished PhD thesis, University of New South Wales: Sydney.

Nolan M, Walker G, Nolan J, Williams S, Poland F, Curran M & Kent B 1996, Entry to care: positive choice or fait accompli? Developing a more proactive nursing response to the needs of older people and their carers, *Journal of Advanced Nursing*, 24, pp 265–74.

O'Brien B & Pope J 1994, Julia Farr Centre Nursing Development Unit. In: Johns C (ed), *The Burford NDU Model*, Blackwell Science: Oxford.

O'Brien B 1996, Developing a practice-based model of nursing. In: Greenwood J (ed), *Nursing Theory in Australia: Development and Application*, Harper Educational: Sydney.

Pearson A 1989, *Optimum Staffing Mix to Obtain Desired Outcomes in Non-government Nursing Homes: A Review of the Literature*, Deakin Institute of Nursing Research: Victoria.

Pearson A 1998, Excellence in care: future directions for effective nursing, *NT Research*, 3(1), pp 25–7.

Pearson A, Hocking S, Mott S & Riggs A 1990, *Optimum Staffing Mix to Obtain Desired Resident Outcomes in Non-government Nursing Homes*, AGPS: Canberra.

Pearson A, Borbasi S, Fitzgerald M, Kowanko I & Walsh K 1997, Evidence-based nursing: an examination of nursing within the international evidence-based health-care practice movement, *Nursing Review*, February: 1–4 (Suppl), pp 1–4.

Pincombe J, O'Brien B, Cheek J & Ballantyne A 1996, Critical aspects of nursing in aged and extended care, *Journal of Advanced Nursing*, 23(4), pp 672–8.

Price B 1983, Just a few forms to fill in, *Nursing Times*, 79(44), pp 26–8.

Rakel B, Titler M, Goode C, Barry-Walker J, Budreau G & Buckwalter K 1994, Nasogastric and nasointestinal feeding tube placement: an integrative review of research, *AACN Clinical Issues in Critical Care*, 5(2), pp 194–206.

Reilly H 1998, Enteral feeding: an overview of indications and techniques, *British Journal of Nursing*, 7(9), pp 510–21.

Retsas A 1997, The use of physical restraints in Western Australian nursing homes, *Australian Journal of Advanced Nursing*, 14(3), pp 33–9.

Roe BH, Griffiths JM, Kenrick M, Cullum NA & Hutton, JL 1994, Nursing treatment of patients with chronic leg ulcers in the community, *Journal of Clinical Nursing*, 3, pp 159–68.

Sackett DL & Rosenberg WMC 1995, The need for evidence-based medicine, *Journal of the Royal Society of Medicine*, 88, pp 620–4.

Sackett DL, Rosenberg WMC, Gray JAM, Haynes RB & Richardson WS 1996, Evidence-based medicine: what it is and what it is not, *British Medical Journal*, 312, pp 71–2.

University of York 1996, *Undertaking Systematic Reviews of Research on Effectiveness*, CRD Report 4, NHS Centre for Reviews & Dissemination, University of York: York.

Wright K 1992, An overview of the nursing process, *Gastroenterology Nursing*, 15(1), pp 14–17.

Young-Meyer V 1992, A two-level approach to the nursing process, *Journal of Nursing Staff Development*, 9(5), pp 230–5.

Ziccardi V, Ochs M & Braun T 1993, Indications for enteric tube feedings in oral and maxillofacial surgery, *Journal of Oral Maxillofacial Surgery*, 51, pp 1250–4.

Zimmer E 1988, Teaching care plans, a five-step approach, *The Journal of Practical Nursing*, 38(4), pp 38–41.

CHAPTER 20

Bedtimes in nursing homes: an action research approach

ANNETTE STREET

INTRODUCTION

The need for research-based practice is articulated in aged-care policy documents and strategic plans but is yet to be seen as relevant or possible for many gerontic nurses. The issues of privatisation, cost cutting, untrained staff and the complexity of care needs for sicker residents have been paramount. Research has been seen as a luxury by most clinical nurses—something that others do. However, the circle is closing, with policy statements and business plans being tied to research productivity and outcomes. Increasingly managers are expecting staff to be able to justify their practice decisions with evidence from the research of others or from their own research.

Gerontic nurses are challenged to develop ways to incorporate research activities into their professional nursing roles. Aged-care facilities are seldom set up to support research which requires a great deal of time, funding, equipment and research assistants. Gerontic nurses rarely have the infrastructure, knowledge, skills, research experience or time to embark on traditional forms of research additional to their regular nursing role. Increasingly nurses are finding that action research enables them to meet the goals of establishing sound evidence that enables them to understand and change a given clinical, educational or management situation (Heslop et al 2000; Kelly & Simpson 2001; Smith et al 2000; Suderman et al 2000).

This chapter highlights the work of nurses, particularly gerontic nurses, who have used action research to improve a situation in aged care. The action research process is explained and explored in conjunction with a common problem for nurses and residents in aged care—bedtime.

ACTION RESEARCH

Action research has been described as a style of research rather than a specific method (Reason & Bradbury 2001a). It is a label that has been loosely applied to a range of participatory research processes that share a common interest in addressing the relationship between theory and practical problems in specific situations (Meyer 2000). With no fundamental consensus about the scope of the participation and outcomes, there has been some agreement in the literature concerning the key values that are central to most action research. These have been distilled by Reason & Bradbury (2001b), who argue for practical knowledge that is useful in the everyday as well as in the larger sociopolitical and economic context. Action research contributes to human flourishing through participatory and democratic processes that enable social, communitarian, ecological, meaning-centred or spiritual goals. Action research has been described as 'a family of research methodologies which pursue action (or change) and research (or understanding) at the same time' (Dick 1999). These methodologies do this through an emergent process which takes shape as understanding increases; it is an iterative process which converges towards a better understanding of what happens. In most of its forms it is also participative (because, among other reasons, change is usually easier to achieve when those affected by the change are involved) and qualitative (Dick 1999).

Thus the name *action research* has come to include action science, action inquiry, action learning, participatory research, cooperative inquiry, soft systems methodology, transparent research, and community development research (Reason & Bradbury 2001b).

A cyclical process

Action research is a form of inquiry that facilitates 'learning by doing'; theory and action are in a continuing interactive partnership. As shown in Figure 20.1, the research generally proceeds through cycles of planning, action, data collection, analysis and critical reflection, followed by re-planning, with the process repeating until the situation improves. In this way there is an evaluation and reflection process after every action has been taken (Street 2002). As has been noted by Cherry (1999), action research has three key strands: an *action strand* directed at making change; a *knowledge strand* which describes collective wisdom about the situation; and a *learning strand* that is focused on improving individual and collective practice. I would extend this and include a *dissemination strand* that includes ongoing information and education to colleagues and stakeholders and various forms of publication.

The interactive process is sometimes depicted as a circle, but more often a spiral shape is adopted. Open-ended spirals illustrate how research, education and action are combined in a process that allows for the novice researcher to understand the effects of small changes before they initiate larger ones. The systematic cyclic process means that the investigation, implementation, evaluation and theorising are linked to reduce the theory/practice gap. Knowledge is tested in action in context, with the resultant new knowledge modifying further action and changing the existing theory (Cherry 1999).

Although there is an integral connectedness between research, action, evaluation and education, as action research projects develop, one or other of these dimensions dominates. Thus at times the inquiry aspect governs the process, while later the focus is on implementing and monitoring action; the evaluative aspect becomes the focus at other points of the spiral; likewise, educating others about the proposed changes or their effects may predominate at another time.

Action research may mean nothing more than research which implements action and evaluates it; or it may mean a long-term process of implementation, evaluation and reflection designed to achieve radical social change. Most action research is situated somewhere between these extremes. Action research in nursing is generally facilitated action research whereby a researcher works alongside a group to investigate and manage change.

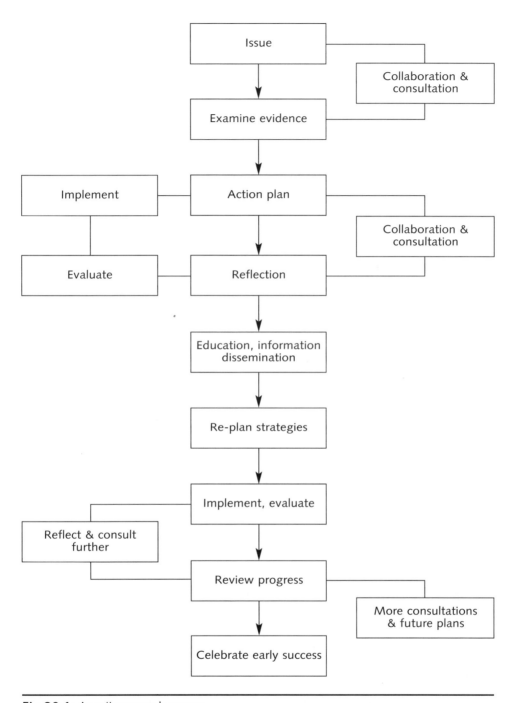

Fig 20.1: An action research process

Topics of interest to gerontic nurses that nurses have investigated using action research include those listed in Table 20.1.

Table 20.1: Topics of interest to gerontic nurses that nurses have investigated using action research

Health concern	Topic	Action researchers
Professional roles & relationships	Developing linkages between aged-care services in a rural context	Robinson 1999
	Identifying and transforming dysfunctional nurse–nurse relationships through reflective practice and action research	Taylor 2001a
	Disabled people in hospital: evaluating the CNS role	Davis & Marsden 2001
Management	Conflict management in a hospital	Skjorshammer 2001
	Implementing audit in palliative care	Cooper 2002
	Developing mental health rehabilitation services in a culturally appropriate context: an action research project involving Arabic-speaking clients	Tobin 2000
	System dynamics and action research in aged care	Walker & Haslett 2001
	Action research from the inside: issues and challenges in doing action research in your own hospital	Coghlan & Casey 2001
Practice	Identifying older people in need	Moyer et al 1999
	Men with diabetes	Koch et al 2000
	Patients' needs in substitutive dialysis treatment	Giacchino et al 2000
	Decreasing polypharmacy in aged care	Beattie 2003
	Action research sets the stage to improve discharge preparation	Suderman et al 2000
Education	Action research: a suitable method for promoting change in nurse education	Smith et al 2000
	Action research in gerontology: faculty, student and community partner perspectives	Silverstein et al 2001

A collaborative and consultative process

Action researchers often describe their collaborative processes using terms like *shared*, *involvement* and *team building*. This is because it is necessary to involve those people, or their representatives, who may be affected by the outcomes of the research. The research relationships can be organised so that nurses and other stakeholders participate in one or more levels of involvement. Figure 20.2 shows the levels of collaboration and consultation.

In gerontic nursing, a participatory relationship may be structured in a partnership that involves staff, volunteers, residents and family members. The partnership itself will be examined as part of the action research process to determine whether its structure is manipulative or enabling. Action researchers are interested not only in what happened, but how it happened, how power was exercised in the process, and the outcomes. Through systematic reflection, action researchers examine and reflect upon their actions and attitudes. Finally, they desire to communicate with each other and their audience in appropriate ways.

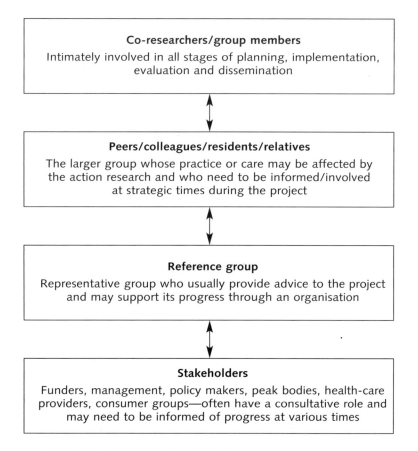

Co-researchers/group members
Intimately involved in all stages of planning, implementation, evaluation and dissemination

Peers/colleagues/residents/relatives
The larger group whose practice or care may be affected by the action research and who need to be informed/involved at strategic times during the project

Reference group
Representative group who usually provide advice to the project and may support its progress through an organisation

Stakeholders
Funders, management, policy makers, peak bodies, health-care providers, consumer groups—often have a consultative role and may need to be informed of progress at various times

Fig 20.2: The consultative process

ACTION RESEARCH IN GERONTIC NURSING

As gerontic nurses begin to search for ways to make their practice more evidence-based, action research is being used to address problems. It is interesting to note that the term 'action research' is being used in the gerontic nursing literature to cover projects that vary from information-gathering exercises with little action involvement to projects with large participation and strong action intent. These differences are sometimes a deliberate design strategy and sometimes develop as a result of circumstances outside the control of the action researchers. An advantage of action research is its flexibility and capacity for action plans to be modified in the light of planned changes initiated by the research and unplanned circumstances such as changes in management structures or government regulations.

An example of the capacity of action researchers to adapt to changed circumstances was evident in an action research project designed to improve inappropriate polypharmacy in nursing homes (Beattie 2003). The initial intention of the project was to develop participative relationships that would shape the structure of the planning and implementation. However, a new accreditation process at the facility and government incentives for staff to move into acute care resulted in staff losses. Although initially nurses were involved in small research groups, the project relied largely on the efforts of the action researcher to facilitate the processes, collect and analyse the interview data with residents, relatives, nurses, pharmacists and general practitioners, and pull together the final conclusions. In this context accreditation processes created a block to the implementation of other change strategies.

Another approach to a similar problem of the quality use of medicines in nursing homes involved two parallel activities: an audit conducted by the researchers and five small action research groups of nurses established to address a number of strategies designed to improve the management of medication (Street & Hunt 1999–2003). In this project, accreditation provided something of an impetus to change because the action research process enabled the aged-care facility to establish a committee for medication management that complied with accreditation expectations. However, the energy invested in accreditation and documentation reduced the capacity for collaborative action related to quality use of medicines in other areas.

These two projects developed different forms of facilitation in order to implement change. Their strategies were largely influenced by the sociopolitical climate of regulation and accreditation that predominated in the Australian aged-care facilities where they were conducted. Similarly, accreditation provided the impetus for another action research project in three English aged-care sites where staff members wanted to critically examine resource allocation, service delivery patterns and outcomes for residents (Chenoweth & Kilstoff 1998).

Each of these projects was able to identify the drivers and barriers to structural and organisational reform and were consistent with the claims made by Kemmis (2001, p 92), who argued that action research 'aims not only at improving outcomes, and improving the self understanding of practitioners, but also at assisting practitioners to arrive at a critique of their … work and work settings'.

Sometimes successful change in action research can set off a string of other changes. As participants become confident with the process and take on co-researcher roles, they can lead the development of a range of smaller projects that fit under the umbrella of the main project. A project designed to improve the networks between acute and aged-care services through changes to the relationships and roles of members of the aged-care assessment teams provided the basis for three smaller networking action research projects in different contexts (Robinson 2001). These projects supported the overall aim but had different target groups. Co-researchers worked to improve their networking relationships with general practitioners and with different acute-care settings (Robinson 1999; Robinson & Street, in press).

Collaborative action research projects provide the opportunity for involvement of older people, their relatives and informal carers in the conceptualisation and implementation of the project, rather than just being the 'subjects' of the study. Positive outcomes were described for day-care staff, family carers and older people with dementia after their engagement in an action research process to design, implement and evaluate a new therapy program for people attending a multicultural dementia day-care centre (Chenoweth & Kilstoff 1998). The involvement in the process was considered valuable in terms of relationships and reduction in distressing symptoms as the actual therapy program. Similarly, action research was effective in enabling Canadian researchers to develop a strategy to identify older people in need. The nurses in the study used a range of quantitative and qualitative tools to assess needs and integrate isolated older people into better health networks (Moyer et al 1999).

These examples of gerontic nursing research highlight the varying levels of participation by nurses, residents and families/carers in studies that have been published under the term 'action research'. The constraints and structures of a given situation will determine how much involvement is possible and appropriate. Residents with cognitive impairment may be able to participate fully in an action research project which requires ongoing rational planning, implementation and evaluation. Research being conducted towards a masters or doctoral degree may have a stronger role for the researcher because of the requirements of their formal study. My own experiences of working with nurses in clinical, management and educational roles (Street 1995) is that when they participate as fully as they desire in a project, the possibility of permanent change is greatly enhanced.

BEDTIMES: DEVELOPING AN ACTION RESEARCH PROJECT

This section has been designed to explore the process of action research and its place in gerontic nursing through an issue of concern to gerontic nurses. Rosalie Hudson, a colleague who was the Director of Nursing of an urban nursing home, provided me with some of her journal accounts of what may seem to be an insignificant issue: bedtimes in aged-care facilities. As gerontic nurses know, this issue is complex, with many people having a vested interest in controlling the bedtimes of residents, including residents and their families.

The practices surrounding resident bedtimes are ritualised and habitual. If more gerontic nurses are to experience mutuality in their care for older people, then traditions, habits and rituals need to be examined and at times jettisoned. Dealing with resident bedtimes is the kind of issue that appears to be straightforward. It may be easy to make a change for the short term but difficult to maintain the new practices unless they become a new form of ritual. Hudson's reflective approach through her journal accounts provides valuable material for us to explore how this topic may become an action research project.

Problem identification

The first step in an action research process is the identification of a problem that needs to be addressed. After identifying bedtimes as the issue for consideration, Hudson has reflected on it by writing in her professional journal. Let's explore the situation with her.

> It's 4.30 pm and the day has begun to wind down. Music therapist and program/activities coordinator have gone home. Residents are being prepared for the evening meal, served no later than 5 pm so that kitchen staff can go before the 6 pm 'penalty rates' deadline. Aware of residents' rights and the important aspect of choice, nursing staff ask each resident, 'Would you like to go to bed before tea?'. 'What's the alternative?' a more assertive resident may ask. Framed in a different way, the nurse's question may be, 'What would you like to do this evening, Mabel?'. With that element of choice, what options are available?

> Who sets the pattern of residents' bedtime? Are residents 'put to bed' at different times each evening, depending on who's on duty? Thorough assessment on admission (and reviewed as required) should indicate the resident's preferred bedtime. However, as one resident replied when asked why he goes to bed at 6 pm each evening: 'There's bloody nothing else to do!'. Or, as another commented: 'I don't like to see the girls (staff) rushed. I like to do all I can to help them. I know there's a lot of us that need help getting to bed.' Furthermore, a more thorough assessment may invite suggestions from the resident and family as to preferred evening lifestyle or activities.

> It's a long time between 4 pm and 7 am, or even 9 pm and 9 am, for a resident whose nursing needs usually include a high risk of pressure sores, incontinence, poor mobility, etc. All these problems are exacerbated by such a prolonged period in bed. The cost implications of the above (incontinence products, assistance with mobility, skin care) have been thoroughly researched but the old problem remains—how to translate objective data into changed practice.

> Much nursing home routine is dictated by meal times—especially the 5 pm 'dinner' with 'supper' at around 7–8 pm. There remain at least 12 hours and in many cases 15 hours between meals (dinner and breakfast). The literature shows that much behaviour attributed to dementia can be 'treated' by a small carbohydrate meal at regular intervals. The importance of regular fluid intake of course cannot be overestimated.

> The sheer boredom of spending so many hours in bed would drive many a calm person to frustration!

Collecting baseline data

To be effective, action research must be able to articulate the complexity of the present problem in order to be able to evaluate whether the situation has improved or been resolved. A well-documented, multifaceted baseline must be established as a foundation for planning action. The toolkit the action researcher uses to collect this baseline data may include the traditional research favourites of surveys or interviews but also may use narrative journal accounts, focus groups or interviews that are analysed and reflected upon. As a manager, Hudson chose to use a professional journal to explore the issue of resident bedtimes. In this journal she has recorded her own experiences along with the relevant stories recounted to her by staff and residents. Hudson's account also demonstrates another important part of the collection of baseline data—an examination of existing evidence. This is usually done in a formal and systematic way, to discover other research on the topic, evaluate its usefulness and identify strategies or recommendations that have been presented as best practice. Hudson continues:

> Recent research shows that over 60% of nursing home residents suffer untreated pain—caused by lack of mobility, arthritis, etc. Spending so many hours in bed does little to alleviate this problem and much to exacerbate it. Night staff (purportedly with the residents' interests at heart) may not wish to disturb a resident to attend to passive limb movements throughout the night—hence the increased potential for contractures.

> Analysis of sleep patterns of the elderly seems to have little impact on the way nursing home routines are organised. If a resident is in bed for 15 hours, how many hours is he or she expected to sleep? Do night staff have an expectation that all residents will sleep from 9 pm to 7 am and that if they don't, the 'problem' must be treated?

Developing an audit

It is common to collect some baseline statistics to justify and define the extent of the problem. This can be done through audit as discussed in the previous chapter.

As she reflected on the situation in her journal, Hudson showed that she had begun to collect information on the situation concerning bedtimes.

> It concerned me [that], when going around the nursing home one day, I counted sixteen residents out of fifty in bed at 4.30 pm. The nurses' logic was clear. 'We always ask them first.' I began to think of the timebound routines and the unwritten law that says all residents must be in bed before the night staff come on duty, and the more that are in bed before tea, the easier it will be to meet the 'night staff deadline'. Such 'deadlines' connote a time when normal life routines are extinguished, when staff actually 'turn the lights out' so that anyone visiting a nursing home after 7 pm must wonder about the dimly lit corridors and what kind of life exists for residents 'after hours'. There seemed to be an impossible gap between ideal and reality when I contemplated asking evening staff to design an alternative 'program' to invite residents to attend each evening—something as simple to organise as a video, game of bingo, cards, or arranging supper in the lounge with the pianola or other music as background atmosphere.

Reflection on the journal account

In this reflective narrative we can see the emergence of a number of undercurrents and questions that affect bedtimes. The meals have to be served at 5 pm so that penalty rates are not incurred. This practice serves the *financial* interests of the institution, not the resident, who may prefer the option of having their meals re-heated later on if they are not hungry at 5 pm.

Central to nursing culture are the unwritten rules about the *moral climate* of nursing (Rodney & Street, submitted 2003). In this case the concern is with what a 'good' nurse does before they leave the shift. A 'good' gerontic nurse is able to get all the residents settled before the night staff members arrive on duty. If this doesn't happen they know that they will be considered a 'bad' nurse. Similarly, in many aged-care facilities a 'good' night shift nurse has all the patients bathed and fed before they hand over to the day shift. When these practices are waived the nurse usually feels the need to justify the change during handover by explaining that the resident had a special need or request. These practices serve the needs of nursing staff to feel that they have accomplished the set of tasks expected of them; they may not necessarily meet the needs of the residents.

The account also highlights the *marketing of choices* to which nurses inevitably subscribe. When there are few real choices, nurses are forced to present the limited choices in such a way as to achieve the best outcome—the question of the best outcome for the resident is often presented in a way that serves the interests of the nurse or the institution.

The practice of turning out the lights at 7 pm gives a message that bedtime is accomplished and any other activity is an interruption to the well-ordered routine. Residents become docile in this process through a number of nursing practices which infer that they need to be fed and in bed early, despite the research evidence that older people need fewer hours of sleep and bed rest (Floyd et al 2000) and that there are a number of strategies that nurses can adopt to manage this (Morgan & Closs 1999).

Finally, these comments highlight the temptation to impose management-devised strategies, no matter how well they can be justified in terms of their value for residents. Action researchers know that if nursing staff are not consulted and included in the decision-making then they will not 'own' the changes and restructure their time and care practices to accommodate them. This final point is crucial. Action researchers acknowledge that changes of this order are in reality changes of culture; nurses are being asked to discard habits and reorganise work priorities to integrate permanent changes to their practice. Changes, even of this magnitude, require ongoing commitment from staff, residents and families to ensure their long-term adoption into the culture of the ward. Resistance will occur and old ways will return if nurses are not active participants in the decision-making process.

Planning action

The problem of bedtimes appears to be a valuable place to begin planning an action research project. In order for Hudson to turn her issue into an action research process she would need to:

- involve all those who are 'stakeholders' in the process of determining the problem—that is, the nursing staff, other staff, residents and family representatives;
- conduct a formal review of the available literature on best practice in sleep promotion for older people;
- collect baseline data, including an assessment of the interests being served by the continuation of the present practices;
- plan systematic action which can be justified;
- educate staff on the purpose of the action plans and the need to monitor the effects of the change;

- initiate appropriate data-collection strategies to monitor the action;
- evaluate the effects of the action;
- reflect on the outcomes in light of the wider sociopolitical situation, including the functioning of power relationships; and
- re-plan, implement, monitor and reflect until the situation is improved.

The first action plan is often investigative, providing more structured baseline data upon which to plan changes. If this were an action research project then at this stage Hudson would ideally involve interested staff, residents and family members in exploring the scope of the problem and the possible options. Together they could organise to conduct an audit of bedtimes for a period of time to see how regularly and consistently this situation is occurring and to determine how many residents or staff were involved. Residents and family members could be asked to discuss their own ideas and preferences. Nurses could be asked to reflect on the way that they present their choices to residents, along with their own habits and preferences.

This initial planning stage could:

- identify the possible options and provide a clear justification for the action plan;
- decide on an implementation strategy through collaborative negotiation;
- involve all those who would be affected by the strategy in the decision-making process; and
- develop tools or data-collection strategies to monitor the effectiveness of the action.

Taking action: implementation and monitoring

It is imperative that evidence is collected concerning the effects of the planned action as it is implemented. This is *systematic research*; it is not just putting a good idea into practice. Monitoring strategies must be designed to collect systematic information about the effects of the implementation. These monitoring strategies need to take account of the dynamic nature of the process. It is difficult to distinguish between fundamental changes that are the direct effects of the particular action, and incidental changes that may have occurred as a result of other changes. Many actions produce initial results, which may not be retained over time. The temptation for the novice researcher is to become disheartened or euphoric about the immediate effects and not allow enough time for a more comprehensive picture to emerge. If the changes are local and only affect a small number of people it can be relatively easy to design a number of strategies to get feedback on the success and value of the action plan. Most action researchers attempt to use more than one data-collection strategy to obtain formal and informal information in order to create a more complete picture of the changing situation.

Evaluation

These data-collection strategies must be matched by appropriate strategies of analysis so that the research team can provide a picture for participants and other interested parties which enables them to understand the effects of the implementation strategy. If a plan was devised to provide an after-dinner entertainment program, then data-collection strategies would need to discover whether this program was meeting the needs of residents and their families. It would need to determine the effects on non-participating residents, the extra workload for staff, the need for extra equipment, or changes to bathing and medication routines. As the information on these and other issues was evaluated, revised action plans could be implemented until all stake-holders were confident that they had created an effective solution or compromise to the issue of bedtimes (Street 1998).

Reflection

Reflection is a central process in action research and it is common for researchers to reflect upon the research processes and not just the research content (Taylor 2001a). The kind of reflective questions a researcher might ask concerning the issue of bedtimes could focus on the issue of whose interests are being served by the changed strategies and the manner of implementation. Are nurses deciding actions 'for the good of the patient' or are they facilitating the participation of residents in the decision-making? Are nurses only involving residents who are manageable and agreeable, or are they deliberately providing space for difficult residents to speak and participate? Are managers taking account of the stresses that nurses experience with change? Are family members being consulted about the proposed changes? Are there oppor-tunities for further research related to specific problems that are becoming evident as the bedtime issue is being addressed, such as sleep disturbance, incontinence, skin breakdown and so on?

Reflection that focuses more on the research process might be concerned with:

- whether the processes are challenging existing power relations;
- whether collaboration is really occurring;
- the ethics of involvement;
- issues of coercion by management to participate; and
- processes of informed consent.

A number of thoughtful nurse researchers have reflected upon their own research roles and processes to provide guidance for the novice action researcher in the dif-ficulties they will need to address (Taylor 2001b).

DILEMMAS AND ADVANTAGES

Action research is not without its problems. Like all research it requires time—a sus-tained time commitment by a number of people over a period of time. But it is not only the amount of time required but the fact that the timing for the proposed activ-ity must also be right. Action research is directed at cultural change, so it is not a quick-fix method. The research endeavour itself consists of a wide variety of data collection analysis and reflective activities, many of which can be tedious and repet-itive to the clinician or manager wanting quick answers to entrenched problems.

CONCLUSION

Learning by doing with action research can bring rewards—the rewards of being involved in a concern that really matters to you and will improve the situation for yourself and others. Many nurses find that the opportunity to collaborate on a shared project with colleagues and residents is very satisfying, particularly in care environments where they can develop a long-term relationship with residents and their families. Action research can be local and specific. The solutions generated are tested and re-tested until they work in the situation. Finally, nurses can see the results of their actions occurring quickly rather than needing to go to journals to read research findings and thinking about how to implement them in a different setting with its own special problems.

References

Beattie J 2003, *Addressing Inappropriate Polypharmacy in Residential Aged Care: An Action Research Study*, unpublished doctoral thesis, La Trobe University, Bundoora, Victoria.

Chenoweth L & Kilstoff K 1998, Facilitating positive changes in community dementia management through participatory action research, *International Journal of Nursing Practice*, 4, pp 175–88.

Cherry N 1999, *Action Research: A Pathway to Action, Knowledge and Learning*, RMIT University Press: Melbourne.

Coghlan D & Casey M 2001, Action research from the inside: issues and challenges in doing action research in your own hospital, *Journal of Advanced Nursing*, 35(5), pp 647–82.

Cooper J 2002, Implementing audit in palliative care: an action research approach, *Journal of Advanced Nursing*, 39(4), pp 360–9.

Davis S & Marsden R 2001, Disabled people in hospital: evaluating the CNS role, *Nursing Standards*, 15(21), pp 33–7.

Dick B 1999, What is action research? Online: http://www.scu.edu.au/schools/gcm/ar/whatisar.html, retrieved 29 May 2003.

Floyd JA, Janisse JJ, Medler SM & Ager JW 2000, Nonlinear components of age-related change in sleep initiation, *Nursing Research*, 49(5), pp 290–4.

Giacchino F, Manzato A, De Piccoli N & Ponzetti C 2000, Patient's needs in substitutive dialysis treatment. Some psychosocial and organizational considerations, *Panminerva Medica*, 42(3), pp 207–10.

Heslop L, Elsom S & Parker N 2000, Improving continuity of care across psychiatric and emergency services: combining patient data within a participatory action research framework, *Journal of Advanced Nursing*, 31(1), pp 135–43.

Kelly D & Simpson S 2001, Action research in action: reflections on a project to introduce clinical practice facilitators to an acute hospital setting, *Journal of Advanced Nursing*, 33(5), pp 652–9.

Kemmis S 2001, Exploring the relevance of critical theory for action research: emancipatory action on the footsteps of Jurgen Habermans. In: Reason P & Bradbury H (eds), pp 91–102, *Handbook of Action Research: Participative Enquiry and Practice*, SAGE: London.

Koch T, Kralik D & Taylor J 2000, Men living with diabetes: minimizing the intrusiveness of the disease, *Journal of Clinical Nursing*, 9(2), pp 247–54.

Meyer J 2000, Qualitative research in health care: using qualitative methods in health related action research, *British Medical Journal*, 320(7228), pp 178–81.

Morgan K & Closs SJ 1999, *Sleep Management in Nursing Practice: An Evidence-based Guide*, Churchill Livingstone: Edinburgh.

Moyer A, Coristine M, Jamault M, Roberge G & O'Hagan M 1999, Identifying older people in need using action research. *Journal of Clinical Nursing*, 8(1), pp 103–11.

Reason P & Bradbury H 2001a, Introduction: inquiry and participation in search of a world worthy of human aspiration, In: Reason P & Bradbury H (eds), *Handbook of Action Research: Participatory Inquiry and Practices*, SAGE: London, pp 1–14.

Reason P & Bradbury H (eds) 2001b, *Handbook of Action Research: Participative Inquiry and Practice*, SAGE: London.

Robinson AL 1999, At the interface of health and community care: developing linkages between aged care services in a rural context, *The Australian Journal of Rural Health*, 7(3), pp 172–80.

Robinson AL 2001, *At the Interface: Developing Inter-sectoral Networks in Aged Care*, unpublished doctoral thesis, La Trobe University: Melbourne.

Robinson AL & Street AF (in press), Improving networks between acute care nurses and an aged care assessment team, *Journal of Clinical Nursing*.

Rodney P & Street AF (in press), The moral climate of nursing practice. In: Starch J, Rodney P & Starzonski R (eds), *Towards a Moral Horizon: Nursing Ethics for Leadership and Practice*, Pearson Education Australia.

Silverstein N, Moorhead J & Murtha J 2001, Action-research in gerontology: faculty, student, and community partner perspectives, *Gerontology and Geriatrics Education*, 22(3), pp 11–32.

Skjorshammer M 2001, Co-operation and conflict in a hospital: interprofessional differences in perception and management of conflicts, *Journal of Interprofessional Care*, 15(1), pp 7–18.

Smith P, Masterson A, Basford L, Boddy G, Costello S, Marvell G, Redding M & Wallis B 2000, Action research: a suitable method for promoting change in nurse education, *Nurse Education Today*, 20(7), pp 563–70.

Street AF 1995, *Nursing Replay: Researching Nursing Culture Together*, Churchill Livingstone: Melbourne.

Street AF 1998, From soulmates to stakeholders: issues in creating quality postmodern participatory research relationships, *Social Sciences in Health*, 4(2), pp 119–29.

Street AF 2002, Action research. In: Schneider Z, Elliott D, Beanland C, LoBiondo-Wood G & Haber J (eds), *Nursing Research Methods, Critical Appraisal and Utilisation* (2nd edn), Mosby: Sydney.

Street AF & Hunt S 1999–2003, *Quality Use of Medicines*, unpublished doctoral thesis, funded by Pharmaceutical Health And Rational Use of Medicines (PHARM).

Suderman EM, Johnson LS, Deatrich JV & Sawatzky-Dickson DM 2000, Action research sets the stage to improve discharge preparation, *Pediatric Nursing*, 26(6), pp 571–84.

Taylor B 2001a, Identifying and transforming dysfunctional nurse–nurse relationships through reflective practice and action research, *International Journal of Nursing Practice*, 7, pp 406–13.

Taylor B 2001b, Overcoming obstacles in becoming a reflective nurse and person, *Contemporary Nurse*, 11(2/3), pp 187–94.

Tobin M 2000, Developing mental health rehabilitation services in a culturally appropriate context: an action research project involving Arabic-speaking clients, *Australian Health Review*, 23(2), pp 177–84.

Walker B & Haslett T 2001, System dynamics and action research in aged care, *Australian Health Review*, 24(1), pp 183–91.

CHAPTER 21

Current and future trends in gerontic nursing research

BILL KOCH AND ADRIANA TIZIANI

INTRODUCTION

Academic staff from schools of nursing across Australia were asked to contribute information about their current funded research in gerontic nursing, and also to provide their thoughts on what issues future research projects within gerontic nursing should address. From a total of 38 questionnaires sent out, 17 (37.8%) containing details of 39 projects were returned (Appendix 1). The purpose of this chapter is to provide a snapshot of these funded gerontic nursing projects in Australia at the time of writing and to suggest future directions for research. It is not an attempt to provide detailed discussion on individual topics; however, where appropriate, mention is also made of recent international nursing publications in the areas of interest cited by respondents.

CURRENT RESEARCH TRENDS

It would appear from the returned questionnaires that most of the research occurring since 2000 has been in either the residential or community setting, collectively accounting for 72% ($n = 28$) of the total projects, with the remainder being in the acute care (8%, $n = 3$), rehabilitation (5%, $n = 2$), or extended-care settings (2%, $n = 1$), or across more than one setting (13%, $n = 5$). While many of the research topics being addressed appear diverse and are treated as discrete for the sake of clarity of discussion, there was, in reality, a degree of overlap. This issue of overlap is also evident in the work of other authors. For example, when addressing challenging behaviours in the residential-care sector, lack of education in dealing with these issues was cited by nurses as a cause of stress and burnout, subsequently leading to dissatisfaction and nurses leaving the profession (Silver et al 1998).

Residential care

Projects occurring in the residential setting addressed a multiplicity of issues including job satisfaction, documentation, challenging behaviours, respite care and the educational needs of nurses.

Job satisfaction

Research projects addressing job satisfaction are in keeping with the report issued by the Nursing Workforce Project (Commonwealth Department of Health and

Ageing 2002) on recruitment and retention of nurses in the residential aged-care setting, which identified a number of factors that contributed to workplace dissatisfaction, nurses leaving the profession and not considering a return to the workforce. These factors included inflexible hours of work, poor rates of pay, staff shortages and lack of support. In addition to these factors, Moyle et al (2003) and Cheek et al (2003) found that other sources of dissatisfaction among nurses included working with unskilled staff, laborious tasks such as documentation, tensions within role expectations, resident care needs becoming increasingly complex, and an increasing need to be available for overtime. In responding to the Nursing Workforce Project (2002), the Commonwealth Government made a number of recommendations to address most of the identified dissatisfactions, including: increased staffing levels; increased rates of pay; improvement in skill mix, generating greater acknowledgement of gerontic nurses' knowledge and skills; and streamlining documentation requirements.

Documentation

Anecdotally it appears that nursing documentation within aged care is a common source of complaint from nurses in this area. In the context of job satisfaction, several projects in both residential care and rehabilitation dealt with issues of documentation. In the latter area one project sought to evaluate the degree to which nurses could improve assessment and care planning outcomes when using an integrated, comprehensive care assessment, care and discharge planning instrument. The project also sought to identify the means of reducing the amount of duplication in nursing documentation and subsequent time spent on documentation.

In residential care another project sought to replace paper-based records with computerised documentation. (These issues are dealt with in depth in Chapter 18.) However, as indicated by Koch (2003), there is already much to recommend the replacement of paper-based approaches in terms of outcomes such as enhanced documentation standards, time savings, the extended range of care possibilities identified for residents, and increased reporting and data-extraction possibilities.

In order to achieve these potential advantages, several precursor issues need to be addressed. These include identifying the relationship of documentation tasks to overall work flow, the specific documentation requirements of residential aged care and the creation of an intuitive computer interface which does not make an already complex task even more difficult (Koch 2003).

Challenging behaviours

Other respondents identified challenging behaviours[1] as the focus of their current research. These behaviours included wandering, aggression, absconding and intrusion into other residents' personal belongings. Aspects of interest included enhancing the quality of life for aged-care residents, and developing a multi-focus care model aimed at improving nurses' management of challenging behaviours, which may in turn improve staff retention rates and well-being by decreasing their stress levels.

Nay, Scherer et al (2003) conducted a small study ($n = 8$) looking at behaviours of concern among people living in residential aged care and found that educating the staff in assessment of the behaviour, developing appropriate goals and interventions

---

[1] The Alzheimer's Association of Australia advocates instead the term 'behaviours of concern' as this has a positive rather than a negative connotation. However, 'challenging behaviours' is used in this paper as much of the literature referred to uses this term.

based on multidisciplinary evidence-based guidelines resulted in seven of the eight clients demonstrating a reduction in behaviours of concern.

Respite care

The use of respite care was the central theme of several projects in both the residential and community settings. Previously, Neville & Byrne (2002) found that over half of respite care admissions (51.4%, $n = 18$) to the residential setting were to give the carer a 'break'. Of these 18 admissions, 13 had a diagnosis of dementia, and this subgroup were also prescribed a greater number of psychotropic medications. Nurses rated 80% of patients entering respite care as exhibiting disruptive behaviours according to the Dementia Behaviour Disturbance Scale (DBDS), with the scores for the dementia sufferers being significantly higher. By way of contrast and despite these nurse ratings, Neville & Byrne indicated that disruptive behaviours accounted for only 28.6% of reported reasons for admission, suggesting that although disruptive behaviour is both common and a major contributor to carer burden, it is not necessarily the major reason for someone to be admitted into residential respite care.

Witt et al (in press) found that although residential respite care was available, it was not the preferred option for many caregivers as they found it inflexible and constraining due to government regulations about length of stay and number of days available. Many caregivers in this study found centre-based programs or in-home respite preferable because these programs appeared to be tailored to individual needs. This project also highlighted the need for improved general practitioner knowledge of general respite options, general evaluation of waiting times for respite services and the needs of carers from non-English-speaking backgrounds.

Another Australian study by Jeon & Chenoweth (2003) had similar findings when looking at the respite needs of patients with mental illness. Their study demonstrated that carers were also commonly not aware of available services and that the problem was compounded as sites providing respite care also had limited availability of beds.

Educational needs of nurses

One of the issues most evident in many of the current projects being undertaken was an attempt to update skills and provide nurses with education and skill development in areas such as pain management, palliative care and management of challenging behaviours. This is in keeping with the findings of Pearson et al (2002), which highlighted the need to improve access to education and training for nurses in order to increase their skills and knowledge, which may in turn improve quality of care and work satisfaction.

Other education projects focused on pain management issues, such as the identification of factors which might be unique to the aged-care setting and which should be considered when planning pain management education programs for nurses. The importance of this area of research was highlighted by Alcock et al (2002), who estimated that two-thirds of people aged 65 and over, and up to 80% of nursing-home residents, suffer from chronic pain. Of the 121 nursing homes in their study, only 25% had a standardised pain assessment tool and 31% had a written pain management policy. These striking data emphasise the need to further explore issues of education or training in pain management strategies.

Educational programs in palliative care for staff working in residential-care facilities were the focus of several projects. The international literature revealed a few similar studies addressing the support needs of staff, residents and relatives in both the United States (Katz et al 2001) and the United Kingdom (Froggatt & Hoult 2002). Wilkes et al (2000) identified a number of similar issues when looking at the future of palliative care nursing research in Australia. In looking at the published and unpublished projects related to palliative care in Australia between 1990 and 1996, most appeared to be focused on nurses' professional issues and pain management for the patient. Little research on families or carers appeared to exist at this time. In response to this recognised deficit in the aged-care sector, the Australian Palliative Aged Care (APAC) project was launched in 2002 and will address the issues of staff training in palliative care as well as producing a standard set of guidelines (APAC 2002).

Community

Projects in the community could be generally grouped under the broad headings of client discharge planning, elder abuse and promotion of well-being among the elderly.

Discharge planning

Several respondents indicated that they were working on projects related to discharge planning. This included specific foci such as post-stroke discharge and carer experiences of discharge planning, with one project seeking to evaluate the efficacy of an individually tailored health support program for people over 65 living alone and discharged to their own homes following surgery. The Cochrane Library review by Parkes & Shepperd (2003) of discharge planning from hospital to home showed that elderly medical patients with a discharge plan had a reduced length of stay and increased satisfaction with their care, but there were no statistically significant differences in health outcomes or readmission rates.

In the area of post-stroke discharge and rehabilitation, Anderson et al (2000) found that when comparing early discharge and home-based rehabilitation to standard care (hospital-based rehabilitation), there was a statistically significant difference in length of stay in favour of discharge planning programs, but no significant differences in general health outcomes or physical and psychological well-being. The study suggested that there may have been some negative impact of early discharge on caregivers' mental health, which provided an interesting alternative view of the data. This appears to be a complex area of research, needing further focus on the possible interrelated nature of prognostic data, strategies for discharge planning and rehabilitation programs.

Elder abuse

One of the projects concerned abuse in the older person with dementia. Koch & Nay stated that

> having dementia and caring for a person with dementia can cause a great deal of stress, and vulnerability. This may lead to physical or verbal aggression by either the person with dementia or their carer. This can escalate the levels of stress and feelings of vulnerability of both the carer and the person with dementia, potentially culminating in a catastrophic abusive situation. Elder abuse can occur in both formal and informal caring situations.
>
> Koch & Nay 2000, p 1

In this study, staff employed to care for people with dementia were asked to identify issues which contributed to them working under difficult situations and they included insufficient staff numbers, lack of education on dementia, lack of professional supports, lack of activities for service users, deficiencies in current practices, inflexible systems and poor environments. These findings are very similar to the issues for the nurse caring for the older person with dementia in the acute setting and the factors identified as contributing to job dissatisfaction (Moyle et al 2003; Cheek et al 2003; Pearson et al 2002; Tolson et al 1999; Eriksson & Saveman 2002; Dewing 2001).

Promotion of well-being

Several of the projects focused on health, maximisation of well-being and the strategies employed to maintain these in community-dwelling people over the age of 65. The literature revealed a number of studies that were interested in the issues of health promotion, disease prevention, nutrition and healthy lifestyles in the elderly. One of the UK studies (Fletcher 1998) advocated a multidimensional assessment in the elderly to reduce mortality, disability and hospital inpatient admissions. Similarly, one of the current projects by Courtney et al (unpublished) focused on comprehensive in-home health assessment as a means of reducing health service utilisation, delaying admission to hospital and/or residential care, and improving quality of life for the older person, whilst another (Edwards et al, in press) looked at information provision as a way of reducing anxiety and clarifying expectations about future residential-care needs.

Acute care

Most projects in acute care were concerned with nurses' knowledge, skills and ability to care for an acutely unwell older person, especially if the person was also cognitively impaired, and the development of nursing care models to meet the specific needs of older patients. A number of studies in this area (Tolson et al 1999; Eriksson & Saveman 2002; Dewing 2001) found that nurses working in the acute-care setting had negative attitudes towards the elderly, did not know how to communicate with patients with dementia, planned care around physical problems, often ignoring the cognitive issues, did not have the skills to deal with behaviours considered to be disruptive, and generally coped by either ignoring the patient altogether or ranking the patient lowest on their list of priorities.

Traditionally, assessing outcome measures for the elderly in the acute-care setting has focused on death, severity of illness, length of stay and cost. However, because the elderly are more likely to have co-morbidities, chronic illness, be frail and have limited activities of daily living, Kleinpell-Nowell & Von Rueden (2000) suggested that research on the elderly in acute care would be better focused on functional outcomes such as health status, quality of life, patient satisfaction with care, and quality of health care received.

One project (Nay, Fetherstonhaugh et al 2003) identified best practice in relation to the admission and discharge of people with dementia from the acute and sub-acute settings. The project identified indicators of evidence-based practice and developed an instrument to assist in the identification of evidence-based practice and the culture and practices that support its development and maintenance within the health-care facility. An evidence-based identification tool was also found to be useful for facility or unit evaluation as well as being an adjunct to educating staff on best practice.

PUBLICATION OF FINDINGS

A search of literature found that nurses generally were reluctant to submit the findings of their results for publication. In the United Kingdom, Hicks (1995) found a very low level of publication by nurses generally (0.4–3%) and a similar result was found among UK nursing academics during the same period (Smith 1994).

A study by Borbasi et al (2002) conducted in Australia concluded that published nursing research from 1995 to 2000 needed to be more closely aligned to health priorities, and published in journals which would reach both specialist and generalist audiences. Only four (10%) of the total projects in the survey described in this chapter had not produced a paper to date. Of those four, two papers had been presented at conferences. The remaining 90% of projects had been widely published in government reports and in both Australian and overseas journals, including the *Journal of Advanced Nursing, Australian Journal of Advanced Nursing, International Journal of Nursing Practice, International Journal of Mental Health, Journal of Nursing Scholarship, Australasian Journal of Ageing, Australian Health Review, Geriaction* and *Gerontological Nursing*.

Although the research was specifically focused on aged-care issues, researchers had their papers published in generalist journals as well as the more specific 'aged-care-focused' journals, in keeping with the comments of Borbasi et al (2002).

THE NURSE AS PRINCIPAL INVESTIGATOR

Of the 39 projects, 38 had nurses as the principal investigator. Furthermore, a quarter of the projects had research teams comprising only nurses, while the remaining projects had multidisciplinary teams that included physicians, psychologists, statisticians, medical administrators and health education personnel.

Gardner (1996, cited in Borbasi et al 2002) wrote that the 'literature suggests that nurse researchers have increasingly adopted qualitative methodologies for research practice and theory development'. However, Borbasi et al (2002) analysed the published research in refereed nursing journals by Australian authors from 1995 until 2000 and found that both qualitative (47%, $n = 230$) and quantitative (41%, $n = 203$) methods were used.

Of the 39 projects reported, only two (5%) were randomised controlled trials. The remaining projects were either mixed methodology (quantitative statistical analysis and theme analysis of open-ended questions) or qualitative methodology employing focus group interviews, staff surveys, descriptive studies, cross-sectional surveys, observational analysis, comparative studies and Delphi method.

THE FUTURE: WHERE TO FROM HERE?

Only a few of the respondents commented on future research, with a total of 11 suggestions being made. Aboriginal and ethnic minorities and hostel residents were identified as groups whose needs had not been sufficiently researched. For example, hostel residents were previously identified as the 'well elderly', with hostels providing low-level care. However, hostel residents today include frail elderly with co-morbidities whose care needs no longer fit with the 'low-level care' model. Therefore, what are the care needs of hostel residents in today's economic climate? The health of Aboriginal and Torres Strait Islander populations has shown very little improvement in the past decade (Ring & Brown 2002), and therefore is an area that merits further research as long as it is focused 'beyond statistical data. For research to have value and to be of benefit, we must try to find out if the strategies referred to are working or not, and why'(Atkinson et al 2002, p 286). For example, what health-care strategies have been put into place with Aboriginals and Torres Strait Islanders? Which have worked? Which haven't and why haven't they? How can the outcomes be improved?

Other issues identified as areas for future research included the continuum of care, nurses' use of computers, the use of assessment tools, increasing evidence-based practice, advanced practice roles in aged care, skills mix and its relationship to providing optimal care, and the completion of further systematic reviews on topics applicable to aged care. These systematic reviews will give nurses access to rigorously reviewed evidence, aiding them in the decision-making process. Furthermore, one of the areas already under review (physical restraint in acute and residential care) has identified another 21 related questions which could be areas for future research (Averis & Pearson 2003).

CONCLUSION

This chapter has overviewed some of the funded gerontic nursing research currently being undertaken across Australia. Many of the areas of concern for Australian researchers are also mirrored in the international literature. Although the research topics appeared initially to be discrete, many of the themes are interrelated. For example, 'quality of care for the resident' also encompasses the themes of nursing skills, knowledge and interventions, organisational culture and staffing levels, which in turn affects job satisfaction. Caring for the older person in the acute-care setting appears to be one area that merits further investigation as the population ages and the average age of patients within the acute-care setting rises.

VIGNETTE

A pilot study testing a multidisciplinary clinical guideline in response to behavioural symptoms in nursing home residents

Anne Pitcher

Behaviours of concern manifested in residents of nursing homes[2] are recognised as a widespread problem with few effective guidelines for management. A collaborative research project between La Trobe University and the Royal Freemasons' Homes of Victoria investigated the management of such behaviours.

---

[2]The term 'nursing home' (rather than 'high care') is used throughout the report as it is internationally used and understood.

The objectives of the project were to:

- evaluate and develop an evidence-based multidisciplinary clinical practice guideline (CG) as the basis of a practical flow chart for dementia care in the residential setting;
- enhance the knowledge and evidence basis for practice in this area in order to promote the consistent and informed implementation of all appropriate and feasible interventions; and
- establish a foundation for further research and learning in this area.

The CG was designed to coordinate the sequence of events associated with the management of behavioural symptoms to support the assessment process with objective observations, and to plan and evaluate processes with evidence-based, measurable interventions.

A review of the literature was conducted in order to inform the development of the evidence-based guideline, and included literature relating to existing instruments used for assessment of behaviours of concern, the impact of the behaviours on the residents' quality of life, and management approaches to behavioural symptoms.

An expert multidisciplinary reference group was established to advise the research team on the various aspects of the project and in particular the development of the CG. Members of this group were from a range of health-related fields such as psychogeriatric medicine, allied health, research, nursing, consumer groups, pharmacy and government. This group met bimonthly for the first 12 months of the two-year project.

The project involved two campuses of the health-care facility, with a pilot of the clinical guideline carried out in one campus (treatment facility), and the second campus serving as a control. Both facilities were randomly selected from an available five. Detailed demographic information was collected to compare and contrast the two facilities in regard to environment, resident mix and staffing.

Implementation of the CG in the treatment facility was preceded by an education program for staff. The education modules were offered, as the literature had shown that staff require education related to recognition and reporting of behaviours, and since the guideline was new, staff would need training in how to use it. The education about behavioural symptoms revolved around the theory that they were an expression of unmet needs. Staff found that this approach helped to give a more objective view of the behaviours and enabled them to look more closely at the reasons behind the behaviours. The program was staged in three phases, beginning with an introduction to the research project, sessions about the identification of behaviours of concern and, finally, action research in the form of case conferencing with a multidisciplinary team using the CG.

Baseline and endpoint psychometric measurements of the participating residents were carried out using validated, reliable tools identified from the literature and approved by the expert reference group. These measurements provided the opportunity to measure any changes that might have occurred during the course of the research.

The CG gave prompts within specific time frames to assess the behaviours from five different categories (environmental issues, psychosocial influences, staffing approaches and pharmacological impact). Appropriate strategies from the same areas were implemented to address the manifestations of unmet needs.

A typical case conference, for example, dealt with the behaviours of one person (Mrs E) referred to the program presenting with disruptive vocalisation at meal times, wandering, and aggressive behaviour during hygiene and toileting procedures. These behaviours had been present for several months and staff had accepted them as the norm, although dealing with them every day caused anxiety and stress for both parties. Application of the guideline prompted staff to look beyond the immediate situation to find out more about the circumstances around the behaviours and to look for reasons behind them. On delving into the resident's history and talking to her family, it was found that not only had she been in the habit of 'eating on the run' for most of her busy life, but also that she had never had a huge interest in food, preferring her cigarettes and coffee. The restraint applied to keep her seated at the meal table exacerbated her frustration, thus contributing to her anger and noise. The aggression surrounding her hygiene and toileting was related in part to a lack of comprehension of what was happening to her, the way in which some staff approached her, and also the inflexible routine imposed upon her. Assessment also considered clinical factors related to her progressing level of dementia and an associated level of irritability.

Goals were set for realistic and achievable outcomes aimed at reducing verbal disruption and aggressive behaviour, stabilising her weight and preventing further loss, and improving communication.

Evidence-based strategies suggested in the guideline advised against the use of restraint, but a perceived conflict arose for staff in deciding between forcing the resident to remain at the table and eat some of her meal or allowing her to roam at meal times and be at risk of dehydration and malnourishment. A compromise was reached, which was to remove the restraint promptly on completion of the meal, and a carer to remain seated with her while she ate. Daily accompanied walks outside the facility were suggested to meet her need for activity. She was commenced on Exelon 1.5 mg twice daily to address the level of irritability and after two weeks on this medication staff reported that her verbalisations were marginally clearer and that more consecutive words could be understood. She was reported to be slightly more irritable, however, and was still pacing. It was thought that the dose of Exelon should be adjusted. Aromatherapy treatments were trialed, which Mrs E appeared to enjoy. Some care staff were giving the directed assistance with meals, and the lap belt was sometimes removed soon after the meal was finished, but there were still times when Mrs E was left restrained at the meal table for an extended time, and so the behaviours of concern prevailed. Mrs E's weight had increased to 51.3 kg. Showering was reduced to second daily, and staff were finding her slightly more cooperative with both hygiene and toileting. The staff made a concerted effort to explain procedures in simple terms and use body language that conveyed goodwill during assistance with procedures. Because Mrs E was less resistive they were able to implement a more effective continence management plan. Wandering continued, but the effect on staff was reported as being less troublesome because she could be redirected more easily than at the beginning of the research project.

The overall findings from this project were positive and the changes in participant behaviours clinically significant. The CG was shown to be an effective tool in providing criteria for the suggestion of assessment and evidence-based strategies. Case conferencing proved to be an effective way of workshopping behavioural problems and providing solutions, and staff expressed satisfaction in being able to participate in the case conferences because it was a way to learn, to share ideas and have the opportunity for debrief.

The CG reduced the frequency and severity of behaviours of concern, and although undergoing continued modification during the research, still needed to be streamlined. Results in the control site were unexpected in that, where methods of management of behavioural symptoms had not changed, there was an across-the-board deterioration in the participants, which was measured by assessing behavioural symptoms, affect, dependency levels and mental status.

Although the sample size of this pilot study was small (eight residents in the treatment facility and seven in the control) and expansion of the project to larger populations is required to ensure confidence in the results, the trends seen from the data were very encouraging and indicated that use of the CG could assist in the care of residents with behaviours of concern, reduce the incidence of such behaviours, and reduce staff stress. (Nay R, Scherer S, Pitcher A, Koch S, Browning M, Flicker L, Nugent N & Ames D March 2003, Responding to behaviours of concern among people living in residential aged care.)

References

Allcock N, McGarry J & Elkan R 2002, Management of pain in older people within the nursing home: a preliminary study, *Health and Social Care in the Community*, 10(6), pp 464–71.

Anderson C, Rubenach S, Ni Mhurchu C, Clark M, Spencer C & Winsor A 2000, Home or hospital for stroke rehabilitation? Results of a randomised controlled trial. I. Health outcomes at 6 months, *Stroke,* 31(5), pp 1024–31.

Atkinson VJ, Graham J, Pettit G & Lewis L 2002, Broadening the focus of research into the health of Indigenous Australians, *Medical Journal of Australia*, 177(6), pp 286–7.

Australian Palliative Aged Care (APAC) 2002, *Project News* No. 2 December 2002.

Averis A & Pearson A 2003, Filling the gaps: identifying nursing research priorities through the analysis of completed systematic reviews, *Joanna Briggs Institute Reports*, 1(3).

Borbasi S, Hawes C, Wilkes L, Stewart M & May D 2002, Measuring the outputs of Australian nursing research published 1995–2000, *Journal of Advanced Nursing*, 38(5), pp 489–97.

Cheek J, Ballantyne A, Jones J, Roder-Allen G & Kitto S 2003, Ensuring excellence: an investigation of the issues that impact on the registered nurse providing residential care to older Australians, *International Journal of Nursing Practice*, 9(2), pp 103–11.

Commonwealth Department of Health and Ageing 2002, *Recruitment and Retention of Nurses in Residential Aged Care—Final Report*, Commonwealth of Australia: Canberra.

Dewing J 2001, Care for older people with a dementia in acute hospital settings, *Nursing Older People*, 13(3), pp 18–20.

Edwards H, Courtney M & Spencer L 2003, Development and evaluation of a consumer's guide to residential aged care, *Australian Health Review* 26(1), pp 145–52.

Eriksson C & Savemen B 2002, Nurses' experiences of abusive/non-abusive caring for demented patients in acute care settings, *Scandinavian Journal of Caring*, 16, pp 79–85.

Fletcher A 1998, Multidimensional assessment of elderly people in the community, *British Medical Bulletin*, 54(4), pp 948–60.

Froggatt KA & Hoult L 2002, Developing palliative care practice in nursing and residential care homes: the role of the clinical nurse specialist, *Journal of Clinical Nursing*, 11, pp 802–8.

Hicks C 1995, The shortfall in published research: a study of nurses' research and publication activities, *Journal of Advanced Nursing*, 21(3), pp 594–604.

Jeon Y-H & Chenoweth L 2003, Respite care: a variation on the theme, *International Journal of Mental Health Nursing* (in press).

Katz JS, Sidell M & Komoromy C 2001, Dying in long-term care facilities: support needs of other residents, relatives and staff, *American Journal of Hospice and Palliative Care*, 18(5), pp 321–6.

Kleinpell-Nowell R & Von Rueden K 2000, Strategies for assessing outcomes in the elderly in acute care, *AACN Clinical Issues*, 11(3), pp 442–52.

Koch B 2003, Advantages of computerised documentation, *Nursing Review*, July, pp 23–4.

Koch S & Nay R 2000, *Overcoming Abuse of Older People with Dementia and their Carers—A Discussion Paper*, Department of Human Services: Victoria.

Moyle W, Skinner J, Rowe G & Gork C 2003, Views of job satisfaction and dissatisfaction in Australian long-term care, *Journal of Clinical Nursing*, 12, pp 168–76.

Nay R, Fetherstonhaugh D, Pitcher A, Closs B & Koch S 2003, *Improving the Admission and Discharge Practices of Acute and Sub-acute Facilities in Relation to People with Dementia*, Department of Human Services: Melbourne.

Nay R, Scherer S, Pitcher A, Koch S, Browning M, Flicker L, Nugent N & Ames D 2003, *Responding to Behaviours of Concern Among People Living in Residential Aged Care*, Gerontic Nursing Clinical School, La Trobe University: Bundoora, Victoria.

Neville CC & Byrne GJA 2002, Behaviour of older people admitted for residential respite care, *Australian Journal of Advanced Nursing*, 20(1), pp 8–12.

Parkes J & Shepperd S 2003, *Discharge Planning from Hospital to Home*, The Cochrane Library, Oxford.

Pearson A, Nay R, Koch S & Rosewarne R 2002, *Recruitment and Retention of Nurses in Residential Aged Care—Final Report*, Commonwealth Department of Health and Ageing: Canberra.

Ring IT & Brown N 2002, Indigenous health: chronically inadequate responses to damning statistics, *Medical Journal of Australia*, 177(11), pp 629–31.

Silver M, Moniz-Cook E & Wang M 1998, Stress and coping with challenging behaviour in residential settings for older people, *Mental Health Care*, 2(4), pp 128–31.

Smith LN 1994, An analysis and reflection on the quality of nursing research in 1992, *Journal of Advanced Nursing*, 19, pp 385–93.

Tolson D, Smith M & Knight P 1999, An investigation of the components of best nursing practice in the care of acutely ill hospitalised older patients with coincidental dementia: a multi-method design, *Journal of Advanced Nursing*, 30(5), pp 1127–36.

Witt E, Chenoweth L & Jeon Y-H (in press), Respite services for older persons and their family carers in southern Sydney, *Geriaction*.

Wilkes L, Tracy S & White W 2000, The future of palliative care nursing research in Australia, *International Journal of Nursing Practice*, 6(1), pp 32–8.

Appendix 1: Summary of reported aged-care research projects (2000–01)

Title of project	Principal investigators	Location
Ensuring quality in aged-care residential facilities: development, trial and evaluation of an Australian National Aged Care Quality Indicator Instrument	M Courtney, H Edwards, U Kellett & J Stephan	Residential aged care
Development and testing of a consumer information system for potential clients of residential aged care	H Edwards, M Courtney & L Spencer	Community
Effectiveness of an in-home preventative health assessment for older adults living alone in the community	M Courtney, H Edwards, U Kellett & J Stephan	Community
Maximising independence and autonomy for vulnerable older people in a residential setting: facilitating best practice	H Edwards, D Gaskill, P Morrison, F Sanders, E Forster, R Fleming & S McClure	Residential aged care

A randomised controlled trial of nursing interventions for managing older people with chronic venous leg ulcers	H Edwards, M Courtney, E Lindsay, M Harris, C Lewis, K Finlayson & G Kempen	Community
Improving the care of dementia sufferers in general practice	D Bruce, G Paley P Nichols, D Roberts, P Underwood & F Schaper	Community
Development of guidelines for palliative care in residential aged care and an education program on palliative care for staff working in aged-care facilities	L Kristjanson, K White, J Parker, D Currow, P Glare & A Larson	Residential aged care
Assessment of the adverse symptoms of elderly people in residential care in Western Australia	L Kristjanson, C Toye, R Hanson & E Nightingale	Residential aged care
Job satisfaction and dissatisfaction in Australian long-term care	W Moyle, J Skinner, G Rowe & C Gork	Residential aged care
A study of family members' and nurses' perceptions of the palliative care provided in aged-care facilities when residents are in the terminal phase of life	C Toye, K White & K Yuen	Residential aged care
Development and validation of a pain assessment tool for use with cognitively impaired adults	E Davies, M Ilu, M Male, V Reimer & M Turner	Extended care unit
Improving and maintaining faecal continence in people with dementia being cared for at home	E Davies, K Joseph, M Bennie & L Clemesha	Community
Association with music and self-actualisation	L Wong	Residential aged care (Chinese)
The impact of residential respite care on the behaviour of older people	C Neville	Community & residential aged care
The development of pain assessment and management skills in regional nurses caring for cognitively impaired older people: a needs analysis	C Neville, A McCarthy & K Laurent	Residential aged care
Toowoomba Community Development Planning Project	D Hegney, K Martin-McDonald, D Gorman, G Pretty, P Fahey & A McCarthy	Acute care interface

Convalescence in the home	M Thomas, M Stokes, S-Y Yap, M Chacko, T Broe & L Chenoweth	Community
Health service needs of older NESB people (Greek, Italian, Hungarian and Chinese) and their family carers on discharge following stroke	L Chenoweth, S Torr, J Price, D Gietzelt & J Sheriff	Community
Discharge planning needs of older patients to the community	K Luck, L Chenoweth, B Brennan, H Antcliff, J Dennis, J Woods & S Jacobson	Community
Efficacy and flexibility of community aged care packages (CACPs)	M Thomas, B Woodhouse, J Rees-Mackenzie & Y-H Jeon	Community
Unplanned respite care needs for older family carers	E Witt, Y-H Jeon & L Chenoweth	Community
Older carers' need for and use of respite care services. Mental health respite care project	Y-H Jeon, C O'Neill & H McIntosh	Community
Outpatient/outreach therapy and education support program for people with Parkinson's disease and their family carers	J Sheriff, N Brennan, L Lim, K Maddill, L Olivetti, J Russell, M Welch, K Taylor & L Chenoweth	Community
Important aspects of nursing care for elderly patients during hospitalisation as perceived by nurses, elderly patients and their family carers	L Hickman, L Chenoweth, E Chang, K Hancock, J Sheriff, Y-H Jeon & J Glasson	Acute care
Understanding behaviour: nursing the acutely unwell, cognitively impaired older patient	H McIntosh, G Fairbrother & L Chenoweth	Acute care
Assessment and care planning documentation for the older patient undergoing rehabilitation	S McIver, T Larkin, N Rynn, H Merkenhoff & L Chenoweth	Rehabilitation
Ageing well for the over-65s	J Sherriff & L Chenoweth	Community
Hospital length of stay for older hospitalised patients	T Farrer & G Greenwood	Acute care
An intelligent mobility assistant	G Dissanayake, L Chenoweth, V Harinath, K Selvarajan, D Graham & B Moulton	Rehabilitation

Rural–urban nursing partnership in dementia care	L McManus, M Goff, A Broadbent, L Chenoweth, P Farrar & Y-H Jeon	Residential aged care
Systematic review of the literature concerning 'behaviours of concern' in elderly people in acute and sub-acute care	R Nay	Acute and sub-acute
Continence Outcomes Suite	R Nay, S Thomas, K Moore, D Fonda & K Watt	Across all settings
A comparison of electronic and traditional mail out survey methodologies for a sample of aged-care facilities	S Koch & G Powell	Residential aged care
Development of an evidence-based multidisciplinary guideline for the management of 'behaviours of concern' in residential aged care	R Nay, S Scherer, A Pitcher, S Koch, M Browning, L Flicker, N Nugent, & D Ames	Residential aged care
Australian aged-care nursing: a critical review	A Pearson, R Nay, S Koch & C Ward	Residential aged care
Nurse returners project—research into strategies for the recruitment and retention of qualified staff in residential aged-care facilities	A Pearson, R Nay, S Koch, C Ward & R Rosewarne	Residential aged care
Elder abuse	S Koch, R Nay & G Powell	Community
Promoting well-being in ageing in the City of Whittlesea	A Pearson, S Koch & W Mitchell	Community
Improving admission and discharge practices for people with dementia	R Nay, B Closs, A Pitcher, S Koch & D Fetherstonhaugh	Acute and sub-acute

Index